MEDICINE AND MEDICAL ETHICS
IN MEDIEVAL AND EARLY MODERN SPAIN
An Intercultural Approach

MEDICINE AND MEDICAL ETHICS IN MEDIEVAL AND EARLY MODERN SPAIN

An Intercultural Approach

Edited by

Samuel S. Kottek and Luís García-Ballester

THE MAGNES PRESS, THE HEBREW UNIVERSITY, JERUSALEM

Distributed by
The Magnes Press, P.O.Box 7695, Jerusalem, Fax 972-2-633370, Israel 91076

ISBN 965–223–930–5

Printed in Israel
by 'Graphit' ('Graph-Chen') Press Ltd., Jerusalem

CONTENTS

PREFACE

DAVID W. WEISS

The joint Israel-Spain symposium on medical-ethical problems in Medieval and Early Modern Spain is one of many events which took place under the aegis of the "Sefarad '92" program. In opening the meeting, I permitted myself a moment of personal reflection, to consider a question I believe many of us ask ourselves: What really is it that we wish to mark during this 500th anniversary year of the cataclysmic expulsion of the Jews from Spain?

That event can hardly be a cause for celebration. Not for us Jews, not for the peoples of the Iberian Peninsula, not for mankind as a whole. Is it rather, then, a celebration of Jewish survival, of resilience, of the seminal vitality among the remnants of the dispersion, of sparks springing from ashes?

In a way, perhaps, yes, in part. But I also see "Sefarad '92" in a different light, from an outlook that is broader, more inclusive, more fundamental: that of memory and its uses.

It has been said that "a man's real possession is his memory; in nothing else is he rich, in nothing else is he poor."[1] I would extend that thought to the collective memory of a people. I would regard it, too, as an apt colophon for the study of history.

The Jewish people's heritage of memories is very old and very rich. Very many of them are not jubilant. But, interspersed, there are also moments of reprieve, moments of grace. They are part of this rich possession. In recalling those moments, we discern affirmation of the constructive and humane in the human situation.

Our deliberations deal with problems and dilemmas of medicine and ethics in Spain's medieval period. But for all the particularity of their time and place and aspect, at their core these problems are *semper et*

1 Alexander Smith, *Of Death and the Fear of Dying* (Dreamthorp, 1863).

ubique. In learning from their circumstantialities we can achieve a sharper delineation of the medicoethical questions that specifically confront us today.

Our discussions are cast in the framework of an interfaith perspective. That perspective was once, too, a reality of the history of Jews, Christians and Muslims in Spain.

It is our intention that this occasion will bring into prominence precisely these elements of our collective memories: the universal, the perennial, the interactive; to bring them into focus as building blocks for the remembrance of things to come.

Introductory Remarks

On December 8–10, 1992, the Departments of History and of the History of Medicine of the Hebrew University, and the Center of Medical Ethics at the Hebrew University-Hadassah Medical School sponsored a special congress: Medical-Ethical Issues in Medieval Spain: An Interfaith Comparative Perspective. It was a unique commemoration, of 500 years since the Expulsion of the Jews from Spain.

The organizing committee selected this subject, which is an extraordinary example of collaboration and mutual trust in Jewish and Christian Spain. A great amount of scholarship was presented by the participants, who came to this gathering from Spain, the United States and Israel. Problems were raised and evaluated in surveying the historical significance of a collaboration which lasted hundreds of years.

In Christian Spain it was unusual not to find a Jewish physician or apothecary in any sizable town. Although the Church pressed hard on the Kings to forbid Jews from practicing medicine, and cautioned Christians not to make use of Jewish doctors even in times of need, it did not succeed.

In times of pestilence, which were common in those days, Jewish doctors excelled in the quality of care they provided to the suffering. For example, the Valladolid edict of January 1, 1412 which prohibited Jewish doctors from practicing medicine or supplying drugs, was abolished after six months. It was common practice for ecclesiastical and civil dignitaries to have their own personal Jewish doctors, as did the royal families. Jewish physicians received a salary from various municipalities, which invited them to come and practice within their boundaries. It was not uncommon for Jewish women to practice medicine as well. There were even ophthalmologists who removed cataracts, using astrological computations in order to determine the appropriate time for the operation.

The forced conversions of 1391 and the century that followed brought physicians to the baptismal font. Many of them were later tried by the Inquisition as Judaizers. Spain lost many Jewish physicians with the Expulsion in 1492, though some returned after converting to Christianity in Portugal. They were granted special permission to keep their Hebrew and Arabic books on medicine in order to attract them back to their former land. One such case is that of the physician Isaac Abuacar (or Abucar), who moved with his family to Portugal, returned after converting, and was granted permission to practice in Toledo and probably in Guadalajara. The Cardinal of Castile, Pedro Gonzales de Mendoza, intervened on his behalf.

This Congress shed light on a special area of mutual trust and coexistence in Spain. The table of contents of this volume indicates the dimensions of this phenomenon, which was uncommon in other places in the Middle Ages. The organizing committee and the participants deserve all praise for having brought to light a little known subject.

H. Beinart
Professor Emeritus of Jewish Medieval History
The Hebrew University of Jerusalem

Ethical Problems in the Relationship between Doctors and Patients in Fourteenth-Century Spain: On Christian and Jewish Practitioners

Luis Garcia-Ballester

Introduction

The lack of attention which historians of medicine have given to the doctor-patient relationship in the ordinary context of the village or parish has recently been the subject of comment.[1] It is extremely difficult to answer with even a reasonable degree of certainty any question about the *precise* nature of this relationship in late medieval Europe. It is not sufficient to provide a detailed description of accumulated, chronologically ordered facts and figures from a particular city, town, geographical region or more or less uniform social context (e.g., the milieu of the court, the members of the civil or ecclesiastic aristocracy, the urban bourgeoisie — the *civi* —, the diffuse and extensive ranks of the poor — the *pauperes*), nor is it enough to explain what a contemporary medical writer might have said about the question. This information may be necessary, but it is not sufficient if we wish to go beyond a mere description and endeavor to determine *why*, from the thirteenth century onward, there is new information in the evidence (both archival material and medical manuscripts) concerning the doctor-patient relationship. The very nature of this relationship obliges us to take into account other elements of an intellectual and social nature, elements which shaped this relationship and endowed it with specific features depending on the place, social milieu and time through

1 L.W.B. Brockliss, review of R. Porter and A. Wear, eds., *Problems and Methods in the History of Medicine* (London: Croom Helm, 1987); *Social History of Medicine*, 1988, *1*:91–92.

the course of one or two centuries. In the thirteenth and fourteenth centuries, an analysis of the different trends in the evolution of social organization is sufficient for a comparison of the countries of southern Europe and their northern counterparts.[2] If the scope is limited to the lands of the western Mediterranean, and more precisely to the arc stretching from Sicily to the south of the Iberian Peninsula, the differences are similarly emphasized. The percentage of religious minorities within the heart of Christendom was by no means uniform. There were fairly substantial Jewish communities in all the lands of the western Mediterranean, but the Christian kingdoms of the Iberian Peninsula also contained Moslem minorities, who, in certain lands (e.g., the Kingdom of Valencia, the Kingdom of Murcia, the south of Catalonia and particular areas of the Kingdom of Aragon) actually formed a majority of the inhabitants. The Jews of Central Europe, including those living in what is today northern France, did not have the same training and esteem for the intellectual way of life as did those living in southern Europe.[3] Even in the latter regions, the intellectual components (natural philosophical or medical) of the doctor-patient relationship were taken into account in a very different way depending on whether or not the Jewish physician was a "rationalist."[4]

It would appear that, from the thirteenth century onward, university institutions (which included medical teaching from the very beginning) provided European lands with a certain intellectual unity. However, this institutionalized intellectual life developed to different levels of organization and complexity in the various European lands (in both the south and the north). Moreover, it was a world closed to the non-Christian members of society. The number of medical students in the thirteenth and fourteenth centuries, though impossible to quantify, must have been very limited and irrelevant in demographic terms. Even so, these students started to become socially noticeable from the

2 This distinction has been made by J. Verger, "Patterns," in *A History of the University in Europe. Vol. I: Universities in the Middle Ages*, ed. H. de Ridder-Symoens (Cambridge: Cambridge University Press, 1992), pp. 35–74.

3 J. Shatzmiller, "On Becoming a Jewish Doctor in the High Middle Ages," *Sefarad*, 1983, *43*:239–250.

4 L. García-Ballester, L. Ferre and E. Feliu, "Jewish Appreciation of Fourteenth-Century Scholastic Medicine," *Osiris*, 2nd series, 1990, *6*:85–117.

first decade of the fourteenth century (with isolated exceptions earlier), at least in the lands of the western Mediterranean.[5]

Furthermore, there was no clear relationship between medical practice and university-based medical teaching. The latter was not the only method of learning medicine available to those members of Christian society who wished to practice medicine. The monopoly on teaching desired by those who designed the new faculties of medicine was one thing; a monopoly over practice, where nobody without university qualifications could work in the field of medicine, which those who were in possession of a university qualification also sought to achieve, was another. The attempt to link both monopolies to the benefit of those practitioners with university qualifications generated social tensions among healers, which in turn had negative repercussions on the doctor-patient relationship. There were no formal qualifications which defined a single, unified medical profession in late medieval Europe, but rather a wide diversity of medical practitioners and a somewhat blurred frontier between "regular" healers (those who possessed a university qualification and/or those who had passed some form of professional test) and "irregular" ones (which does not necessarily mean that they lacked some sort of medical and/or surgical training), among both men and women. In addition, there was no uniform or constant social control of medical practitioners (whether or not university trained) by the rulers and social and political leaders in the various countries of southern Europe where some effort at control was made. The degree of control could not have been particularly high, given the constant flow of summonses from the civil authorities (the king and/or the town councils) to those individuals who practiced medicine without undergoing a legal test. These summonses were accompanied by substantial fines, which were yet another method of collecting income. There are examples of this procedure throughout

5 Ridder-Symoens, ed., *Universities in the Middle Ages* (cit. n. 2). Two studies of a western Mediterranean country are L. García-Ballester, M. McVaugh and A. Rubio, *Medical Licensing and Learning in Fourteenth-Century Valencia* (Philadelphia: The American Philosophical Society, 1989) [Transactions of the American Philosophical Society, vol. 79, part 6], and M.R. McVaugh, *Medicine Before the Plague. Practitioners and Their Patients in the Crown of Aragon, 1285–1345* (Cambridge: Cambridge University Press, 1993).

the fourteenth century, at least in the territories of the Crown of Aragon, the Mediterranean coast and Ebro valley of the Iberian Peninsula. This control was part of the struggle for power between the various governing authorities, including the king, the nobility, the town councils, and pressure groups such as the incipient guilds of physicians and/or surgeons. The municipal contracts reveal the strength of popular support for technical medicine based on rational principles with well-trained physicians, both Christians and Jews; something then not incompatible with popular beliefs concerning demons and regarding the magical causes of mental and/or bodily illnesses.[6]

The doctor-patient relationship was related to all the factors which have already been mentioned. In fact, the doctor-patient relationship is, and also was in late medieval Europe, something more than the relationship between healer and patient together in a room. Non-medical scholars of the second half of the thirteenth century and university physicians who reflected upon the doctor-patient relationship in their writings were aware of this complexity. The norms of behavior which the physician was supposed to observe when treating his patient (medical etiquette) obviously formed part of this relationship, but they were not the only aspect. Later medieval medicine could draw on a written tradition of medical etiquette clearly identifiable in twelfth-century medical literature from Salerno.[7] Medical writers of the late thirteenth and the first half of the fourteenth centuries limited themselves to maintaining this tradition. However, during the thirteenth century, the doctor-patient relationship incorporated various elements of an intellectual nature which gradually complicated its medical contents. At the same time, these elements provided a doctrinal basis which enabled the doctor-patient relationship to adapt to the new social and economic circumstances which gradually appeared in thirteenth- and fourteenth-century Europe, especially in the lands of the south. I am aware that the common stock of values and rules of

6 L. García-Ballester, *Historia social de la medicina en la España de los siglos XIII al XVI* (Madrid: Akal, 1976), pp. 7–75; idem, *La medicina a la València medieval. Medicina i societat en un pais medieval mediterrani* (València: Edicions Alfons el Magnànim, 1988).

7 See note 21.

which *all* members of any society are, consciously or not, participants are also present in the doctor-patient relationship.[8]

In this article, I offer a restricted sample of the social and intellectual complexity involved in the study of the doctor-patient relationship in later medieval Latin Christendom, together with the ethical repercussions. With this aim in mind, I shall analyze some of the underlying doctrinal elements in that part of the doctor-patient relationship which is connected with the fees due to the physician. I shall try to demonstrate that the doctor-patient relationship was supported by university institutions and learned circles in doctrinal terms, and not just in its medical-doctrinal contents.[9] Concepts and doctrines which were introduced by natural philosophers and jurists were incorporated into medical practice within a short space of time. I refer, on the one hand, to the relationship between health/illness and political power presented in Aristotle's *libri naturales* (in the widest sense of the expression) and especially in the *Politics*. On the other hand, the spread of Roman Law (or the "Romanization" of later medieval society) made it possible, among other things, for concepts such as *salarium seu pensio* to take hold in private law, and for contracts dealing with the economic aspects of the doctor-patient relationship to be drawn up before a notary as standard practice. Jewish medical practitioners also took part in this process, as they formed part of the network of medical care which gradually developed in later medieval Christian Europe. They did so despite the prohibitions on their practice, which were totally ineffective, though personally and socially disturbing. Many members of this group, at least those belonging to the "rationalist" faction, also shared the socio-medical consequences of the Aristotelization and Romanization of the European society to which they belonged.

8 F. Kudlien, "Medical Ethics and Popular Ethics in Greece and Rome," *Clio Medica*, 1970, *5*:91–121, on p. 91.

9 Part of the material in this article was used in an earlier article. See "Medical Ethics in Transition in the Latin Medicine of the Thirteenth and Fourteenth Centuries: New Prospects on the Physician-Patient Relationship and the Doctors' Fee," in *The History of Medical Ethics*, eds. A. Wear, R. French and J. Geyer-Kordesch (Amsterdam: Rodopi, 1994), pp. 38–71.

I

Starting in the 1280s, the intellectual movement which has been called the "new Galen" took hold in university medical circles in Montpellier, Bologna and Paris.[10] This movement not only broadened the horizons and aroused the scientific curiosity of the university physicians and surgeons, but also enabled them to re-interpret texts and concepts (e.g., fever, *complexio*, grade, pain) which were already well known, and led them to express the diagnosis in increasingly technical language. The doctor-patient relationship itself was affected by this movement, including the problem of the doctors' fee. In addition, some Jewish physicians saw scholastic medicine (i.e., university Galenism) as a model to be imitated and as a resource to be exploited through the translation of the most representative medical works of the Christian university medical professors into Hebrew.[11]

An intellectual appreciation of the "new Galen" required that the university physician or surgeon should previously have a detailed knowledge of the Aristotelian natural philosophical corpus. This knowledge provided the methodological guidelines, the terminology and the biological and social doctrine without which it was impossible to understand the confused and complex world of Galen's writings, even with the aid of such doctrinally highly structured books as the *Canon*, the *Pantegni*, or the *Viaticum*. The students did learn about Aristotle, as between 1240 and 1275, the Aristotelian *libri naturales*, as well as works dealing with personal or social behavior such as the *Politics*, became firmly established in the schools of arts.[12]

10 N. G. Siraisi, *Taddeo Alderotti and His Pupils. Two Generations of Italian Medical Learning* (Princeton, N.J.: Princeton University Press, 1981); L. García-Ballester, "Arnau de Vilanova (c. 1240–1311) y la reforma de los estudios médicos en Montpellier (1309): el Hipócrates latino y la introducción del nuevo Galeno," *Dynamis*, 1982, 2:97–158; D. Jacquart and F. Micheau, *La médecine arabe et l'occident médiéval* (Paris: Editions Maisonneuve et Larose, 1990), pp. 176–185.

11 See note 4.

12 For the role played by Aristotle's *libri naturales* in the schools of arts of the mid-thirteenth century, see J.A. Weisheipl, "The Parisian Faculty of Arts in Mid-thirteenth Century: 1240–1270," *American Benedictine Review*, 1974, *25*:200–217.

II

In his commentary on the first of Hippocrates' aphorisms, Arnau de Vilanova asks himself what one must do in order to become a good physician. The third of his prerequisites, the need of the physician to express a series of judgments in the performance of his true medical activity, raises the problem of the intellectual and technical (*secundum artem medicam*) organization of the doctor-patient relationship.[13]

His replies to this problem include the presentation of more than twenty works by Galen to his pupils.[14] The judgments which the physician was obliged to make while treating the patient had to be made within a technical or rational scheme, which was that of the *rerum naturalium, non naturalium* and *contra naturam*,[15] to which the *externa accidentia* or *res extraneae et diversae* was added.[16] The first three factors were familiar to university physicians of the thirteenth century through their reading of Johannicius' *Isagoge*.[17]

This four-factor scheme was applied to the physician-patient relationship and endowed it with the rich doctrinal contents derived from the knowledge of the complicated works of Galen which these physicians had in the opening years of the fourteenth century. It was not enough to win the confidence of the patient, however important that might be,[18] nor was the mere examination of the urine sufficient,[19]

13 *Repetitio Arnaldi de Villanova super canonem 'Vita brevis,'* ed. M. McVaugh, in *Arnaldi de Villanova Opera Medica Omnia*, vol. XIII (Barcelona: Universidad de Barcelona, forthcoming). The second part of the commentary deals with this question. It was written in 1300.

14 *Ibid.*

15 "Bonitas autem...iudicii [medici] consistit in recta cognitione et consideratione rerum naturalium et non naturalium et contra naturam." *Ibid.*

16 "ea que de se nullo modo requiruntur ad opus [medicine] sed accidentaliter superveniunt ei et possent eius impedire processum." *Ibid.*

17 See the edition by G. Maurach, "Johannicius, Isagoge ad Techne Galieni," *Sudhoffs Archiv*, 1978, *62*:148–174.

18 "Confidentia de medico plus confert ad curam morbi quam medicus cum suis omnibus instrumentis." See J.L. Pagel, ed., *Die Chirurgie des Heinrich von Mondeville* (Berlin, 1892), p. 114.

19 "medicus non potest cognoscere per urinam omnia..., scilicet causam morbi et accidens." *Ibid.*, p. 112.

although the physician occasionally had no other alternative if he wanted "to give the impression that he is doing something."[20]

These university physicians went further: everything connected with the conduct of the physician, from strictly technical matters (for example, the exact identification of the patient's *complexio*, how to take the pulse correctly, the structure of the anamnesis or the enquiries into the patient's symptoms) to the question of fees or the problems of etiquette (in technical language the *res* or *accidentia extraneae* or *exteriores*) was derived from this technical organizational scheme.[21] The morality of the practitioner was thus derived from his being a technically trained healer, and was essential if he was to be considered an expert in medicine.

These university physicians were fully aware that the doctor-patient relationship was more than a relationship between two abstract individuals or an intellectual problem. The overall approach to the physician-patient relationship detailed by these writers (e.g., Arnau de Vilanova or Henry de Mondeville) is permeated with what could be called social and psychological aspects which condition the technical structure of this relationship. Such aspects include fear of failure, problems derived from fame, lack of comprehension by the laity, the structure of the social circles in which the physician moved, problems with fees and the contractual relationship between the physician and his patient, the complex world of the relationship between healers at the patient's bedside, poverty, passing fashions within the world of medicine and treatment, and the problems of etiquette. In addition, there are personal difficulties as age, the type of professional activity or treating female patients. In my opinion, a most interesting aspect is that both Arnau de Vilanova and Henry de Mondeville included these social and psychological connotations in the fourfold organizational scheme of the physician-patient relationship. They are not problems

20 "Et non in omnibus dictis morbis medici inspiciunt ad urinas non propter necessitatem, sed ut videatur aliquid facere." *Ibid.*

21 Arnau de Vilanova expressed both of the opinions circulating in academic circles: "Una opinio est quod ideo dicuntur accidentia extrinsecus vel extra quia cadunt extra limitem regulationum artis,... [alia opinio] supponit quod cadunt sub regulatione artificis, quoniam necessario pertinere dicit ad eius considerationem." *Repetitio super canonem 'Vita brevis'* (cit. n. 13). He finally adopted the latter: "pro tanto quisque sapiens medicus se debet in eis diligenter exercitare." *Ibid.*

"added to," but rather are "derived from" the technical nature of this relationship. This scheme was much more complicated than the straightforward explanation of Johannicius' *Isagoge*, and became even more complicated with the new contributions which gradually enriched university medical teaching and medical practice during the thirteenth century.

The pre-Salernitan and Salernitan writings, which enjoyed wide circulation throughout the thirteenth and fourteenth centuries, were not sufficient to satisfy the new demands. These short medical writings, though increasingly complex, were no more than simple and direct advice on how to take the pulse, examine the urine, gain the patient's trust, or manage the delicate subjects of the relationship with other colleagues and the collecting of fees.[22] However, the new doctor-patient relationship demanded a process of technical education and implied a complex intellectual background. Arnau took pains to warn his pupils, physicians-to-be:

> The problems involved in the training of the physician, those connected with the obedience of the patient, and the characteristics which those who surround the patient and attend him should possess, and everything which is connected with the external circumstances which bear upon the physician and the patient... are not self-evident, nor do they become apparent to us without any effort on our part; once again, they are the result of intellectual effort and reflection. Not everyone finds it easy to know what a physician has to do and to bear [these things] in mind in order to accomplish his task... Moreover, I have not read what I am about to explain to you in either the works of Hippocrates or those of any of his commentators.[23]

22 For descriptions of manuscripts and the Latin texts, see S. de Renzi, *Collectio salernitana* (Naples, 1852–59), Vols. II, pp. 73ss., and V, pp. 102ss., 333ss.; E. Hirschfeld, "Deontologische Texte des frühen Mittelalters," *Archiv für Geschichte der Medizin*, 1928, *20*:353–371; L.C. MacKinney, "Medical ethics and etiquette in the early middle ages: the persistence of Hippocratic ideals," *Bull. Hist. Med.*, 1952, *26*:1–31.

23 "Recoligamus ergo genera istorum considerabilium que dicit necessitati ceteris medicis ad opus nostram perfectionem et videamus in generali que sunt observanda circa unumquodque illorum. Sunt ergo illa quatuor in genere: diligentia

III

The salary of the physician, surgeon, or any other healer who took part in the treatment, was to be derived from the medical or technical structure of the doctor-patient relationship, which had been so deeply affected by the so-called "new Galen" and the earlier reception of the Aristotelian *corpus*. As Nutton has pointed out, practical administrative procedures derived from the application of some passages of Roman law which deal specifically with the civic salary given to doctors affected this aspect of the doctor-patient relationship.[24] During the thirteenth and fourteenth centuries, Roman law spread throughout what are today the French Midi and Catalonia.[25] The reception of those of Aristotle's works which deal with the social function of the healer in urban communities and the results of the adoption of Roman law by such communities deserve a careful examination.

The views of the nature of the doctor-patient relationship were also connected to the reception of Aristotle's works on social organization and the role which the healer should play in an urban context. Aristotle expressed his opinion on this topic in his *Politics* (1258a 10ff.). From the point of view of economic theory, medicine would belong to the so-called art of acquisition, which was related to exchange or barter, with the result that it became a form of "labor for hire" (*mistharnía*,

medici, obedientia infirmi, ydoneitas ministrorum, et quartum congruitas extrinsecorum accidentium... Sed certam est quod non sunt per se nota, quia nec offerunt se sensui nec etiam apprehenduntur ab intellectu nisi per discursum rationis et studiosam meditationem. Similiter patet quod non sunt omnibus nota etiam medico; non enim omnes prompte cognoscunt ea que medicus habet agere vel observare ad sui directionem in finem operis medicinalis... Sed que sint hec considerabilia et ordinabilia in speciali non explicat Ypocras nec etiam eius expositores." *Repetitio super canonem "Vita brevis"* (cit. n. 13).

24 V. Nutton, "Continuity or Rediscovery. The City Physician in Classical Antiquity and Medieval Italy," in *The Town and State Physician in Europe from the Middle Ages to the Enlightenment*, ed. A.W. Russell (Wolfenbüttel: Herzog August Bibliothek, 1981), pp. 9–46, on pp. 27–28.

25 A. Gouron, "The Training of Southern French Lawyers during the Thirteenth and Fourteenth Centuries," in *Post Scripta. Essays... in Honor of Gaines Post* (Rome, 1972), pp. 219–227 (Studia Gratiana, XV), repr. in A. Gouron, *La science du droit dans le Midi de la France au Moyen Age* (London: Variorum, 1984).

1258b 25).[26] Thus, medicine was not only a source of health, but also of wealth for those who practiced it. Throughout the thirteenth and in the early fourteenth centuries, particularly in southern Europe, a social group developed which made trade and commercial exchange the most significant factor for social progress. This group came to dominate the European cities. This development was not merely a way of doing things, but also a new philosophy which affected human relations.[27] The doctor-patient relationship adapted to this norm of behavior and became an item of barter, subject to a contractual relationship between physician and patient. Moreover, the academic training of the physician or surgeon had a direct effect on the amount involved in the contract. Thus the activities of the medical practitioners were adopted to the commercial customs of the bourgeois groups which governed thirteenth- and fourteenth-century cities. This adaptation was perceived and criticized by both Christian and Jewish patients and physicians.

Aristotle's writings were of particular interest to the scholars of the faculties of arts in the mid-thirteenth century.[28] His *Politics* was the subject of commentaries by natural philosophers (among them Albert the Great and Thomas Aquinas), especially those parts dealing with the economic side of medical activity.

In the opinion of Albert the Great (d. 1280) in his commentary on the *Politics* (c. 1261),[29] the aim of medicine is to maintain health and recover it when lost, though the social circumstances of the mid-thirteenth century implied that those who practised medicine made

26 L. Edelstein, "The Professional Ethics of the Greek Physician," *Bull. Hist. Med.*, 1956, *30*:391–419, on p. 397 n.12.

27 A. Rubio-Vela, "Ideologia burgesa i progrés material a la València del Trescents," *L'Espill*, 1981, *9*:11–38, on pp. 24–28; Idem, *Epistolari de la València medieval* (València: Universitat de València, 1985), pp. 14–21, 133–134.

28 Weisheipl, "The Parisian Faculty of Art," (cit. n. 12), and J.A. Weisheipl, ed., *Albertus Magnus and the Sciences* (Toronto: Pontifical Institute of Mediaeval Studies, 1980).

29 Albertus Magnus, *In octo lib. Politicorum Aristotelis commentarii, Opera Omnia*, ed. P. Petrum Iammy, Vol. IV/2 (Lugduni, 1651). On the redaction date, see James A. Weisheipl, "Albert's Work on Natural Science (*libri naturales*) in Probable Chronological Order," in Weisheipl, ed., *Albertus Magnus* (cit. n. 28), pp. 565–577, on p. 575.

money.[30] A few years later, in 1272, Thomas Aquinas made matters more precise in a critical commentary, and stated that medicine is *neutra* with regard to earning money through its practice, but that the power of money has actually converted medicine into an *ars ad pecuniam.*[31] In the second decade of the fourteenth century, the university physician and surgeon Henry de Mondeville would already include the salary as an intrinsic element of the doctor-patient relationship.

Albert the Great identified three ways of acquiring money in the urban European society of the second half of the thirteenth century: merchandise (*mercatura*), usury (*usuraria*), and services (*ministrativa*). Medicine belonged to the last.[32] Thomas Aquinas classified medical practice as mercenary (*mercenaria*), as it involves hiring services in exchange for money, although its "useful" nature placed it in a special category.[33] The physician offered his technical knowledge in exchange for money. The salary of the physician or the surgeon was not an addition to the doctor-patient relationship, but an inseparable part of it. Fifty years later, Henry de Mondeville said that to practice free of charge could only be justified as an act of charity (*pro amore Deo*) for the poor, but not as a general situation for the entire population. The nature of medical practice as a "service" provided him with a justification to charge those who could afford to pay.[34] Arnau de Vilanova, a contemporary of Henry de Mondeville, stated that the physician achieves the two most important goals of a medieval Christian of the urban bourgeoisie: he secures eternal salvation through the practice of charity and he earns money from his work.[35] The conflicts between the

30 *In octo lib. Politicorum*, lib. I, c. 6 , ed. Iammy (cit. n. 29), p. 37.

31 "Medicinalis [ars] propter sanitatem, neutra tamen est propter pecuniam: sed quidem... medicinalem convertunt ad acquirendum pecuniam, et ita faciunt... esse pecuniativam, id est acquisitivam pecuniae, ordinantes huiusmodi artes ad pecuniam, sicut ad finem ad quem oportet ordinari omnia alia." Thomas Aquinatis, *In octo libros Politicorum Aristotelis expositio*, ed. P.R.M. Spiazzi (Taurini-Romae, 1966), li. I lect. viii no. 128, p. 40. On the date, see the Introduction, pp. xxiv–xxv.

32 *In octo lib. Politicorum*, lib. I, c. 8, ed. Iammy (cit. n. 29), p. 41.

33 *In octo lib. Politicorum*, lib. I, lect. ix, no. 141, ed. Spiazzi (cit. n. 31), p. 44.

34 See below.

35 "tunc splendebit pericia medici et erunt omnia opera eius meritoria postquam ex caritate fiant; nam apud Deum merebitur gratiam et ab hominibus et emolumentum." *Repetitio super canonem "Vita brevis"* (cit. n. 13).

mandate to give charity (valid for both Christians and Jews), the supposed "neutrality" of medicine in relation to the earning of money, and a pecuniary conception (*pecuniativa*) of medical activity appear to have been real problems in the thirteenth and fourteenth centuries. All of these issues were collected in the form of *quaestiones* in the commentaries of the university professors on Aristotle's *Politics*, and were also a part of the contents of some rabbinical *responsa*. Additional evidence that the problem of the earnings of medical practitioners was also of great concern to non-university laymen and medical people at this time are the criticisms which this topic aroused among both Christians and Jews. Among these criticisms are significant paragraphs in *The Book of the States* by the Castilian aristocrat and scholar Don Juan Manuel (1281–1348), a younger contemporary of Henry de Mondeville and Arnau de Vilanova,[36] and the harshly self-critical and courageous words written by learned Catalan and Provençal Jewish physicians such as Maimon Gallipapa (*fl.* 1353–1384)[37] and Leon Joseph of Carcassone (*c.* 1350–*c.* 1418).[38]

In addition to the commentaries on Aristotle, there is another type of evidence from university circles which is connected with the reintroduction of Roman law to medieval Latin Europe. These are the commentaries which the professors of the law school of Bologna wrote on the newly rediscovered Roman law texts, the *Digest* and the *Code* of Justinian. Some passages of these Roman legal texts deal with the rights and privileges of doctors, and members of the law school commented upon them in the early thirteenth century.[39] These commentar-

36 *El libro de los estados*, book I, c. 96 (Madrid: Castalia, 1991), p. 288.

37 See the English translation by H. Friedenwald, "The Physician's Aphorisms: A Medieval Hebrew Satire," in *The Jews and Medicine*, vol. I (Baltimore: The Johns Hopkins University Press, 1944), pp. 69–83. The chronology and biographical sketch given by Friedenwald are wrong, see E. Feliu and J. Riera, *Poemes hebraics de jueus catalans. Segles XI–XV* (Barcelona: Fundació Vives-Casajuana, 1976), pp. 151–152; E. Gutwirth, "En Maymon Galipapa: texto y contexto de un intelectual ilerdense," in *Actes Ir. Col.loqui d'Història dels Jueus a la Corona d'Aragó* (Lleida: Institut d'Estudis Ilerdencs, 1991), pp. 339–348.

38 Prologue to his Hebrew translation of Gerard de Solo's *Practica super nono Almansoris*. Hebrew text and English translation in García-Ballester *et al.*, "Jewish Appreciation" (cit. n. 4), Appendix D, pp. 106–117.

39 Nutton, "Continuity or Rediscovery" (cit. n. 24) p. 27 and the references cited therein.

ies reveal that the idea of a *salarium* contracted between a doctor and a private patient or a public institution such as a municipal council began to be known in university circles at this time.[40] The first documentary evidence of a city in the Po valley hiring a doctor to attend to its citizens is roughly contemporary, from 1211–1214 (Reggio, Bologna). From the end of the thirteenth century and during the fourteenth century, the position of the public doctor spread to several cities and even small towns throughout Italy,[41] the south of present-day France, and eastern Spain.[42] All of these factors may have provided a stimulus for the social acceptance of the concept of *salarium* and for the employment of doctors by local governments. *Salarium seu pensio* is the technical term used in contracts from the Crown of Aragon from the late thirteenth century onward to indicate the money and other benefits which doctors (physicians or surgeons, Christian or Jewish) received for their hired practice.

Henry de Mondeville, who studied in northern Italy and Montpellier,[43] derived the contractual nature of the medical activity from the medical structure of the doctor-patient relationship. One of the elements of this relationship, which belongs to the fifth *res non naturalis* (movements or accidents of the soul, *accidentia anime*), is the mutual confidence which should exist between doctor and patient. Without such confidence, the curative process would be much less efficient. "Without confidence rarely will the treatment have any effect."[44] The confidence of the physician or surgeon in his patient was demonstrated by two conditions of equal significance: the first was that the patient should carry out the instructions of the healer; the second that the patient should pay the fee agreed upon. The fee was the objective and tangible expression of the doctor's relationship with the patient and that of the patient with the doctor. At the same time, it guaranteed continuity in treatment. The following words of Henry de Mondeville

40 *Ibid.*, p. 28.

41 *Ibid.*, pp. 26 and 28–29.

42 Gouron, "The Training of Southern French Lawyers" (cit. n. 25), pp. 220–226.

43 D. Jacquart, *Supplément* to E. Wickersheimer, *Dictionnaire biographique des médecins en France au moyen age* (Genève: Librairie Droz, 1979), pp. 117–118.

44 *Die Chirurgie*, ed. Pagel (cit. n. 18), p. 114, where he cites Avicenna's commentary on book VI of Aristotle's *Naturalia*.

reflect the particular social and moral values prevailing in the society in which he practiced: "The patient mistrusts whatever is given free of charge. He does not believe that he will be given something of value for nothing."[45]

This process was reciprocal, and the contractual relationship also involved a series of obligations on the part of the physician, obligations which society came to subject to legal norms. The patient had legal means derived from Roman law to defend himself against increasingly aggressive treatment and an increasingly complex and expensive network of practitioners and medical care (physicians, physician-surgeons, surgeons, barbers, apothecaries). These practitioners displayed a high degree of adaptability to the laws of an already sensitive market, to the law of supply and demand, and also to the practical administrative laws which were derived from Roman law. In addition, the explanation by university physicians of the nature of the physician-patient relationship supplied interesting material to potential patients, and allowed the latter to check whether daily practice really corresponded to these explanations.[46]

Medicine was something more than individual practice, and the responsibility of the qualified healer had to go beyond the relationship between two individuals. Health came to be seen as a good in itself, as a positive factor for the community; it therefore had to be protected and encouraged. At the same time, health acquired political and moral

45 "Et vere nihil confert, aut parum patienti, quia minus confidit ex quo mente concipit, quod vix datur gratis aliquod pretiosum, et similiter medicina data gratis nihil confert cyrurgico penitus, immo nocet," *Ibid.*, p. 98.

46 The number of copies of thirteenth- to fifteenth-century manuscripts on medical etiquette belonging to the pre-Salernitan and Salernitan period which have survived is evidence of the popularity of this medical literary genre; see note 22 and the literature cited therein. Many times, these words, written by Arnau de Vilanova at the end of his commentary on the first of Hippocrates' *aphorismi*, turned against the daily behavior of the medical practitioners: "Medicus debet esse in cognoscendo studiosus et in precipiendo cautus et ordinatus, in respondendo circumspectus et providus et in pronosticando ambiguus, in promitendo iustus ut non promittat sanitatem quia tunc usurparet divinum officium et faceret Deo iniuriam; sed promittat fidelitatem et diligentiam in visitando et sit discretus et diligens, in sermone modestus, in affectione benevolus... Extrinsecus autem accidentalia convenit esse ne corpus patientis inde ledatur aut animus perturbetur." *Repetitio super canonem 'Vita brevis'* (cit. n. 13).

connotations. The preservation of health was perceived by normal citizens to be a moral obligation on the part of the public authorities (royal or municipal). The political authorities regarded the physician or surgeon who had been trained in medical science as an element which contributed to the better health of the *res publica*, and also considered that the physician's actions not only defended but also extended the demand for health care among the civil population of thirteenth- and fourteenth-century Mediterranean Europe.[47] This social aspect, which went beyond the personal relationship between physician and patient, acquired social validity during this period.

From the first third of the thirteenth century and throughout the fourteenth century, there is documentary evidence from Italy,[48] the south of France,[49] and the Crown of Aragon that in the cities and even in small towns, ordinary people understood sickness in rational terms. The town councillors left its treatment and possible cure in the hands of the physicians and surgeons who were under contract to take care of the people.[50] The concern which the municipal councils showed in obtaining medical assistance may be seen in the conditions they demanded from the medical practitioners. The conditions were stipulated more or less in detail in public contracts before a public notary, and constituted a form of recognition of the social responsibilities of the physician, something peculiar to the late medieval European world.

What gave rise to this concern on the part of the municipal authorities for the preservation of health and the cure of diseases? I agree with Nutton[51] that one of the factors which led to these contracts, in which the practitioner agreed to a series of socio-medical obligations as dictated by the municipal authorities, is the reception of Roman law.

47 García-Ballester, *et al.*, *Medical Licensing* (cit. n. 5), pp. 3–4.

48 Nutton, "Continuity or Rediscovery" (cit. n. 24), pp. 24ff and the references cited therein.

49 J. Shatzmiller, *Médecine et Justice en Provence Médiévale. Documents de Manosque, 1262–1348* (Aix-en-Provence: Université de Provence, 1989).

50 See Nutton, "Continuity or Rediscovery" (cit. n. 24), pp. 24ff. Michael McVaugh and I are working on this topic with materials from the archives of the Crown of Aragon from 1280–1400. See a partial approach in McVaugh, *Medicine Before the Plague* (cit. n. 5). The assertion that there was a rational understanding of sickness does not exclude the receipt of medical care from empirical healers and the use of magic procedures.

51 Nutton, "Continuity or Rediscovery" (cit. n. 24).

The contract itself and the intervention of the notary are consequences of this reception.[52] However, there is another type of evidence which provides an additional explanation of the attitude of the municipal councils, at least from the last third of the thirteenth century onward. This is the doctrine resulting from the commentaries on works by Aristotle such as the *Politics*, which, as I have already mentioned, were widespread in the schools of Arts of the mid thirteenth century. The responsibility of the authorities for the health or illness of the citizens is one of the themes of this work. When Henry de Mondeville wrote the dedication of his *Cirurgia* in 1306, he referred to this responsibility and cited Aristotle's *Politics*.[53]

Albert the Great's commentaries on Aristotle's *Politics* in the 1260s, together with the commentaries by Thomas Aquinas in 1272, impressed upon university circles, and through them on society in general, that "the urban authorities should be particularly concerned about the health (of the body) of their citizens."[54] The governors of society should also understand the problems of health and illness.[55] They added an important detail: the problems of the preservation of health and the treatment and cure of diseases were to be resolved by the doctor. Albert the Great believed that the medicine of his period had a technical foundation based on Galenism.[56] This opinion led him to

52 J. Plescia, "The rise of modern jurisprudence: Roman law, glossators and commentators," *Annals of the Archive of Ferran Valls i Taberner Library*, 1989, *6*:193–210.

53 "insuper ad utilitatem communem, quae secundum philosophum XI politicorum praeponenda est utilitati singulari," *Die Chirurgie*, ed. Pagel (cit. n. 18), p. 10.

54 "[Conditor civitatis] primum quidem tanquam necessarium ad sanitatem, scilicet quod cives in ea sani permaneant," "legislator qui curat de vita hominis, prius debet ordinare vitam secundum corpus quam secundum animam," Albertus Magnus, *In octo lib. Politicorum*, lib. VII, c.9 and 14, ed. Iammy (cit. n. 29), IV/2, pp. 433 and 459; "primo dicit quoniam conditorem civitatis oportet esse solicitum multum de sanitate inhabitantium civitatem," Thomas Aquinatis, *In octo libros Politicorum*, lib. VII, lect. 3, ed. Spiazzi (cit. n. 31), p. 377.

55 "principis enim oeconomi est providere ut habeatur medicus in sanitate conservans familiam, et curans aegrotos, et hoc modo pertinet medicina ad oeconomum et principem." Albertus Magnus, *In octo lib. Politicorum*, lib. I, c.7, ed. Iammy (cit. n. 29), IV/2, p. 37.

56 "Unde sciendum, quod Augustino in his quae sunt de fide et moribus plus quam philosophis credendum, si dissentiunt. Sed si de medicina loquitur, plus ego

believe that if the civil authorities were obliged to provide a doctor for the community, the doctor alone was responsible for both his technical training and the decisions which result from his medical work. He should identify the causes of diseases and the mechanisms which produce them, and also the function and correct use of drugs in the healing process.[57]

There remained at least two problems not directly touched upon by the commentators on Aristotle. The first was the methods which the civil authorities — the nobility in feudal dominions, the king in his realms, or the municipal authorities — would use in order to be sure that the practitioner (physician or surgeon) was well qualified. The other problem was that of the doctors' fee, or more generally, the economic part of the doctor-patient relationship. Despite the existence of university qualified doctors, or perhaps because of the lack of them, the civil communities established methods of examining the skills of medical practitioners, university trained or not, Christian, Moslem or Jew. Health was under municipal and also royal control, at least by law.[58] The problem of the salary, and of the economic factor in relation to the patient, did not at the outset appear to present any problem. A contract where the doctor's fee was clearly stated in annual, biannual, quinquennial, decennial, or life-long terms sufficed. It did not matter

crederem Galeno vel Hippocrati, et si de naturis rerum loquatur, credo Aristoteli plus vel alii experto in rerum naturis." *Super II Sententiarum*, d.13, C, a.2, *Opera omnia*, ed. A. Borgnet (Paris, 1890–1899), vol. XXVII, p. 247, cited by Albert Zimmermann, "Albertus Magnus und der lateinische Averroismus," in *Albertus Magnus Doctor Universalis, 1280–1980*, ed. G. Meyer and A. Zimmermann (Mainz: Matthias-Grünewald, 1980), pp. 465–493, on p. 475 note 41.

57 "sed medici [pertinet] cognoscere causas morborum et curarum, utrum purgativis et alterativis sit utendum in morbis, hoc est medici," Albertus Magnus, *In octo lib. Politicorum*, lib. VII, c. 14, ed. Iamny (cit. n. 29), p. 459. Thomas Aquinas, in answering a question, said: "Quare ars medicinalis nos est pars economicae, sicut pecuniativa? Et respondendum, quod ad dispensatorem domus et ad principem civitatis pertinet quodammodo considerare de sanitate, scilicet utendo consilio medicorum ad sanitatem subiectorum: alio autem modo non pertinet ad eos, sed ad medicos, considerando scilicet ex quibus rebus sanitas conservetur vel restituatur." *In octo libros Politicorum*, lib. I, lect. 8 no. 132, ed. Spiazzi (cit. n. 31), p. 40.

58 García-Ballester, *et al.*, *Medical Licensing* (cit. n. 5).

whether the medical practitioner made the contract with individuals or families, or with a civil or ecclesiastic community.[59]

I have not yet studied the contents of the rabbinical *responsa* on this matter, but at least from the Christian side, the ambiguity in Albert the Great's and Aquinas' commentaries on Aristotle when they declare the technical autonomy of the physician (in my opinion a way of washing one's hands of the issue), together with the blatant accumulation of money by individuals who belonged to social groups which had prospered through the commercial activities of the cities of Mediterranean Europe, introduced exceptions to the commandment to give charity and to the contractual demand for equality (free medical service for all the citizens of the municipality). In addition, there was of course the greed of certain physicians and surgeons, both Christian and Jewish, who converted the exception into general practice.

Leon Joseph of Carcassone (*c.* 1350–*c.* 1418), a Jewish doctor who practiced medicine in Languedoc and in the north of the Crown of Aragon (Perpignan), spoke out harshly against this situation:

> The majority of those who practice the art of medicine among my people do not intend to fathom the depths of their object; even if they were able to go into it in greater depth, they do not wish to tire their intelligence with this, and they mutter: this science is not a true science, but rather a skill; and with a 'sound of tumult' (Ezek. 1:24) everybody wishes to turn it into a means of existence; and they say that a learned physician is he who asks for a large sum of money and does not heal free of charge.[60]

59 For instance, the contracts between the bishop and the chapter of canons and the physician for medical attention for their persons and families. There are many examples in the Crown of Aragon: in Vic (Catalonia), Arxiu Curia Fumada, *Liber primus vitae*, 1288–1345, fols. 39r-v, contract with *Magister* Johannes de Portugal, *fisicus*, Kal. June 16, 1312 = May 17; another contract (fol. 49) with *Magister* Bernardus, *cirurgicus*, Idus July 8, 1315 = July 8. The bishop of Valencia signed a contract with *Magister* Mironus de Corça, *magister in artibus et in medicina*, Arxiu del Regne de València, Notarial records, Reg. 2923: Domingo Moliner, Nonas October 6, 1341 = October 2.

60 Prologue to his Hebrew translation of Gérard de Solo's *Practica super nono Almansoris*. See García-Ballester, *et al.*, "Jewish Appreciation" (cit. n. 4), Appendix D.

Two hundred years previously, around 1180, the Catalan Jewish physician Joseph ben Meir ibn Sabara gave a relentless description of the greed of the physicians in his work *The Book of Delights (in Teaching)*, written in Barcelona. He finished his arguments against bad physicians by citing a cynical epigram: "Be a physician, because by killing people you will become a wealthy man."[61] Three decades after the Black Death (around 1380) in Lérida, the only medieval university city in Catalonia with an operational faculty of medicine, Maimon Gallipapa, another Catalan Jewish physician, wrote a pitiless satire under the title "The Physician's Aphorisms." One of them states: "Whoever practices medicine without getting fees deserves to be stoned" (III,7).[62] Jewish medical practitioners were especially self-critical, as I have not found similar evidence among their contemporary Christian colleagues, whose clinical behavior certainly moved patients to fury.

The polemic character of the work of Maimon Gallipapa and of the *Prologue* by Leon Joseph (both written in the 1380s) reveals the intellectual and social tensions over both medical education and the crisis of moral values within the Catalan and Provençal Jewish communities. Gallipapa says:

> The sick are foolish and put their trust in a physician, a heretic or an atheist (I,1). The foundation of medicine was brilliant wisdom and its ways were upright. Recently, however, new people have come; the present doctors, who have learned little, boast: 'We are wise and know all the secrets of science,' but they are ignorant and empty-headed. They only take the gold, the silver, the coin. They corrupt and do evil, but how to do good they know not (I,3); to increase his fee is his only thought (I,2). This is the way the present doctors slaughter, in order to get large fees and to be regarded as experienced... Be ready to visit the patients, but not for mere talk or to be their aid and protector; only for a large compensation and not for nothing!... Be careful in your practice... and do not leave the patient's house with empty hands, or with

61 *Sepher Shaashuim*, Hebrew critical edition by Israel Davidson, 2nd ed. (Berlin, 1925). Catalan translation by I. Gonzàlez-Llubera (Barcelona: Editorial Alpha, 1931), pp. 152–154.

62 Friedenwald, "The Physician's Aphorisms" (cit. n. 37), p. 91.

> only some eggs or a piece of bread (III,7). In the valley of weeping on the night of the Ninth of Ab, when Lamentations is being read, the doctors of the present day prepare the oil...(IV,4).

Gallipapa concludes his book:

> [Forgive me] if I have spoken badly about the physicians, for I meant well! To wake their conscience; to make them study better their medical books [is my sole purpose]...; from this day on there shall be peace [between us] (V,1). Let us make peace between us and become friends... And you physicians, do your work diligently and with clean hands; and take for yourselves silver or gold, for the living must die and the dead shall be restored to life. Seize fortune when it deals pleasantly with people. I have found a noted proverb, and it shall be as a sign to you: 'Good fortune comes not to the faithful man' (V,2).[63]

In 1380 and 1387, when Maimon was writing his *Aphorisms*, Na Bellaire and Na Pla, the widows of two members of his family, Samuel and Jafuda Gallipapa, both physicians who had practiced in Lérida, asked the King for permission to practice medicine, and both received it.[64]

I do not know how many Christians and Jews were attended by Jewish practitioners. Indirect and very provisory figures indicate that in the second half of the fourteenth century (just before 1391) in north-east Spain (Catalonia, Aragon, Valencia and Majorca), between twenty and thirty per cent of the medical and surgical manpower which took care of the Christian population was Jewish.[65] Therefore the medical care of the Christian majority would be greatly influenced by the troubles affecting a minority of Jewish medical practitioners, as revealed in Maimon Gallipapa's *Aphorisms* and Leon Joseph of Carcassone's Prologue. It would thus be very useful for a comprehensive approach to the doctor-patient relationship, including the obvious

63 Friedenwald's translation, *Ibid.*, pp. 85ff.

64 Archive of the Crown of Aragon, Barcelona, C, reg. 1891 (1387 March 5), fols. 90v–91r, where the king confirms the permission given them in 1380 (October 10).

65 "Jewish medical practitioners in a Christian society: Catalonia and Majorca after the Black Death" (work in progress). The figures are derived from the evidence preserved in Christian archives.

ethical repercussions, in the context of the villages and towns of this part of Spain (where there is relatively abundant documentation) to have a better understanding of the intellectual and social life of the Jewish communities, especially the medical training and education of their practitioners and the relationship of the latter with their Christian patients and colleagues.

As I said at the beginning, I have endeavored to offer a sample of the social and intellectual complexity, together with the ethical repercussions, involved in the study of the doctor-patient relationship in later medieval Latin Christendom, with specific references to East Mediterranean Spain. Part of this complexity arose from the presence of two religious minorities (Moslem and Jewish) together with the Christian majority. In this article the Moslem minority has not been considered, as their healers were not hired by Christian municipal councils. At the same time, members of the Christian and Jewish communities relied on both Jewish and Christian healers for their medical care. The latter groups did not limit their medical practice to individuals of their own communities.

Acknowledgement

I am indebted to Eduard Feliu, who helped me in several steps of this chapter. Funding for this research was provided by the CICYT grant no. PB/89–0066 from the Spanish Ministry of Education and Science.

Jewish Physicians and Medicine in Medieval Spain

Yom Tov Assis

Introduction

For a variety of reasons medieval Jewish scholars found medicine a most attractive science. It offered them obvious advantages. It combined practical utility and theoretical speculation while providing a respectable livelihood and prestigious status. Moreover, it was considered religiously safe as, in the opinion of many, it did not contradict the Jewish faith and precepts. Even the ban of Barcelona of 1305 against the study of philosophy and secular sciences before the age of twenty-five specifically excluded medicine. Many Jewish scholars and rabbis were therefore students of medicine and practicing physicians.

Notwithstanding certain restrictions, such as the prohibition of autopsies, Judaism contained certain principles which promoted the medical sciences and hardly any injunctions similar to canon 22 of the IV Lateran Council of 1215, which forbade all physicians to attend to patients without first consulting the ecclesiastical authorities, and many restrictions decided upon in the Church Councils of Reims in 1131, Lateran in 1139, Montpellier in 1162 and 1195 and Paris in 1212.[1] The circumstances that prevailed in medieval Spain, particularly during the *Reconquista*, permitted many Jewish physicians to attain positions of power and influence both inside and outside the Jewish communities.

1 For the decision of 1215, see K. J. von Hefele, *Histoire des conciles*, V, Paris 1907–1952, pp. 1351ff. (This is the expanded French translation by H. Leclerq & others of the German original).

Spanish Jews in Medicine

The medieval physician differed in several respects from his modern counterpart. The distinction between quacks or magical healers and physicians was not clear. Despite Maimonides' opposition to the former category, eminent Catalan rabbis like R. Moshe ben Naḥman (Naḥmanides) and R. Shelomo ben Adret (Rashba) of Barcelona were not against magical healing. The former was himself a doctor.[2] Adret was asked on several occasions about the different magical cures which were prevalent among Iberian Jews. The use of figures, magical solutions and recipes, superstitious formulas and amulets was tolerated and even condoned by Adret and some of his Iberian colleagues.[3] Little children, men, women and even rabbis acted as magical healers.[4] For emergency cases, amulets were written on Shabbat with rabbinic consent.[5] Despite the popularity of a large variety of non-medical recipes for curing purposes, Jewish physicians in Spain were very much in demand and enjoyed a special status in all the Hispanic kingdoms.

Jewish Physicians in Muslim Spain

In Muslim Spain, the Jews were deeply involved in various fields of medical science and practice. Jews took part in translation projects of medical works into Arabic. They were students as well as teachers of medicine. Even when anti-rationalist trends caused the decline of the medical profession in Muslim society, Jewish medical tradition was not affected and even an anti-rationalist like R. Yehudah ha-Levi was a physician.[6]

2 S. Kottek, "Naḥmanide, médecin (1174–1270)," *Revue d'Histoire de la Médecine Hébraïque*, Mars 1965, *LXVII*: 23–28.

3 R. Shelomo ben Adret, *Responsa*, Bologna, 1539 [henceforth Adret I], Nos. 167, 413, 548, 825; idem, *Responsa*, Leghorn, 1657 [henceforth Adret II], No. 281; idem, *Responsa*, Leghorn, 1778, [henceforth Adret III], Nos. 82, 100.

4 Adret III, No. 318; Adret I, Nos. 418, 548.

5 R. Shelomo ben Adret, *Responsa*, Vilna, 1881 [henceforth Adret IV], No. 245.

6 D. Margalit, "R. Yehudah haLevi as Physician," *Koroth*, 1953, I: 94–97 (Hebrew); IV–V (English).

Jews were also prominent in medical literature. A number of medical treatises were written by Jews in Muslim Spain. Jonah ben Isḥaq ibn Biklarish of Almería (d. ca. 1100) wrote the *Kitāb al-Musta'ini,* a book on remedies, the names of which were given in six languages. The well-known grammarian Jonah ibn Janaḥ prepared a medical dictionary. Most productive in medical works was Yusuf ben Aḥmad ibn Ḥisdai, who was, however, to leave Spain and abandon Judaism. The Jewish influence in the Faculty of Medicine on Montpellier, which has been pointed out by several historians, can be traced mostly to the activities of Jewish immigrants from the Iberian peninsula, following the Almohadic invasion. The inclusion of Montpellier within the territories of the Crown of Aragon facilitated the integration of the immigrants in the region.[7]

Under Muslim rule, Jewish physicians in Spain played an important role in the Jewish community and in society at large. The propaganda of Muslim extremists did not deter people from turning to Jewish physicians. Many held important positions in politics, finance, science and culture thanks to their medical expertise. While taking care of the ruler's health, many Jewish physicians gained his confidence and were sometimes entrusted with important political posts. The most famous Jewish physician who attained political prominence was Ḥasdai ibn Shaprut who may be considered the founder of Spanish Jewry. He was sent by the Caliph Abd al-Raḥman III to cure the king of Leon. His medical mission was highly praised by his proteges Dunash ben Labrat and Menaḥem ben Saruq.[8]

Jewish Physicians between Andalusia and Christian Spain

Our information on the Muslim period is derived primarily from literary sources and medical literature, as we lack archives from the period. The situation is completely different for the kingdoms of

7 M. H. Halevy, "Contribution à la proto-histoire de la médecine montpelliéraine: Ibn Zabarra et les relations hispano-languedociennes au XIIe siècle," *Revue d'Histoire de la Médecine Hébraïque*, Juillet 1960, *XLVIII*: 63–79; G. Sarton, *Introduction to the History of Science*, II, pt. 1 (Baltimore, 1931), p. 235.

8 E. Ashtor, *The Jews of Moslem Spain* (Philadelphia, 1973), vol. I, pp. 155–227.

Christian Spain, and particularly for the Crown of Aragon and Navarre, where central archives preserve invaluable material on Jewish physicians. The Hebrew sources, especially the responsa of great halakhists of the thirteenth and fourteenth centuries, provide additional data on the status and activities of the Jewish physicians.[9]

Jewish physicians found refuge in the Hispanic kingdoms following the Almohadic invasion and the progress of the *Reconquista*. Many Jewish scholars who were expert in philosophy and science and versatile in Arabic took part in translation projects in the Christian kingdoms of Spain between the end of the eleventh and the end of the thirteenth centuries. The transmission of scientific works of the classical age and of the Arabic period to Christian Spain and then to Europe through their translation from Arabic into Latin, Romance languages and Hebrew totally transformed the study and practice of the sciences in Christendom. Whilst the Jews' contribution to other sciences was very significant, in medicine the number of medical works written or translated by Jews is relatively small.[10] Jews of Andalusian origin in the kingdoms of Christian Spain and local Jews raised in the Judeo-Arabic tradition continued to promote Andalusian science and study scientific works in Arabic, including medical books.[11] Jewish scholars in the Hispanic kingdoms also benefited from medical literature in Romance and Hebrew.[12]

9 On Jewish physicians in the territories of the Crown of Aragon, see J. Rubió y Balaguer, "Metjes y cirurgians juheus," appendix to A. Rubió y Lluch, "Notes sobre la ciencia oriental a Catalunya en el XIVen sigle," *Estudis Universitaris Catalans*, 1909, *III*: 389–398; 489–497; and more recently J. Danon, "La medicina judía en la Corona de Aragón," *Medicina e Historia*, 1987 (third series) *XIX*: I–XVI.

10 D. Romano, "Le opere scientifiche di Alfonso X e l'intervento degli ebrei," *Oriente e Occidente nel Medioevo: Filosofia e Scienze* (Rome, 1971), pp. 677–711; *idem*, "La transmission des sciences arabes par les Juifs en Languedoc," *Juifs et Judaïsme de Languedoc* (Toulouse: Edouard Fayard Editeur, 1977), pp. 363–386; *idem*, "El papel judío en la transmisión de la cultura," *Hispania Sacra*, 1988, *XL*: 955–978.

11 A. Rubió y Lluch, *Documents per l'història de la cultura catalana mig-eval*, vol. II (Barcelona, 1921), pp. 13–14.

12 L. García-Ballester, L. Ferre & E. Feliu, "Jewish Appreciation of Fourteenth-Century Scholastic Medicine," *Osiris*, 1990, 2nd series, *VI*: 85–117.

Many medical works were translated from Arabic into Latin, Romance and Hebrew in Castile, Catalonia and Aragon. Jews from Toledo, Saragossa, Barcelona, Gerona and Montpellier took part in these medical translations which, despite their relatively small number, contributed much to medicine. In 1134, Abraham bar Ḥiya translated into Romance the treatise *Aeneas de pulsibus et urinis* of Hunain ibn Isḥaq (Johanitius), whose Arabic compilation of the ninth century was based on Greek sources. Shemuel ben Yehudah ibn Tibbon, inhabitant of Barcelona, translated the *Comentarios al Tegni de Galeno* of Ali ibn Ridwan.[13] Shem Tov ben Yisḥaq, originally from Tortosa, was the translator of al-Zahrawi's *Liber servitoris* into Hebrew.[14] His son Abraham ben Shem Tov translated this work into Latin in collaboration with the Genoese Simon Cordo. At the beginning of the fourteenth century Jahuda ben Astrug Bonsenyor translated *Arabico in romancio*, a treatise of al-Zahrawi. Jaime II's physician Benvenist Samuel or Ozmel was commissioned to translate several medieval works, one of which was Maimonides' *Treatise on Asthma*. In 1349, maestro Shelomo de Mallorca translated a book of medicine into Catalan.[15]

Jews in Medical Literature

Reference must also be made to original medical works written by Jews. Sheshet Benvenist's treatise on gynecology, written at the end of the twelfth century, was subsequently translated into Hebrew by Yehudah ben Shelomo al-Ḥarizi. Abraham de Castlar from Besalú was the author of various medical treatises in Hebrew, one of which was *'Aleh Ra'anan*. In Castile, at the beginning of the fourteenth century, an anonymous work appeared in Arabic, entitled *Al Tibb al-Gastalli* (Castilian Medicine). Shemuel ibn Waqar wrote in Arabic a book on medicine. Shem Tov ben Falaquera wrote a book on diet and ethics. A

13 B. Z. Dinur, *Israel in the Diaspora*, vol. II, Book VI (Tel Aviv: Devir, 1972), p. 215 (Hebrew).

14 For an excerpt from his introduction to al-Zahrawi's work, see *Ibid.*, pp. 213–214.

15 For medical works translated from Arabic into Hebrew, see *Ibid.*, pp. 214–215. On Jahudah Bonsenyor, see A. Cardoner Planas, "Nuevos datos acerca de Jafuda Bonsenyor," *Sefarad*, 1944, *V*: 287–293.

treatise on hemorrhoids was written by Shelomo ibn Ayub the Spaniard.[16] Moshe ben Yisḥaq ibn Waqar, who lived at the beginning of the fifteenth century, was a prolific writer and wrote several books on medicine.[17]

The participation of Jews in medical research and the publication of original and translated books of medicine is vitally important but is only one aspect of the Jews' contributions to medicine in medieval Spain. Jewish physicians enjoyed the highest reputation among all sectors of society. Their work at the courts is the most eloquent illustration of their status. Although they were barred from the medical faculties of the Hispanic kingdoms, the kings who engaged the best physicians invariably had Jewish physicians at their courts.[18] The records from the *Archivo de la Corona de Aragón*[19] provide a comprehensive picture for the Crown of Aragon that was equally true in the other Hispanic kingdoms.

Privileges and Advantages

The royal families were particularly interested in ensuring that Jewish physicians and surgeons should not be prevented from attending to the sick in their households. The physicians' freedom of movement was not to be restricted for any reason.[20] During Jaime II's reign, Vidal Roven, a Jewish doctor from Barcelona, was guaranteed freedom of

16 *Ibid.*, p. 223. Shem Tov Falaquera, *Batte Hanhagat haGuf haBari*, ed. S. Muntner, 1950.

17 B. Richler, "Medical Treatises by Moses b. Isaac ibn Waqar," *Koroth*, 1989, *IX*, No 9–10: 700–707 (English); 253–264 (Hebrew).

18 A. Cardoner Planas & F. Vendrell Gallostra, "Aportaciones al estudio de la familia Abenardut, médicos reales," *Sefarad*, 1947, *VII*: 303--348; J. Miret y Sans, "Les médecins juifs de Pierre, roi d'Aragon," *Revue des Etudes Juives*, 1909, *LVII*: 268–278; A. de la Torre, "Un médico de los Reyes Católicos," *Hispania*, 1944, *XIV–XVII*: 66–72.

19 The following are the abbreviations used in connection with sources from the archives referred to in this article: ACA = Archivo de la Corona de Aragón; R = Registro; f = folio.

20 ACA, R 218, f 42v [see J. Régné, *History of the Jews in Aragon, Documents and Regesta 1213–1327*, ed. Y. Assis, (Jerusalem: Magnes, 1978), No. 3130 [henceforth Régné followed by the number of the document; R 206, f 123v–124 [Régné 2904].

movement. His means of transportation could not be confiscated so that his visits to his patients would not be disrupted. His patients should have free access to his house in the *call* (the Jewish Quarter). His Muslim servant was not to be detained either.[21] On the whole, Jewish physicians, including those from foreign lands, were permitted to settle in any locality they chose.[22]

Jewish physicians enjoyed various privileges and were often under special royal protection. Apart from their privilege not to wear the special clothes which the rest of the Jews did, Jewish physicians received a variety of benefits which sometimes aroused the opposition of the community no less than that of the local authorities. They were both frequently ordered not to act against Jewish doctors.[23] Some of the privileges granted to the Jewish doctors separated them from their brethren in their obligations vis-à-vis the royal family and other factors.[24] The physicians valued the charters they received from the king for their protection.[25] On the whole, Jewish doctors enjoyed preferential treatment. Abraham de Castlar, for instance, was authorized to marry a second wife in 1320.[26] Others benefited from different protective measures for services rendered.[27]

Exemption from taxation was the most frequent privilege granted to Jewish doctors in royal service. Alfonso III, wishing to show his appreciation to his physician Juceff de Orta for his excellent care, granted him an annual income and an exemption from the taxes paid by the Jews of Calatayud.[28] During the Sardinian campaign in 1323, while on an official mission, the Jewish doctors Azaria Abenjacob, from Saragossa, and Mosse, from Huesca, were exempted from paying

21 ACA, R 211, f 337v [=Régné 3020]; R 213, f 267 [=Régné 3059]

22 ACA, R 204, f 34 [=Régné 2870] see J. Miret y Sans, "Le massacre des Juifs de Montclús en 1320," *Revue des Etudes Juives*, 1907, *LIII*: 257–258; R 205, f 245 [=Régné 2893].

23 ACA, R 74, f 43 [=Régné 1843]; R 75, f 28v [=Régné 1780]; R 204, f 48 [=Régné 2869]; R 223, f 160v [=Régné 3250].

24 ACA, R 205, f 152 [=Régné 2882].

25 ACA, R 199, f 31 [=Régné 2769].

26 ACA, R 218 , f 29 [=Régné 3129].

27 ACA, R 89, f 169 [=Régné 2607]; R 219, f 236 [=Régné 3173]; R 223, f 160v [=Régné 3250].

28 ACA, R 75, f 33v [=Régné 1804–5].

taxes with their respective communities.[29] Juceff Almuli, the doctor of the *infante* Alfonso, obtained tax exemption for ten years.[30] Abraham de Castlar, who lived in Besalú since his immigration from southern France, had taken care of various members of the royal family and especially the *infante* don Pedro. Jaime II granted him several privileges to express his appreciation. In 1327, he exempted him and his heirs from any taxes and subsidies. The exemption from indirect taxes, customs and other duties was for thirty years.[31] Privileged physicians were sometimes freed from the collective responsibility which the entire community bore in the payment of taxes.[32] This privilege was meant to facilitate the doctors' work and advanced training.[33]

Some Jewish physicians serving the nobility, churchmen or the general population obtained easy terms for their tax payments. Such was the case of Alaçar, a doctor of Huesca, whose payment of the tax in 1280 was postponed by three months by Alfonso III at the request of the lord of Ayerbe.[34] Salomon, son of en Çahen, a physician from Egea, received a reduction on the same tax at about the same time.[35] In 1301, at the request of the Dominicans of the city of Valencia, Jaime II freed the Valencian Jewish doctor Omar from the collective tax responsibility of the *aljama*.[36]

Doctors' Fees and the Poor

The fees of the physicians varied from place to place and from time to time. The king and the *infante* often paid their Jewish physicians with benefits and income due to them from various sources. Regular income from economic enterprises and institutions as well as payments to the

29 ACA, R 223 , f 272 [=Régné 3264]; R 224, f 56 [=Régné 3274].
30 ACA, R 226, f 48v; R 229, f 214v–215 [=Régné 3310, 3412].
31 ACA, R 229, f 292v–293; R 230, f 96v–97 [=Régné 3433, 3447].
32 ACA, R 201, f 21 [=Régné 2820]; R 205, f 243v [=Régné 2892]; R 211, f 254 [=Régné 3011].
33 ACA, R 210, f 46 r&v [=Régné 2973–4].
34 ACA, R 66, f 75 [=Régné 1550].
35 ACA, R 67, f 25v [=Régné 1574].
36 ACA, R 196, f 296 [=Régné 2750].

royal treasury were often used to pay for medical services.[37] There are records showing that Jewish physicians were paid for the expenses they incurred whilst attending to the needs of the royal family.[38] In some instances the payment was made in kind. In 1285, Pedro III of Aragon gave special clothes to Samuel, the physician of the king of Castile.[39]

As usual, the lower classes had difficulties in paying for the doctor and the medicines. For some families these expenses were heavy.[40] The creation of confraternities for medical aid was designed primarily to meet the needs of the sick among the poor. These societies were formed in various regions on the peninsula.[41] The first records are from the first half of the fourteenth century. The functions of some of these societies or *ḥaburot* were to visit the sick and to provide food and medicines to those who could not afford them. In the case of the very ill, the members of the society undertook to recite psalms and prayers beside their beds. The *biqur ḥolim* societies received their income from the regular payments of their members and from the contributions of generous Jews. In some wills *biqur ḥolim* was promised a certain sum. In several communities, such as that of Perpignan, donations were regularly offered to *biqur ḥolim* societies.[42]

In some communities the *biqur ḥolim* society became a most important institution in the life of the community. In fourteenth century Saragossa, the *biqur ḥolim* society developed considerably. In the 1380s, it obtained permission to establish a synagogue of its own which became fairly soon a center of communal life in the city. In the last decade of the fourteenth century, the poorer classes concentrated their

37 See, for instance, ACA, R 14, f 143 [=Régné 505 [F. Bofarull y Sans, *Los judíos en el territorio de Barcelona (siglos X al XIII, Reinado de Jaime I, 1213–1276* (Barcelona: 1910), No. CXI]; R 71, f 59 [=Régné 1747]; R 75, f 33v [=Régné 1804]; R 74, f 43 [=Régné 1844].

38 ACA, R 85, f 182 [=Régné 2365].

39 ACA, R 58, f 22 [=Régné 1343].

40 R. Asher ben Yeḥiel, *Sheelot u-Teshuvot* (Venice, 1607), LXXXV, 2; R. Yehudah ben Asher, *Zikhron Yehudah* (Berlin, 1846), No. 38.

41 For a general description of these confraternities in Spain, see Y.T. Assis, "Welfare and Mutual Aid in the Spanish Jewish Communities," in *The Sephardi Legacy*, ed. H. Beinart (Jerusalem: Magnes, 1992), pp. 327–330.

42 *Responsa of R. Nissim Gerondi*, ed. L. A. Feldman (Jerusalem: Institute Schalem, 1984), Nos. 1, 75.

activities in the *biqur ḥolim* synagogue.[43] In the Aragonese towns of Huesca and Teruel, similar *biqur ḥolim* societies operated. In the former city, the society had its own *bet midrash*.[44]

Another confraternity which worked for the sick was *shomre ḥolim*. Such a confraternity operated in Santa Coloma de Queralt in the first half of the fourteenth century. Its revenues came from members' payments and individual bequests and donations. It functioned as a mutual aid society which also promoted religious life. Its primary function was the care of the sick. Its members undertook to take turns by the bedside of the sick person.[45] A *shomre ḥolim* society was set up in Saragossa in 1387. Its purpose was to ensure that someone was present day and night at the bedside of the sick. Its members agreed to teach Hebrew and Torah to the sick.[46] In Murviedro, in the Kingdom of Valencia, a confraternity by this name took care of the sick.[47]

All of these societies catered first and foremost to the needy sick people who lacked the money for doctors and medicine and who had no one to look after them while they were confined to bed. The hospice, the hospital in the Latin and Romance sources, was a shelter for poor sick Jews but catered to other categories as well. The hospices developed in the fourteenth century parallel to a similar development in Christian society.[48]

The Status of Jewish Physicians

The physicians belonged to the upper and middle classes of Jewish society. Some families had more than one physician among their

43 A. Blasco Martínez, "Instituciones sociorreligiosas judías de Zaragoza (siglos XIV–XV) — Sinagogas, cofradías, hospitales," *Sefarad*, 1990, L: 27–29.

44 J. L. Lacave, "Las juderías aragonesas al terminar del reinado de Fernando I," *Sefarad*, 1979, XXXIX: 221–222; F. Baer, *Die Juden im christlichen Spanien, I, Aragonien und Navarra* (Berlin, 1929), pp. 531–2, No. 351.

45 Secall i Güell, *La comunitat hebrea de Santa Coloma de Queralt* (Tarragona: Institut d'Estudis Tarraconenses, 1986), pp. 153–156, Notes 56, 69–71, 79.

46 Blasco, "Instituciones" (cit. n. 43), pp. 277–278, doc. 6.

47 A. Chabret, *Sagunto — Su historia, sus monumentos*, vol. II (Barcelona, 1888), p. 344.

48 Assis, "Welfare and Mutual Aid" (cit. n. 41), pp. 330–333; E. Gutwirth, "Jewish Hospitals in Spain," *Pe'amim*, 1989, XXX: 140–150 (Hebrew).

members.[49] These doctors possessed real estate and substantial assets. Samuel, for instance, the king's physician, owned houses in Tarrazona and was engaged in extensive moneylending in addition to his medical occupation.[50] The Valencian physician Vives was among the rich Jews of the community as he was one of the few who were asked in 1287 to rescue Alfonso III from his financial difficulties by lending him money. Vives was not the richest in the list but he must have been among the wealthy of the community.[51] The position of the physician in Jewish society depended on his reputation and the public's need for his services. In 1302 the municipal authorities and the community of Saragossa declared the services of R. Salamon Avenjacob, a local Jewish physician, to be indispensable. The king was asked to free him from all responsibility for the non-payment of taxes. He was also exempt from the obligation to assume any post in the communal administration so that he would be free to attend to the sick at any time of the day.[52] About a year later, another Jewish physician from Saragossa, Baron Almelich, obtained the same benefits.[53] As in the case of R. Salamon Avenjacob, some physicians enjoyed an even greater prestige owing to their rabbinic and general erudition. Such was the case of R. Azaria Abenjacob, most probably a relative of R. Salamon, who also acted as notary and scribe and who was authorized to appoint someone to assist him and replace him when necessary.[54] As in many communities members were obliged to accept any appointment or nomination, the privilege granted to physicians not to fill any official post was significant. Both Omer Tahuyl and Abraffim Tahuyl, father and son physicians from Valencia, enjoyed such a privilege.[55]

The number of Jewish physicians in any Jewish community was usually very high. Their number in small communities such as Besalú, Santa Coloma de Queralt and Valls is striking. In Besalú, there were a

49 For the case of the Portella family from Tarazona, for instance, see ACA, R 194, f 208v–209 [=Régné 2609]; R 197, f 144 [=Régné 2743]; R 204, f 108 [=Régné 2883].

50 ACA, R 61, f 106 [=Régné 1048]; R 70, f 190v [=Régné 1774].

51 ACA, R 71, f 49v [=Régné 1726].

52 ACA, R 199, f 120v–121 [=Régné 2794].

53 ACA, R 201, f 21 [=Régné 2820].

54 ACA, R 477, f 147; R 860, f 213 [=Régné 2985]; R 211, f 220 [=Régné 3001].

55 ACA, R 211, f 235v [=Régné 3005]; R 215, f 185v, 254v [=Régné 3075, 3083].

number of well-known families of doctors, such as de Castlar or Caslari. In Santa Coloma, the list is very long and impressive and includes at least two women.[56] The practice of medicine by Jewish women is noteworthy from several aspects. It is indicative of the status of women in Jewish society and also of the popularity of, and need for, Jewish doctors. The names of Na Ceti from Valencia, Na Floreta Ça Noga from Santa Coloma, Bonanada are all known because of their services to the royal family in the second half of the fourteenth century. The two Jewish women doctors who received their licenses from Pedro IV of Aragon, Na Bellaire wife of Samuel Gallipapa and Na Pla wife of Jafuda Gallipapa, had their licenses confirmed in 1387. These women doctors were very likely trained by a family member.[57]

Medical Training

We are still very much in the dark concerning the training of Jewish physicians. As there are no records indicating that Jews studied in Christian institutions, it is reasonable to assume that most Jewish physicians and surgeons were coached privately. Some were certainly trained by their own fathers or relatives. Many doctors had at least one of their sons follow in their footsteps.[58] Leon Cohen, from Puigcerdà, and his sons Bonet and Bonjuach were all surgeons.[59] With the introduction of medical examinations in 1289 at the *Cortes* of Monzón, provisions were made for Jews to take the examination and obtain a license. In the same *Cortes* of 1363, it was decided that a Jewish (and Muslim) candidate had to be examined by two physicians, a Jew and a

56 Secall i Güell, *La comunitat hebrea* (cit. 45), pp. 77–94; M. Grau i Montserrat, "Metges jueus a Besalú, (s. XIV)," in *I Assemblea d'Estudis sobre el Comtat de Besalú, 1968, Actes*, (Olot, 1972), pp. 29–33; G. Secall Güell, "Els metges jueus de Valls," *Cultura*, 1978, *CCCLXVIII*: 11–14.

57 A. Cardoner Planas, "Seis mujeres hebreas practicando la medicina en el reino de Aragón," *Sefarad*, 1949, *IX*: 441–445; A. Lopez de Meneses, "Cinco catalanas licenciadas en medicina por Pedro el Ceremonioso (1374–1382)," *Correo Erudito*, 1957, V, No 37: 152–154.

58 See, for instance, ACA, R 215, f 254v [=Régné 3075, 3083] and R. W. Emery, "Jewish Physicians in Medieval Perpignan," *Michael*, 1991, *XII*: 113–134.

59 ACA, R 219, f 236 [=Régné 3173].

Christian, and in the absence of a Jewish examiner, by two Christians. The Jewish candidates had to be examined by Jewish physicians and one Christian. They had to take an oath *per Deum et decem praecepta habitas quam Deum dedit Moysi in Monte Sinay*.[60] In Montpellier, which was under Catalan rule in the thirteenth century, the obligation to pass an examination before practicing medicine applied to both Jews and Christians, according to a ruling issued by Jaime I in July 1272. The ruling was subsequently repeated many times.[61] Davit Abrahem of Cervera, Vidal Abib, David Bonet Bonjorn of Perpignan, Mair Caravida of Besalú were among those who took the medical examination in the fourteenth century. Some Jews like Mosse des Portal of Camprodón were allowed to practice medicine without taking an examination. It was only after the 1391 massacres that the number of Jewish examinees rapidly declined.

Christian Patients in Jewish Hands

The physicians' responsibility for the health of their patients depended on several factors, of which the most important was the status of the patient. The death of a patient who was a member of a powerful family could cause serious problems for the physician who failed to cure him. Jewish physicians were especially vulnerable. Jewish physicians and surgeons were liable to prosecution even when their dead patients were Jewish. In 1283, Bonastruch Baco, a Jewish surgeon from Saragossa, was arrested following the death of his Jewish patient. The *infante* ordered that the charges be dropped if there was no evidence against Bonastruch, who was also to be released.[62] Legal actions against Jewish physicians for incompetence and failure in their profession were a frequent occurrence.[63] In 1321, a Jewish surgeon from Arbós, Abraham Carbo, was held responsible for the death of one of his patients. Jaime II intervened on his behalf.[64] Additional dangers awai-

60 A. Cardoner Planas, "Seis mujeres" (cit. n. 57), p. 444.
61 See Régné 525 for bibliography.
62 ACA, R 61, f 135 [=Régné 1065].
63 ACA, R 84, f 17v [=Régné 2296].
64 ACA, R 220, f 17v [=Régné 3186].

ted Jewish physicians who were asked to visit sick members of noble or rich families. The risks during these journeys were very real. There were instances of premeditated attacks against Jewish doctors, which were designed to obtain ransom money.[65]

Despite the decision of the Council of Béziers to forbid Christians to turn to Jewish physicians for treatment, no sector of Christian society was prepared to forego the services of Jewish physicians, who were highly esteemed. Kings and members of the royal family, the rich and poor, and even churchmen turned to Jewish doctors when their health was at stake. The great benefits which the inhabitants of a city derived from Jewish doctors is made explicit in many royal documents. The king insisted that Jewish doctors not be disturbed in the exercise of their profession or in their efforts to improve their medical expertise.[66] Churchmen also availed themselves of the services of Jewish physicians despite the prohibitions issued by many Church Councils. The Dominican friars in Valencia employed a Jewish doctor at the end of the thirteenth and the beginning of the fourteenth century.[67]

Jewish Physicians in Royal Service

Almost every ruler in Christian Spain availed himself of the services of a Jewish physician. The list of Jewish physicians at the courts is too long to be given in full. Açach Avenbenvenist from Barcelona was Jaime I's physician and was highly appreciated. Another physician in the service of Jaime I was Jucef Abencredi from Saragossa. Both enjoyed various privileges for their loyal services.[68] Samuel Alfaquim from Valencia was Pedro III's doctor and secretary. In his double capacity he accompanied the royal family on all its travels. He was exempted from wearing the special mantle which the Jews were ordered

65 ACA, R 44, f 235v [=Régné 1182].

66 For the case of Vidal from Barcelona see ACA, R 210, f 46 r&v [=Régné 2973–4]. Other cases have been referred to elsewhere in this article.

67 ACA, R 196, f 296 [=Régné 2750].

68 ACA, R 16, f 170v [=Régné 430]. See Bofarull y Sans, *Los judíos* (cit. n. 37), No. XCIII; R 14, f 143 [=Régné 505] Bofarull y Sans, *Los judíos* (cit. n. 37), No. CXI.

to wear.[69] Even after the dismissal of all Jews from official positions in the Crown of Aragon in 1283, Jewish doctors continued to serve the royal court. Maestre Samuel was the physician of Alfonso III and was supported by the king in recovering his loans to Christian debtors.[70] Another Jewish doctor who attended to Alfonso III was Juceff de Orta, who was handsomely recompensed for the good treatment he provided the king.[71] Jahuda Almeradi was the physician of the *infante* Pedro, Alfonso's brother.[72] Jaime II had several Jewish doctors in his service. Omar Abnarranhel or Abnacahuel, Abraham Toroç, Alazar, Azariah Abenjacob, Mosse, Juceff Almuli attended to Jaime II and his family. They all benefitted from a special status and were granted certain privileges, sometimes at the expense of the community.[73] Although from the end of the thirteenth century, in general, Jews were no longer in the service of the Aragonese kings, throughout the fourteenth century Jewish physicians continued to serve the royal court.[74] During the reign of Alfonso IV several Jewish physicians were mentioned: Juceff Baron, Mayr Alatzar, Ezdra Alaçar, Salamon and Jucef Almuli (or Almali), all from Saragossa, and Jucef Almujuciel from Lérida. Alatzar Abenardut, Bonhuha Cabrit, mestre Cresques, mestre Salamo, Benvenist Salamo and R. Nissim Gerondi acted as physicians to Pedro IV. There were also some women physicians who catered to the female members of the royal household. They were Na Ceti, Na Floreta wife of Jucef Ça Noga from Santa Coloma de Queralt and Bonanada, all mentioned above.[75]

Samuel ibn Waqar, physician of Alfonso XI, don Zag and don Salamon, in the service of Juan Manuel and Meir Alguades, physician

69 ACA, R 46, f 178v [=Régné 1117]. See J. E. Martínez Ferrando, *Catálogo de la documentación relativa al antiguo reino de Valencia*, vol. II (Madrid, 1934), No. 1903.

70 ACA, R 70, f 190v [=Régné 174].

71 ACA, R 75, f 33 [=Régné 1804].

72 ACA, R 85, f 24v [=Régné 2128].

73 ACA, R 200, f 210 [=Régné 2813]; R 204, f 48 [=Régné 2869].

74 J. Rius Serra, "Aportaciones sobre médicos judíos en Aragón en la primera mitad del siglo XIV," *Sefarad*, 1952, *XII*: 337–350; A. Cardoner Planas, "El linaje de los Cabrit en relación con la medicina del siglo XIV," *Sefarad*, 1956, *XVI*: 357–368; A. Cardoner Planas & F. Vendrell Gallostra, "Aportaciones al estudio de la familia Abenardut, médicos reales," *Sefarad*, 1947, *VII*: 303–348; Miret y Sans, "Les médecins juifs" (cit. n. 18), pp. 268–278.

75 Miret y Sans, "Les médecins juifs" (cit. n. 18), pp. 268–278.

of Juan I, all in Castile, are just a few names of Jewish physicians serving the Castilian crown.

Conclusion

The medical profession remained very popular among the Jews of Spain from the Muslim period until the Expulsion. The situation did not change among the *conversos*. Numerous were the physicians of *converso* origin who practised the profession and fulfilled an important role in teaching it in Spanish universities in the sixteenth and seventeenth centuries.[76]

The Castilian and Aragonese kings granted their physicians numerous privileges, many of which were at the expense of the Jewish community. Jewish physicians in the service of the crown enjoyed some advantages, such as tax exemptions and reductions. In many instances, relatives of the Jewish physicians also benefitted from tax exemptions. Some of these privileges were granted at the request of the *infantes*, noblemen, municipal authorities and even churchmen, including members of the Dominican order.

Extensive freedom of movement was granted to many Jewish physicians and surgeons so that they could perform their tasks without obstacles. Even when the gates of the Jewish quarter were closed as a means of punishment, Jewish doctors were permitted to move in and out in total freedom. In the case of the Crown of Aragon, many could travel throughout its territories without any restrictions. The Jewish communities which usually controlled the emigration of their members were ordered to respect the freedom of movement of Jewish physicians.

In view of all this, it is remarkable that there are few records indicating a widespread feeling of resentment within the Jewish community against physicians. This may be due to the fact that their

76 See, for instance, Y. Kaplan, *From Christianity to Judaism: The Story of Isaac Orobio de Castro*, Oxford, 1989; Y. Kaplan, "The Sephardim in North-Western Europe and the New World," in *The Sephardi Legacy*, II, ed. H. Beinart, Jerusalem, 1992, pp. 279ff. M. de Lozoya, "Andrés Laguna y el problema de los conversos segovianos"; L. Martin Marcos, "El médico segoviano Andrés Laguna, figura universal del siglo XVI" in *Estudios Segovianos*, 1960, *XII*.

services in the Jewish community were also greatly appreciated. Nevertheless, there were some clashes between the community and Jewish physicians. This was particularly the case when certain Jewish doctors, acting in overconfidence, disregarded the rules of the Jewish community and in their extreme misbehavior left the community no choice but to react. Contrary to ordinances which were in force in their communities, some Jewish doctors were permitted to refuse any communal office, a privilege that was widely resented by the Jewish public.

If Jewish physicians and surgeons continued to command the respect of Jewish society in general, it was most probably due to their special task of curing the sick members of the community. The Jewish doctor, after God Almighty, was revered and feared and no man or woman who could at any time fall into his hands could afford to be on bad terms with him.

Medical Licensing and Practice in Medieval Spain: A Model of Interfaith Relationships?

Etienne Lepicard

Golden Age Spain has often been seen as an example of the ideal multicultural society.[1] According to this view, in late Middle Age Spain, there were great interactions between Christians, Moslems, and Jews, each group making its contribution to the whole. The legends about the founding of the medieval medical schools show a related conception. A Greek, a Latin, an Arab, and a Jew are claimed to have founded together the medical school of Salerno, and similarly, the founders of the University of Montpellier are supposed to have been an Arab, a Jew and a disciple of Constantine the African.[2] Historical research has shown that these claims are but "fanciful legends," as the nineteenth-century historian De Renzi concluded in his study of the founding of the school at Salerno. Despite this, from the point of view

1 This essay is a tentative complementary viewpoint on the religious question as it appears in the documents presented in Luis García-Ballester, Michael R. McVaugh, and Augustín Rubio-Vela, "Medical Licensing and Learning in Fourteenth-Century Valencia," *Transactions of the American Philosophical Society*, Vol. 79, Part 6 (1989). For other primary texts, see *Estudios de Edad Media de la Corona de Aragón*, 10 vols. (Zaragoza: Escuela de Estudios Medievales, 1945–1975), and for Jewish sources, see Jean Régné, *History of the Jews in Aragon, 1213–1327* (reissued Jerusalem: Magnes Press, 1978).

2 For the legend of Salerno, see P.O. Kristeller, "The School of Salerno," *Bulletin of the History of Medicine*, 1945, *17:* 138–194; Harry Friedenwald, *The Jews and Medicine*, 2 vols. (Baltimore: The Johns Hopkins University Press, 1944), Vol. I, p. 223; Charles Singer, *From Magic to Science, Essays on the Scientific Twilight*, (New York: Dover, 1958), chapter VII, pp. 240–248; for Montpellier, see Vern L. Bullough, *The Development of Medicine as a Profession: The Contribution of the Medieval University to Modern Medicine* (Basel: S. Karger, New York: Hafner, 1966), p. 53.

of the History of Medicine in its connections to Ethics, it is interesting to examine the interfaith relationships which are claimed to have existed at the time.

In order to study these relationships, I will focus this essay on medical licensing and practice in the fourteenth-century Crown of Aragon. I have made this choice despite the fact that I am not a specialist in the history of Aragonese, or even of medieval Spanish medicine. Recently, however, a book was published which presents primary sources on the licensing of physicians in fourteenth-century Valencia. When I read this book, I was fascinated by the fact that each physician swore an oath according to his faith. What did this indicate? Was it a sign of interfaith relationships, or not? This question brought me to think of the oath which I myself swore. It was drawn up by the O.M.S. after the Second World War, in 1948, and contains an article stating that "I will not let considerations of religion, nationality, race, or other factors come between my duty and my patient."[3] I had always connected this article with the gross abuses of human rights carried out during the War, and the idea of human rights in general was linked, in my mind, to the Enlightenment. My reading of the book, however, indicated to me that things were not that simple. More precisely, the medieval regulation of medical licensing may have something to say about the place of interfaith relationships in medical ethics.

First of all, some general background. The Crown of Aragon was created in the twelfth century as the result of a dynastic union between the Kingdom of Aragon and the County of Catalonia. In the thirteenth century, it lost most of its trans-Pyrenean possessions, but gained Valencia and the Balearic Islands as the Reconquista proceeded southward. In the fourteenth century, the Crown of Aragon became a political and economic power in the Mediterranean, with control over Sicily, the South of Italy, and parts of Greece. The citizens of the Crown, as in all of Spain, were a mixture of Christians, Jews, Moslems, and *Conversos* of various kinds. In contrast to the situation in the Balearic Islands, the Moslems were not expelled from Valencia after

3 Etienne Lepicard, *A propos de trois problèmes quotidiens d'éthique médicale (Avortement, Contraception, Euthanasie), réflexion d'un médecin chrétien sur les sources juives*, MD diss. (Paris, 1986).

the conquest, despite the opposition of the Aragonese barons and against the express counsel of the Papacy, and were even allowed to retain their own institutions. At the same time, however, the Moslem élite did not remain in Valencia, since Islamic orthodoxy dictated that it was not proper to live under Christian rulers. The right to emigrate was one of the few privileges which was always allowed to the Moslem community by the kings.[4]

How, then, did the Kings of Aragon act in relation to medical education and licensing? James II (1291–1327), who ruled at the start of the fourteenth century, has been called "the greatest among the governors of the Crown." By contrast, his grandfather was called "the Great Conqueror," and his father "the Great Defender."[5] James II advanced the royal interest in higher education with the founding of a University at Lerida in Catalonia in 1300, which included a medical faculty.[6] His biographers also state that he had a "passionate devotion to medicine." He brought some of the greatest physicians of the time, such as Arnau de Vilanova, to his court, and Moorish and Jewish physicians were also to be found there. He also encouraged the professors at Lerida to translate medical texts from Arabic to Latin. A recent summary of his connections to medicine concluded that "he has been a visible patron of medicine, especially of learned medicine."[7]

Alfonso IV (1327–1336), who inherited the throne from James II, enacted the Valencian *furs* of 1329, which I will soon discuss. A *furs* was a piece of legislation ratified by the king. The first *furs* of Valencia, that of 1238, affirmed complete freedom for any cleric or other man to teach medicine in the city "without service or tribute."[8] A further

4 T.N. Bisson, *The Medieval Crown of Aragon, A Short History* (Oxford: Clarendon Press, 1986); L.P. Harvey, *Islamic Spain* (Chicago: The University of Chicago Press, 1990); John Boswell, *The Royal Treasure, Muslim Communities under the Crown of Aragon in the Fourteenth Century* (New Haven: Yale University Press, 1977).

5 Bisson, *The Medieval Crown of Aragon* (cit. n. 4), p. 96.

6 Michael R. McVaugh and Luis García-Ballester, "The Medical Faculty at Early Fourteenth Century Lérida," *History of Universities*, 1989, *8*: 1–27; F.H. Rashdall, *The Universities of Europe in the Middle Ages*, 3 vols. (reissued London: Oxford University Press,1969).

7 García-Ballester et al., *Medical Licensing* (cit. n. 1).

8 *Ibid.*, p. 41.

mention of medical regulation appears not in Valencia but in the Kingdom of Aragon, in the *fueros* of Monzon in 1289, which gave the municipal authorities the legal right to examine and license physicians and surgeons. However, the 1329 *furs* of Valencia details the licensing process, for the first time. Candidates for licensing had to have "followed the art of medicine for at least four years in a *Studium Generale*." They would then be examined by two leading physicians elected annually for this purpose. If they were found competent, the municipal agent would issue a license.

The *furs* of 1329 does not directly discuss the interfaith issue. The only mention of religion, and one which also appears in the *furs* of 1238, is a quite long clause which specifies that each practitioner, whoever he might be, "shall swear each year... that he will not treat anyone who is seriously ill or wounded... if the patient has not first made confession." If the illness was such that "a delay would be dangerous," this prohibition was waived, but only for the first visit, as "the practitioner will not make a second visit until the patient had confessed." This *furs* does not mention the licensing of non-Christians, even though a survey of 28 fourteenth-century licensing documents recently published indicates that seven Jewish physicians and one Moslem barber were licensed. These documents also indicate that each faith had its own oath. Each candidate swore that "he would engage well and loyally in the said art." The Christian oath was taken "on the four holy Gospels of our Lord God," while he was "physically touching them with his right hand." A Jew swore "on the ten commandments of the Law that our God gave to Moses on Mount Sinai," and a Moslem, "turning his face toward the south, swore by God and the *quibla*, by the *zuna* and the *xara* of the Moslems."

Later, in the *fueros* of Monzon of 1363, the candidate's religion was explicitly taken into account. Here, "Jewish and Saracen physicians are to be examined by physicians of their law or sect, if there are any, although one Christian should assist in their examination; and, if there are no physicians of their law or sect, they should be examined by two Christian physicians; and once the examination is carried out, if they are found qualified, they must swear publicly to practice well and loyally before they are admitted to practice." Some may understand these passages as indications of a flourishing *convivencia*, while others will see them as indicating carefully executed control over minority groups.[9] This is the issue which I would now like to discuss.

In the Crown of Aragon, the three religious communities were, at least theoretically, ruled by their own laws. On the Christian side, the second half of the thirteenth and the beginning of the fourteenth centuries were marked by a strong tendency toward interfaith relationships visible in the work of Ramon Lull and in the efforts made by Dominicans and Franciscans to learn Hebrew and Arabic. This opening was closely connected to the hope that the Moslems and Jews would soon convert to Christianity. The Kings of Aragon and the Church hierarchy encouraged conversion, but socio-economic factors often dictated a much more pragmatic approach to the subject. The Kingdom of Valencia is a special case in this respect, because the Moslem majority it retained provided the labor force vital to an agriculturally-based economy.

There was considerable interaction between the three groups in day-to-day life, despite the fact that, according to the Church, this was not supposed to happen. Jews and Moslems were to live in separate quarters, and only their shops could be outside these areas. Despite the laws, the communities were never entirely separated. There was also a difference between the three constituents of the Crown. In Aragon, the communities were less separated, as the Moslem minority was more assimilated into Christian society, and by the fourteenth century only a few of them could read or write Arabic. In Valencia, on the other hand, Moslem society remained relatively unchanged. Even after the conquest, few Christians moved to Valencia, and those that did remained largely in the towns. The Christians seem to have had mixed feelings about the Moslems, as they were economically necessary, yet at the same time posed a threat to their safety.[10]

What, then, can be found out about the relations between the physicians of the three religions? First of all, the documents on which I

9 *Ibid.*, pp. 25–29; Boswell, *The Royal Treasure* (cit. n. 4), pp. 58–59.

10 For all the interreligious relationships, see the references in note 4 and J.N. Hillgarth, *The Spanish Kingdoms 1250–1516*, 2 vols. (Oxford: Clarendon Press, 1976–1978), especially chapter V : "A Land of Three Religions," Vol. I, pp. 155–214. For the Jews of Aragon, see Yitzhak Baer, *A History of the Jews in Christian Spain*, 2 vols. (Philadelphia: The Jewish Publication Society of America, 1961), especially Vol. I, pp. 177–185 for the thirteenth century and Vol. II, pp. 1–34 for the fourteenth century.

have based this paper are all derived from the dominant Christian community. They provide information only on those Jewish and Moslem physicians who wished to cross cultural-religious lines and practice medicine among the Christians. Thus, they only indicate one point of view. The Church had mixed feelings about such practitioners, as without interaction it would be harder to reach the goal of conversion, but, at the same time, the non-Christian practitioners were a potential "bad influence" on the Christian population. The Moslem religious elite, as I have noted, also had problems with the interaction of the populations. Only the Jews seem to have been in favor of integration, perhaps because they had nowhere else to go. The reaction of the Jews seems to me an important point, and I will return to it in my discussion of why non-Christians wished to practice among Christians.

On the more intellectual level, Jacquart and Micheau, in their discussion of the influence of Arabic medicine on the medieval West, describe two paths for the spread of such knowledge: an Italian path and a Spanish one. In the case of the latter, they give the example of how Gerard of Cremona and his co-workers translated medical works from Arabic into Latin via a vernacular language. The work was done with the aid of a translator from Arabic to the vernacular, who was usually a Jew. Thus, translation formed an important point of collaboration and interaction between physicians of different faiths. Most of these translations were done in the thirteenth century, after the conquest of Toledo at the end of the twelfth century. In the Kingdom of Aragon, translations were also done at the beginning of the fourteenth century. James II issued an order in 1302, two years after the founding of the University of Lerida, in which he asked to borrow "certain Arabic works of medicine which various Jews of our kingdom possess, in order to correct the incomplete volumes which are in the *Studium Generale* of Lerida."[11]

Does this order indicate interfaith collaboration in the new University? The "fanciful legends" about the founding of Salerno and Montpellier were found by de Renzi in a work from the end of the seventeenth

11 Danielle Jacquart and Françoise Micheau, *La médecine arabe et l'Occident médiéval* (Paris: Maisonneuve & Larose, 1990), especially chapter 4. On the request of King James II, see Cecil Roth, "The Qualification of Jewish Physicians in the Middle Ages" in *Speculum*, 1953, *28*: 834–843, especially pp. 835–836.

century. Friedenwald, in his work on Jews and Medicine, came to the conclusion that the legendary four founders were symbolic representations for general influences active in tenth- through twelfth-century medicine in southern Italy and France. In practice, however, medieval universities were generally closed to non-Christians.[12] Some individuals, such as Abraham Avigdor of Arles, may have heard lectures, but they did not receive degrees. The only known exception is the case of a Jew who received a medical degree from Perpignan in 1390, an act expressly prohibited by the statutes of the University.[13] In addition, it has recently been argued that not only in theology and canon law, but even in medicine, the content of the curriculum itself was specifically Christian in nature. According to this view, one of the first purposes of medical teaching was to prove that medical knowledge proceeded deductively from simple propositions about the nature of God.[14]

It is thus difficult to reconcile the granting of medical licenses to Jews and Moslems with the demand of the 1329 *furs* that the student spend four years in a university *Studium Generale*. At first glance, the requirement of the *furs* made the practice of medicine a Christian monopoly, but any question about licensing also requires a look at medical training. The common view among the first historians and sociologists who investigated the development of the professions was that the development of medical licensing and university medical training were closely connected, and were part of the process of professionalization. In the last fifteen or twenty years, however, many scholars have suggested that university-trained physicians were only a minority among the whole community of medical practitioners: physicians, surgeons, barbers, apothecaries and empirics.[15] Even among

12 Siraisi, Nancy : "The Faculty of Medicine" in *Universities in the Middle Ages*, ed. Hilde de Ridder-Symoens (Cambridge: Cambridge University Press, 1992). This work is volume one of the four volume *A History of the Universities*, ed. Walter Ruegg.

13 Roth, "The Qualification of Jewish Physicians" (cit. n. 11), p. 835; Joseph Shatzmiller, "On Becoming a Jewish Doctor in the High Middle Ages," *Sefarad*, 1983, *43*:239–250, especially p. 245.

14 Cornelius O'Boyle, "Medicine, God, and Aristotle in the Early Universities: Prefatory Prayers in Late Medieval Medical Commentaries," *Bulletin of the History of Medicine*, 1992, *66*:185–209.

15 Katherine Park, *Doctors and Medicine in Early Renaissance Florence* (Princeton, New Jersey: Princeton University Press, 1985), especially pp. 11–13 and the

those who attended a university, only a minority ever received a doctorate. The lack of university training does not necessarily indicate that the practitioner was unlearned, even though this was true in many cases, especially among barbers and other practitioners of surgery. The requirement for practical skills in surgery can be seen in the documents from Valencia, which indicate that licences were sometimes granted for specific operations, usually cataract, bladder stone, and hernia. These operations were among the most complicated performed, and the fact that they were left in the hands of the practically experienced rather than in those of the formally trained surgeons indicates the pragmatic attitude of the medical examiners, an attitude clearly in contradiction with the letter of the *furs*.

In fact, there seem to have been two different kinds of licenses. One was granted by the universities, or in the case of Montpellier by the local bishop, and the other by the guilds in coordination with the local authorities. The latter seem to have been more in tune with the medical needs and the political situation of the time. The Valencian guilds sometimes favored a "Christianization" of the profession, while at other times they were more flexible. The former attitude can be seen in the formulation of the 1329 *furs* and in the letter sent by physicians to the King during the rebellion of the Union in 1356. At that time, they complained about "the constant intervention of the King in licensing Jews, Saracens and apostates despite the *furs*." In contrast, the flexibility of the system can be seen in the licensing of seven Jews and one Moslem between 1378 and 1396, according to the documents examined for this paper.

This ambiguous position requires an examination of the role of the Valencian medical guilds. There is a curious paradox between the

references therein. These pages pushed me to suggest further directions for work on the Aragonese case. See also Vern L. Bullough, "Training of the Nonuniversity-Educated Medical Practitioners in the Later Middle Ages," *Journal of the History of Medicine and Allied Sciences*, 1959, *14*:446–458; Pearl Kibre, "The Faculty of Medicine at Paris, Charlatanism and Unlicensed Medical Practice in the Later Middle Ages," *Bulletin of the History of Medicine*, 1953, *27*:1–20; Margaret Pelling and Charles Webster : "Medical Practitioners" in *Health, Medicine and Morality in the Sixteenth Century*, ed. Charles Webster (Cambridge: Cambridge University Press, 1979), pp.165–235.

refusal of the guilds to restrict the teaching of medicine by founding a *Studium Generale* in Valencia and the continued enforcement of the *furs*. It seems that, despite their personal interest in the founding of a *Studium*, they were afraid that its existence would open the door to increased episcopal control. They may also have been influenced by Lullian philosophy, which called for a more popular sort of medicine. In my opinion, it would be also interesting to study the effect of the plague on the reactions of the physicians.[16]

The King also played a role in medical licensing. I have already mentioned the presence of Jewish and Moorish physicians at the court. In addition, the 1356 document indicates that the King often granted medical licenses despite the requirements of the *furs*. One example of this process was the granting of a license to a Jew after an examination carried out by a Christian and a Jewish physician. The Christian one is known as a Valencian, but not as one of the two elected to the position of examiner for that year. Other reports suggest that the King even dispensed with examinations altogether, as in the case of two Jewish women from Aragon. The royal prerogative was derived from Roman law, which states that the King is above all the laws and rights of the land, and seems to have been used to help Jewish and Moslem physicians against municipal and episcopal authorities.[17]

This intervention raises several questions. Were the Jewish and Moslem physicians who received royal aid only court physicians, or were there also others? Was the siding of the physicians against the King in the rebellion of 1356 indicative of the position of elite physicians, or were those who practiced among the general community also involved? More important, what was the relationship between Jewish and Moslem practitioners who primarily served their own communities and potential Christian patients? It is difficult to answer such questions, as the surviving documents which I have examined relate only to the Christian community. Collective biographies of medical practitioners,

16 For attempts to evaluate the effects of the plague on medical demography, see García-Ballester et al., *Medical Licensing* (cit. n. 1), chapter 5; Park, *Doctors and Medicine* (cit. n. 15). For the effects of the plague on the Jewish community of Aragon, see Baer, *A History of the Jews* (cit. n. 10), vol. II, pp. 24–28.

17 See García-Ballester et al., *Medical Licensing* (cit. n. 1); Roth, "The Qualification of Jewish Physicians" (cit. n. 11); Shatzmiller, "On Becoming a Jewish Doctor" (cit. n. 13).

such as those written about medieval Italy, France and England, might help to answer these questions. I do not know, however, if the relevant documents survive in the case of the Crown of Aragon, or if the long arm of the Inquisition may have made such a research impossible.[18]

Finally, there are two examples which may indicate the beginning of a limited answer to these questions. In one case, a Jewish woman was accused of practicing medicine without a license. She appealed to the King, who ruled that she did not need a license, as she worked only within the Jewish community. This example suggests that different rules were indeed applied to different communities, and also that the King provided a court of appeal in the case of local problems. The King may thus have acted as a buffer of sorts between the communities, a role which was to vanish a century later.

An additional example, and one which indicates a difference of opinion between the Church hierarchy and the populace, comes from the nearby County of Provence. In 1337, the Council of Avignon "forbade Christians to employ Jewish physicians and surgeons or to take their medicines, except in case of danger when it was impossible to secure experienced Christian physicians." The same year, Robert of Provence promulgated "an order revoking all earlier authorization to Jewish physicians to practice." These attempts to restrict the activity of Jewish physicians did not succeed. Despite the interdictions, and because of the popularity of Jewish physicians, the Synod of Avignon lifted the prohibition after only four years, citing a lack of medical care. The Synod also revoked the sentence of excommunication imposed on those who had been treated by Jewish physicians.[19] Thus, the wishes of the populace may have played a role in the licensing of non-Christian practitioners.

18 See note 15. For the French practitioners, see Ernest Wickersheimer, *Dictionnaire biographique des médecins en France au Moyen Age* (Paris, 1936). This work was reissued in two volumes with a Supplement by Danielle Jacquart (Geneva: Droz, 1979). For England, see C.H. Talbot & E. A. Hammond, *The Medical Practitioners in Medieval England, A Biographical Register* (London: Wellcome Historical Medical Register, 1965). For works based on collective biographies, see Danielle Jacquart, *Le milieu médical en France du XIIè au XVè siècle* (Geneva: Droz, 1981); and Edward J. Kealey, *Medieval Medicus: A Social History of Anglo-Norman Medicine* (Baltimore: The Johns Hopkins University Press, 1981).

19 Friedenwald, *The Jews and Medicine* (cit. n. 2), vol.II, p. 675.

In conclusion, it is difficult to define precisely the significance of the fact that Aragonese physicians swore their oaths each according to his faith. The teaching of medicine in the Crown of Aragon went from an informal process to the organized and controlled teaching of medicine within the university. A connected phenomenon was the simultaneous effort made by both the guilds and the Church, each for its own reasons, to limit the practice of Jewish and Moslem physicians among the Christian population. At the same time, the kings and the real or perceived needs of the populace often acted to protect the position of the non-Christian physicians in the Christian community.

All of these conclusions are preliminary, as more information is needed to fill in the broader picture of the interrelationship and possible cooperation between physicians of the different religions. The existing sources I have examined are all from the Christian side, and there is a severe lack of information on the internal regulation of medical affairs in the other two communities. In addition, collective biographies of physicians would help in understanding the social and professional role of the various medical practitioners. It would also be interesting to determine if the Jewish physicians were more interested in crossing the cultural-religious lines, and if so, for what reasons. Was it because of their uncertain social position between two vastly larger groups, or did they have a particular vision of man which enabled them to envision a more pluralistic society?[20]

Finally, I would like to come back to the legend of the foundation of Salerno. Folk historians have pointed out that legends are the outcome of people's inability to agree on the exact point in time at which something originated. This may explain the legend of Salerno, a symbol of interreligious understanding. The story appeared at the end of the seventeenth century, so it is not surprising to find in it some humanistic elements. There exists, however, a long history of interfaith contexts of medical practice; fourteenth-century Spain provides a case in point, but much more research is needed on this topic.

20 See, for example, Abraham A. Neuman, *The Jews in Spain, Their Social, Political and Cultural Life during the Middle Ages*, 2 vols. (Philadelphia: The Jewish Publication Society of America, 1942), Vol. I, p. 108f.

The Ideal Medical Practitioner in Counter-Reformation Castile: The Perception of the Converso Physician Henrique Jorge Henriques (*c.* 1555–1622)

Jon Arrizabalaga

1. Introduction

The many changes (economic, social, religious, political and cultural) which Europe experienced during the late Middle Ages transformed it into a repressive society. As R.I. Moore has shown, during the eleventh and twelfth centuries there was a transformation of Western society: persecution became habitual. Not only were individuals subjected to violence, but also a

> deliberate and socially sanctioned violence began to be directed *through established governmental, judicial and social institutions*, against groups of people defined by general characteristics such as race, religion or way of life; and that membership of such groups in itself became to be regarded as justifying these attacks.

If heretics, lepers, Jews and sodomites were the earliest victims of persecution, during the following centuries this xenophobia also affected many other social groups. This persecution in all its manifestations was an essential part of a program implemented to strengthen the

This study has been partly funded by the research fellowship PB89–0066 of the CICYT (Spanish Ministry of Education and Science). I am deeply indebted to Annie Oakes for her care in revising my text and in improving its English style. I also thank Luis García-Ballester, Alvar Martinez-Vidal, Guillermo Olagüe de Ros, Ole Peter Grell and Andrew Cunningham for their advice and material assistance. I wish to dedicate this article to the cause of a just and lasting peace in the Middle East.

power and influence of a literate élite whose culture and institutions penetrated deeply and sharply into the European society of the high medieval period.[1]

This process showed specific traits in each community depending upon its particular social structure and political situation. An important characteristic of medieval Spain was the presence of Moslem and Jewish minorities alongside the Christian majority. The coexistence between Christians and Jews began to break down in the late thirteenth century. There was serious deterioration from the mid fourteenth century onward until the final collapse in 1492, when the so-called "Catholic Kings" promulgated the edict which was responsible for the expulsion of about 90,000 Jews from the Crowns of Castile and Aragon who were not prepared to convert to Christianity. Moreover, from the fourteenth until well into the eighteenth centuries, this conflict was extended to the "new Christians," who were Jewish converts and their descendents (*Conversos*). In about 1480, the Catholic Kings launched a new Inquisition intended to expose those who supposedly had remained secretly loyal to their former faith (*Judaizantes*). Starting in the sixteenth century, the Inquisition, which was not formally abolished until 1834, extended its mandate to the persecution of other groups, among them Lutherans, Erasmists, Calvinists, *Alumbrados* and *Moriscos*. The coexistence between Christians and Moslems gradually deteriorated during the sixteenth century, but its final collapse did not come until 1609, when King Philip III signed the order which provoked the expulsion of about 300,000 *Moriscos* (members of the Moslem minority who had converted to Catholicism) by 1614, irrespective of whether they were sincere Catholics.[2]

1 R.I. Moore, *The Formation of a Persecuting Society. Power and Deviance in Western Europe, 950–1250* (Oxford: Blackwell, 1987) pp. 5, 135, 152–153.

2 On these issues, see, *inter alia*, Y. Baer, *A History of the Jews in Christian Spain*, 2 vols. (Philadelphia: Jewish Publication Society of America, 1961–66); L. Cardaillac, *Morisques et Chrétiens. Un affrontement polémique (1492–1640)* (Paris: Klincksieck, 1977); J. Caro Baroja, *Los judíos en la España moderna y contemporánea*, 3 vols., 2nd ed. (Madrid: Istmo, 1978); J.M. Monsalvo Martín, *Teoría y evolución de un conflicto social. El antisemitismo en la Corona de Castilla en la Baja Edad Media* (Madrid: Siglo XXI, 1985); H. Kamen, *Inquisition and society in Spain* (London: Weidenfeld & Nicolson, 1986) [henceforth citations refer to its Sp. trans.: *La Inquisición española*, 4th ed. (Barcelona: Crítica, 1992)]; A. Alcalá,

It is not surprising, then, that the new political order which the Catholic Kings inaugurated in the late fifteenth century promoted the development of a new pattern of medical practice in early modern Spain. In this paper, I would first like to make some general comments on the evolution of this pattern in sixteenth- and early seventeenth-century Spain, with particular attention to the fortunes of Converso and Morisco practitioners. Second, I would like to supply a brief reconstruction of the life of the Converso physician Henrique Jorge Henriques (*c.* 1555–1622), a Portuguese national whose professional training and career took place mostly in Castile. Finally, I would like to deal with the image of the ideal medical practitioner as stated by Henriques. I would claim that his "perfect physician" (male, Catholic and university-trained) fits, to a great extent, the image of the medical practitioner promoted by the Spanish Counter-Reformation, but it also illustrates the impact of the general crisis of the late sixteenth century on this image.[3] Needless to say, Henriques' status as a "Converso," a special social status in early modern Castile, must be kept in mind in order to fully understand his views.

2. Medical practice in sixteenth-century Spain: toward a new pattern

In the field of medicine, the gradual development of the Spanish state bureaucracy starting from the time of the Catholic Kings involved the reinforcement of those procedures of control which were already established as well as the setting up of some new procedures. The former included the process through which, after the fourteenth century and particularly from the late fifteenth century onward, the universities were given a monopoly on granting titles to practice medicine. This process caused the model of medical teaching characteristic of late medieval Spanish society, which García-Ballester has called an "open model," to be suppressed and to be replaced by a "closed" or institu-

ed., *The Spanish Inquisition and the inquisitorial mind* (Highland Lakes, N.J.: Atlantic Research and Publications, 1987).

3 For a general historical framework for early modern Spain, see the recent synthesis of H. Kamen, *Spain 1469–1714: a society of conflict* (London: Longman, 1983).

tionalized one.[4] The most obvious case of new mechanisms for controlling medical practice was the setting up of the *Tribunal del Protomedicato*, an institution which continued working until 1799, and was legally abolished only in 1822. In contrast to Aragon and Navarra, where the authority of this Tribunal was limited by the confraternities (*Cofradías*) of physicians, surgeons and apothecaries which had previously settled in the cities and towns, in Castile the *Protomedicato* had the sole right to exercise a great number of specific powers, among them the regulation and control of the professional practice of physicians, surgeons and apothecaries, the punishment of offenses and the resolution of professional conflicts.[5]

In 1477, the Catholic Kings dictated a law (*pragmática*) which, along with the further acts of 1491 and 1498, has been considered the foundation of the Castilian *Tribunal del Protomedicato*.[6] This law gave those "protophysicians" (*protomédicos*) and "head examining officers" (*alcaldes examinadores mayores*) who had the appropriate royal authorisation the power to

> examine physicians, surgeons, enchanters (*ensalmadores*), apothecaries, herbalists and other people working in these jobs full- or part-time, as well as in others connected to them, whether they are men or women, of whatever [religious] law, status, pre-eminence and dignity; to give letters of examination, approbation and license to freely practise such jobs without any trouble

4 L. García-Ballester, *La medicina a la València medieval. Medicina i societat en un país medieval mediterrani* (València: Edicions Alfons el Magnànim, 1988), pp. 42–45.

5 The history of the Spanish *Protomedicato* is mostly to be written, except for the case of Spanish Colonial America. See J.T. Lanning, *The Royal Protomedicato. The regulation of the medical profession in the Spanish Empire*, ed. J.J. TePaske (Durham, N.C.: Duke University Press, 1985). Among the few printed reference works on this topic are Miguel Eugenio Muñoz, *Recopilación de las Leyes, Pragmáticas reales, Decretos, y Acuerdos del Real Protomedicato...* (Valencia, 1751), (facs. repr.: Valencia: Librerías París-Valencia, 1991); Pascual Iborra, *Memoria sobre la institución del Real Proto-Medicato...* (Madrid, 1885–1886), in *Historia del Protomedicato en España (1477–1822)*, eds. J. Riera and J. Granda-Juesas (Valladolid: Universidad de Valladolid, 1987), pp. 17–285; G. Albi Romero, *El Protomedicato en la España ilustrada. (Catálogo de Documentos del Archivo General de Simancas)* (Valladolid: Universidad de Valladolid, 1982).

6 Iborra, *Memoria* (cit. n. 5), pp. 23–24.

> or slander to those who are judged to be suitable; and to order those who are judged to be unsuitable for the said jobs not to practice them, as well as to make sure that the order has been observed.[7]

This act represents a royal attempt to regulate the practice of a wide number of sanitary occupations in a comprehensive manner by introducing a single restriction to licensing, the suitability of the applicants for the performance of their duties. Yet, this *pragmática* left untouched the "open model" characteristic of late medieval Spanish society. The range of practitioners whom this disposition addressed could hardly have been wider. It included physicians, surgeons, enchanters, apothecaries, herbalists and other related occupations; both sexes; the three religions; full- or part-time workers; and there was no evident discrimination on the grounds of social status.

The importance of the *Tribunal del Protomedicato* in the control of sanitary practitioners was gradually reinforced during the sixteenth and early seventeenth centuries, but the tone of the subsequent legal acts which the Spanish kings dictated for this institution was radically opposed to that of the first *pragmática*. The whole series of laws taken together makes it obvious that the Habsburgs were intent on setting up a hierarchy among sanitary occupations, as well as reducing their number and the variety of social groups involved in them.[8]

7 R. Muñoz Garrido, "Normativa legal española sobre la enseñanza facultativa de las ciencias médicas," in R. Muñoz Garrido and C. Muñiz Fernández, *Fuentes legales de la medicina española (Siglos XIII–XIX)* (Salamanca: Universidad de Salamanca, 1969), pp. 21–22: "Mandamos que los Protomedicos, i Alcaldes Examinadores Mayores, que de Nos tuvieren poder, lo sean en todos nuestros Reinos, i Señorios, que agora son, o fueren de aqui adelante, para examinar los Fisicos, i Zurujanos, i Ensalmadores, i Boticarios, i Herbolarios, i otras personas, que en todo, o en parte usaren en estos oficios, i en oficios a ellos, i a cada uno dellos annexo i connexo, ansi hombres, como mugeres, de qualquier lei, estado, preeminencia, i dignidad que sean: para que si los hallaren idoneos, i pertenescientes les den cartas de examen, i aprobacion, i licencia para que usen de los dichos oficios libre, i desembargadamente, sin pena, ni calumnia alguna: i que los que hallaren que no son tales para poder usar de los dichos oficios, o de alguno dellos, los manden, i defiendan que no usen dellos."

8 See L. S. Granjel, *La medicina española renacentista* (Salamanca: Universidad de Salamanca, 1980), pp. 63–83, 133–150; J.M. López-Piñero, "The medical profes-

During the sixteenth century, the range of sanitary occupations which required some sort of royal legitimation was reduced to university physicians, surgeons (university and non-university or *romancistas*), barbers, blood-letters, apothecaries and a number of surgical specialists: bonesetters (*algebristas*), hernia-setters (*hernistas*), stone-pullers (*sacadores de piedra*), cataract-beaters (*batidores de la catarata* or *oculistas*), tooth-pullers (*sacamuelas*) and midwives (*parteras*), among others. Philip II's *pragmáticas* of 1563, 1588 and 1593, and those of Philip III from 1603 and 1617, make it clear that the *Protomedicato* tended to give general and unlimited licenses to physicians, surgeons (university and non-university) and apothecaries. Other sanitary practitioners, whose practices had hitherto been regulated at a similar level, received only particular and limited licenses.[9] At the same time, the Habsburgs' intention to limit the variety of social groups involved in sanitary activities is well illustrated by the gradual marginalization of women (except for midwifery [*parteria*])[10] and of Converso and Morisco practitioners within those sanitary occupations which required royal legitimacy.

Converso and Morisco practitioners were thus potentially liable to a double legal threat. On the one hand, they were members of minorities whose religious beliefs and practices were persecuted by the Tribunal of the Inquisition; on the other, they practiced their sanitary occupa-

sion in 16th-century Spain," in *The Town and the State Physician in Europe from the Middle Ages to the Enlightenment*, ed. A. W. Russell (Wolfenbüttel: Herzog August Bibliothek, 1982), pp. 85–98; Muñoz Garrido, *Normativa legal española* (cit. n. 7), pp. 21–61; Iborra, *Memoria* (cit. n. 5), pp. 23–73; D. Goodman, *Power and penury: government, technology and science in Philip II's Spain* (Cambridge: Cambridge University Press, 1988) (Sp. trans.: Madrid: Alianza, 1990), pp. 242–259.

9 Muñoz Garrido, *Normativa legal española* (cit. n. 7), nos. 23, 24, 45, 46, 54, 59. The "midwives" (*parteras*) were not examined by the "Protomedicato" until 1750. See Iborra, *Memoria* (cit. n. 5), p. 68.

10 Muñoz Garrido, *Normativa legal española* (cit. n. 7), Nos. 12, 17, 25. Philip II's *Pragmática* of 1593 states: "That no woman can possess or possesses a pharmacy, even if she has employed an examined official at it" ("Que ninguna mujer pueda tener ni tenga botica, aunque tenga en ella oficial examinado"). See *Novísima Recopilación de las Leyes de España*, 6 vols. (Madrid, 1805–1807) [facs. repr.: Madrid: Imprenta Nacional del BOE, 1975, vol. IV, p. 107 (lib. VIII, tt. XII, ley III.6)].

tions within a legal framework which was becoming increasingly restrictive as a result of the development and politics of the Tribunal of the *Protomedicato* during the sixteenth and early seventeenth centuries.

In addition, from the mid fifteenth century onward, the cult of the "purity of blood" gave rise to a profusion of statutes (*Estatutos de limpieza de sangre*) where this requirement was legally regulated. As a result of a royal *pragmática* (1501), Inquisitorial condemnation not only disqualified the condemned from jobs such as medicine, surgery and apothecary, but also mandated professional disqualification for his or her descendants until the second generation.[11] This rule was later extended to all descendants of Conversos and Moriscos. In consequence, a discrimination which had been founded on purely religious grounds during the late Middle Ages gradually came to rest on the origins of the members of these minorities. Thus, the stigma did not end with their conversion to Christianity, but extended potentially to all those who lacked "old Christian" lineage.[12] One of the major implications of this cult was that the access of the "new Christians" from both of these minorities to the universities was made difficult, if not blocked. They found it difficult to prove that they were descended from "old Christian" lineage and that they had "clean," uncontaminated blood. The rigidity of the "purity of blood" statutes in the colleges of the sixteenth-century Castilian universities (particularly Valladolid, Salamanca and Alcalá) was notorious.[13] Those who could not manage to prove their origins had no choice but to become second-class students at these universities, to try another university with less strict

11 Muñoz Garrido, *Normativa legal española* (cit. n. 7), p. 72: "Mandamos que los reconciliados por el delito de herejía, y apostasía, ni los hijos, y nietos de quemados, y condenados por dicho delito, hasta la segunda generación por vía masculina, y hasta la primera por vía femenina no puedan ser, ni sean ... ni fisico, ni cirujano, ni boticario..."

12 On the "purity of blood" in early modern Spain, see H. Ch. Lea, *A History of the Inquisition of Spain*, 4 vols. (facs. repr.: New York: AMS Press, 1966), vol. II, pp. 285–314; A. A. Sicroff, *Les controverses des statuts de "pureté de sang" en Espagne du XVè au XVIIè siècle* (Paris: M. Didier, 1979); Kamen, *Inquisition and society* (cit. n. 2), pp. 159–181.

13 R.L. Kagan, *Students and society in early modern Spain* (Baltimore-London: The Johns Hopkins University Press, 1974), pp. 90–92.

statutes, or simply to give up on getting any university training at all.

In conclusion, from the late fifteenth to the late seventeenth centuries, a dominant political tendency in Spain consisted of gradually "closing" the Christian majority to the Converso and Morisco minorities. This "closing" seriously affected the chances of these minorities for both medical training and professional practice. Even so, some individuals from both minorities succeeded in studying medicine at university, and achieved enough prestige in their careers to become practitioners to kings, noblemen and urban patricians. In addition, some Christian authorities (civil and ecclesiastic) and social groups ("Erasmists," some religious orders) came up with alternative routes to education in order to integrate the members of these minorities into Christian society.[14]

3. Henrique Jorge Henriques (*c.* 1555–1622): a biographical note

In the Iberian kingdoms, as in other late medieval European societies, the university model of medical training was in competition with other models within an open system. However, the political authorities gave the university pattern of medical training and practice resolute support from the fourteenth century onward. As a result, during the following centuries it gradually became the dominant model throughout Europe, and even played a very influential role in the making of early modern European states.

The social hegemony of the university model was substantially strengthened in sixteenth-century Castile. At the same time, there was an unparalleled development of the bureaucratic apparatus of the Spanish state. Moreover, at least from the late sixteenth century, university medical knowledge appears to have increasingly played a prescriptive role in the politics of the Spanish Crown. Indeed, in the late sixteenth and early seventeenth centuries, a number of university physicians assumed that the medical system, on both the educational

14 For the case of the Moriscos, see L. García-Ballester, *Los moriscos y la medicina. Un capítulo de la medicina y la ciencia marginadas en la España del siglo XVI* (Barcelona: Labor, 1984), pp. 60–64.

and professional levels, was part of the general crisis of the Spanish Empire, and therefore it also had to be part of the solution. In these circumstances, a great number of prescriptive works, partly or fully focusing on medical education and practice, were published. Some of them also included proposals for solving the misfortunes of the "republic" which might justify their being considered as some sort of *arbitristas avant-la-lettre.*[15] Among them were Pedro Mercado, Juan Huarte de San Juan, Henrique Jorge Henriques and Rodrigo de Castro.[16] In this paper, I would like to focus upon Henriques and his *Retrato del perfecto médico.*

Most of the scarce information known about Henrique (Henrico, Anrrique) Jorge (Iorge, Ieorge) Henriques (Anrriquez, Anriquez, Henriquez) comes from his own writings.[17] He was born in the Portuguese city of Guarda (Beira Alta),[18] halfway between Coimbra and Salamanca, in about 1555. Henriques was of Jewish lineage, and was most probably a Converso. After his death in 1622, his relatives and servants were denounced to the Inquisition as having buried his corpse

15 On the seventeenth-century Spanish *arbitristas*, see H. Kamen, *Vocabulario básico de la historia moderna. España y América 1450–1750* (Barcelona: Crítica, 1986), pp. 13–16; G. Anes, ed., *Memoriales y discursos de Francisco Martínez de Mata* (Madrid: Ed. Moneda y Crédito, 1971), pp. 28–33.

16 See Pedro Mercado, *Dialogos de Philosophia natural y moral...* (Granada, 1558 and 1574); Juan Huarte de San Juan, *Examen de ingenios para las ciencias* (Baeza, 1575 and 1594, profusely reprinted during the sixteenth to eighteenth centuries); Henrique Jorge Henriques, *Retrato del perfecto médico* (Salamanca, 1595 and 1603); Rodrigo de Castro, *Medicus-politicus: sive de officiis medico-politicis tractatus* (Hamburg, 1614 and 1662).

17 Bio-bibliographical sketches of Henriques are provided by Antonio Hernández Morejón, *Historia bibliográfica de la medicina española*, 7 vols. (Madrid, 1842–1845) (facs. repr.: New York-London: Johnson Reprint Corp., 1967), vol. III, pp. 386–393; Anastasio Chinchilla, *Anales históricos de la medicina en general y biográfico-bibliográficos de la española en particular*, 4 vols. (Valencia, 1841–1846) (facs. repr.: New York-London: Johnson Reprint Corp., 1967), vol. II, pp. 85–88; J.M. López-Piñero *et al.*, *Diccionario histórico de la ciencia moderna en España*, 2 vols. (Barcelona: Península, 1983), vol. I, pp. 299–300; M. Betes de Toro, *La ética médica renacentista de los judeoconversos peninsulares* (Barcelona: Uriach, 1982), pp. 12–15.

18 Henriques, *Retrato del perfecto médico* (cit. n. 16) (henceforth *Retrato*), p. 295. Hereafter, all my references and quotations from this work refer to the first edition, unless otherwise stated.

according to Jewish rites; they were jailed for two years before being absolved for lack of evidence.[19]

In about 1568, Henriques seems to have begun his studies in arts at the University of Coimbra under the guidance of "Cardoso" (perhaps the Latinist Jeronimo Cardoso or the physician Fernando Rodrigues Cardoso) in logic and Lorenzo de Freitas in natural philosophy, among others. He later studied medicine, first in Coimbra with Tomas Rodrigues da Veiga, and then in Salamanca with Ambrosio Núñez, Cosme de Medina and Juan Bravo de Piedrahita (medicine), Agustín Vázquez (anatomy) and Andrés Alcázar (surgery).[20]

After his medical studies and before 1594, Henriques was successively ordinary lecturer in the faculty of arts of Salamanca (probably in dialectics, since he seems to have written a handbook on this topic, as we will see later on), and "substitute" lecturer in the chair of Avicenna and "first elected" lecturer in the chair of practical medicine at the University of Coimbra. He finally became the court physician of Antonio Alvarez de Toledo, the fifth Duke of Alba (1582–1639).[21]

To the best of my knowledge, Henriques wrote five works (four on medicine and one on dialectics), at least two of them published in the 1590s. The earlier one was a *regimen sanitatis* entitled *De regimine cibi atque potus et caeterarum rerum non naturalium nova enarratio...* (Salamanca: Michael Serranus de Vargas, 1594), and contained a commentary on Avicenna's *Canon* book I, fen iii. It was dedicated to the Archduke of Austria, Cardinal Albert of Habsburg (1559–1621), who was governor of Portugal (1583–1593), General Inquisitor of Portugal (1586–1596?), archbishop of Toledo (1594–1598), governor

19 Kamen, *Inquisition and society* (cit. n. 2), pp. 223–224.

20 *Retrato*, pp. 116–117, 129, 212, 222, 232, 291-292. For information on these professors, see M.T. Santander, *Escolares médicos en Salamanca (Siglo XVI)* (Salamanca: Universidad de Salamanca, 1984), *passim*; V. Beltrán de Heredia, *Cartulario de la Universidad de Salamanca*, 4 vols., vol. IV: *La Universidad en el Siglo de Oro* (Salamanca: Universidad de Salamanca, 1972), *passim*. See also the relevant entries in Hernández Morejón, *Historia bibliográfica* (cit. n. 17), *passim*; Chinchilla, *Anales históricos* (cit. n. 17), *passim*; López-Piñero *et al.*, *Diccionario histórico* (cit. n. 17), *passim*; G. Díaz Díaz, *Hombres y documentos de la filosofía española*, 4 vols., vol. IV: *H-LL* (Madrid: CSIC, 1991), *passim*.

21 See the title page of the *Retrato* and pp. 247, 280. In the second edition of this work there is no trace of the last academic position he claimed to have occupied.

of the Low Countries (1595–1598) and finally sovereign of the Low Countries from 1598 until his death in 1621. The dedicatory letter is dated 1584, which is ten years before the work was published.[22] The later work was the *Retrato del perfecto medico...*, which Henriques claimed to have written between 1581 and 1582,[23] but which was not published until 1595. Its first edition (Salamanca: Juan and Andrés Renaud, 1595) was dedicated to his master the Duke of Alba, while he addressed the second edition (Salamanca: Juan and Andrés Renaud, 1603) to King Philip III.

Henriques received a single royal license in August 1592 to print and sell these two books, together with another entitled *Compendium dialecticum*. It seems logical that the latter book was also printed at about the same time, although it seems that no copies have survived.[24] As to Henriques' other medical works, his comments in the *Retrato* indicate that he addressed an epistle, supposedly on the use of music as a medical remedy, to the *vihuela* player Jorge Ruiz de Acosta. In this work, he dealt with the importance of musical knowledge for any physician, among other topics.[25] He also wrote a Latin *oratio* to the staff of the medical faculty at Salamanca asking them to encourage the good students, rather than treating them in the same way as the bad ones.[26]

The contents of the *Retrato* suggest that Henriques' academic career

22 Henriques, *De regimine cibi atque potus et caeterarum rerum non naturalium nova enarratio* (Salamanca, 1594), signat. $6r.

23 *Retrato*, pp. 240, 323.

24 For the contents of the royal license, see Henriques, *De regimine* (cit. n. 22), signat. $2v: "Por quanto por parte de vos el Licenciado Anrique Iorge Medico natural de la ciudad de la Guarda en el reyno de Portugal, nos a sido fecha relacion que vos aviades compuesto un libro de Medicina intitulado de Regimine cibi atque potus, y otro de Artes intitulado Compendium dialecticum, y otro en romance intitulado Retrato del perfecto Medico, en los quales aviades puesto mucho estudio y trabajo, y aviades gastado muchos años, y los dichos libros eran buenos y provechosos...."

25 *Retrato*, pp. 267–270. I have found no mention of this vihuela player in the standard reference works on the history of Spanish music and musicians.

26 *Ibid.*, p. 110: "Acuerdome que quando estuve en Salamanca hize una oracion en lengua Latina al Claustro de los Medicos, encargandole que no lo hiziessen assi, y que no premiassen al ruyn estudiante, tanto como al bueno que siempre estudiava, mas veo que no aprovecha nada, y deve de ser porque se mete de por medio un poco del triste interes."

was cut short, first in Salamanca and then in Coimbra. This was probably due to his Converso origins, as the University of Salamanca was well known in sixteenth-century Spain for its strict application of the purity-of-blood statutes to its potential lecturers. As to Coimbra, a very harsh Inquisition was introduced by Philip II after the annexation of Portugal to the Spanish Crown in 1580. Many descendants of those Jews expelled by the Catholic Kings who had taken refuge in Portugal and who had been obliged to convert formally to Christianity in 1497 escaped back to Spain, where the Converso question had already lost relevance.[27]

Other features also suggest that Henriques' professional career was never easy. In 1595, Henriques was about forty-five and had held three different lectureships in Salamanca and Coimbra, but he still signed the first edition of the *Retrato* as "licenciate" (*licenciado*). He only appears as a "doctor" in the second edition (1603). I think that, despite his close ties to such powerful and influential noblemen as the Duke of Alba and the Cardinal-Archduke of Austria, Henriques did not manage to receive his doctorate during the reign of Philip II, and that he only succeeded in doing so under Philip III, when he could take advantage of the more favorable political climate which the new king had introduced toward the Portuguese Conversos who had immigrated to Castile.[28] In addition, Henriques apparently did not get a royal license to print and sell the works he had written in 1582 (*Retrato*) and 1584 (*De regimine*) until 1592, and he did not publish them until 1595 and 1594 respectively. This delay strongly suggests that he had not been able to overcome the obstacles which prevented him from publishing his works, despite his close ties to the above-mentioned noblemen and his former status as a university lecturer. Finally, the contents of Henriques' dedicatory letters, the identity of their addressees and the continuous criticisms and complaints he made in the *Retrato* about the knowledge, skills and behavior of his colleagues (at one point he claimed that there was no profession where there was more envy than in medicine)[29] suggest a figure who felt that he had been badly treated

27 Kagan, *Students and society* (cit. n. 13), pp. 90–92; Kamen, *Inquisition and society* (cit. n. 2), pp. 288–301.

28 *Ibid.*, p. 291.

29 *Retrato*, pp. 71–76.

in his career, and who had only succeeded in making his voice heard through the protection of powerful people.

Henriques was eventually able to make his way as a court physician, a position to which most contemporary academic doctors aspired as the culmination of their careers. By the two last decades of the sixteenth century, Henriques was court physician to the Duke of Alba, who was head of one of the most influential noble houses of Spain, if not the most influential. The contents of the *Retrato* also suggest that Henriques belonged to the intellectual circles which were under the patronage of the Duke of Alba. Lope de Vega, the Duke of Alba's personal secretary, even wrote two sonnets for the *Retrato*, which Henriques included in its presentation.[30] Henriques also seems to have had particular ties to Coria, a city belonging to the Alba family, where he maintained close contact with its bishop and canons. In the dedicatory letter of the *De regimine*, he mentioned that he had accompanied the bishop of Coria when the latter went to some Portuguese walled cities as the envoy of King Philip II "to negotiate the peace and tranquility between Portugal and Spain."[31] This bishop could well have been Pedro García de Galarça (1579–1604), whom Henriques praised in the *Retrato*.[32] In addition, the five fictitious dialogues which make up the *Retrato* were held in the countryside around Coria between the author, *Licenciado Henríquez Lusitano*, and Doctor Palomares, archdeacon of the cathedral of Coria under the same bishop.[33]

30 *Ibid.*, fols. ++2v–++3r. In the presentation of the work there are two more sonnets which are signed by the author's brother, the lawyer Gaspar Fernández, and by Luis Henríquez de Monroy, "regidor" of Alba (fols. ++2r, ++3v).

31 Henriques, *De regimine* (cit. n. 22), signats. $5r-v: "...cum episcopum Cauriensem comitarer, qui missus erat ab eodem Christianissimo rege [Philippo II] ad aliqua huius regni oppida, ut cum oppidanis tractaret de pace et tranquillitate Lusitaniae cum Hispania...." On the Portuguese crisis of 1578–1580, which eventually brought the annexation of the kingdom of Portugal to the Spanish Crown, see J. Hermano Saraiva, *Historia de Portugal* (Madrid: Alianza, 1989), pp. 194–199.

32 *Retrato*, p. 10 (see next footnote).

33 *Ibid.*: "Era el Theologo el doctor Palomares Arcediano de Coria muy privado y querido del Illustrissimo y sapientissimo don Pedro Garcia de Galarça, Obispo dignissimo de Coria, y el Medico era el Licenciado Enriquez Lusitano; lo que entre ellos se finge que passo, para que se entienda mejor y parezca estar los dos presentes, se propone en esta forma."

4. Henriques' portrait of the perfect physician

Written in Spanish so that "everybody can take advantage of it,"[34] the five dialogues of the *Retrato del perfecto médico* were between the author, acting as a physician, and Doctor Palomares, acting as a theologian and canonist. According to Henriques, both of them would leave Coria in the early morning and walk across the green fields to enjoy the wonders of nature, to thank God for "so many things He has created because of mankind," and "to philosophize on the mysteries of nature."[35] As the title of the work suggests, the dialogues deal with medical ethics and etiquette, although Henriques' quick, fresh and lively style is not always compatible with systematic order.

Explicitly building on the Platonic theory of ideas,[36] Henriques drew the portrait of the perfect physician by describing the physical aspect and personality, training, knowledge and practical behavior which any practitioner must possess to approach such a condition. He openly expressed his deep concern over the situation of medical practice in Castile at the time,[37] and claimed to have written the *Retrato* with the intention that it would be useful to the "republic."[38] According to his brother's foreword, this public usefulness was twofold. It was

34 *Ibid.*, signat. ++1v. These words and others justifying the writing of this work in Spanish and not in Latin appear in the foreword which was written by the author's brother, the lawyer Gaspar Fernández. Henriques himself also dealt with this topic on p. 76.

35 *Ibid.*, p. 1. I have not been able to document the life of Doctor Palomares, who, according to Henriques, was archdeacon of Coria during the reign of Bishop Pedro García de Galarça (1579–1604), whom he also praised (*Ibid.*, p. 10). On the latter, an outstanding bishop of the city, see Q. Aldea-Vaquero *et al.*, *Diccionario de Historia Eclesiástica de España*, 5 vols., vol. I: *A-C* (Madrid: CSIC, 1972), p. 627.

36 *Ibid.*, pp. 29–30: "... no pretendo otra cosa, sino mostrar la perfection de un poeta, a imitación de los quales trabajare por proponer un perfecto medico, que sera como una figura traçada en el entendimiento, la qual Platon llama Idea, y no como retrato de los medicos que agora ay, de los quales, aunque muchos sean muy habiles, ingeniosos y sabios, no son sino como sombra de lo que pienso dezir."

37 *Ibid.*, pp. 109–110.

38 *Ibid.*, signat. +3r: "Y esto con intento de ver si puedo aprovechar a la Republica"; p. 9: "...declarar esto sera servicio muy accepto a la Republica digno de muy gran galardon."

meant to offer a medical model which those practitioners who were desirous of improving their art could emulate, and also a way for potential patients to identify those physicians to whom they could entrust their health.[39] In his dedicatory letter to the Duke of Alba, Henriques emphasized this second purpose by claiming that he wished to allow people to distinguish real medical practitioners from false ones, those to whom "princes, lords and republics should not entrust their diseases."[40] He was convinced that he was dealing with a very controversial issue, and showed his anxieties about the reception the *Retrato* might have among his colleagues in several pages.[41] He asked his master and addressee for protection against any attacks he might eventually receive from them.[42] He insisted that his aim was not "to offend anybody, but to give rules and advice through which each one can improve his knowledge and skills in this art."[43] Henriques claimed to be the first to write a work on such a topic, and his initiative was celebrated by his brother, who saw the *Retrato* as destined to cover a hitherto unexplained gap in a "science" such as medicine which was "so noble and necessary" to mankind. Henriques anticipated possible criticisms for having resorted to instances from "authors of several sciences" to illustrate his position, and claimed that in doing so he merely followed in the footsteps of Galen, who used to report "stories, verses and adages of wise authorities in other sciences to confirm his own doctrine."[44]

39 *Ibid.*, signat. ++1v: "No menos, por cierto, sera util y provechoso este retrato, para que los Medicos vean las partes requisitas para su perfection, y trabajen por alcançarlas, y los que no lo son, sepan de que Medicos han de confiar su salud."

40 *Ibid.*, fols. +3r-v: "Y esto con intento de ver si puedo aprovechar a la Republica. Porque bien veo, quan dubdosa y llena de peligros sea la facultad que professo. Y lo que me da grande pena, es ver, que acaece en nuestros tiempos lo que dezia de los suyos Plinio, que a cada cual que se finge Medico se le da credito, no aviendo mentira mas peligrosa. Y por tanto pense que haria cosa muy provechosa, si diesse a entender en este libro, los que son Medicos solo en el vestido, y enseñasse quales son los Medicos que mas lo quieren parecer, que serlo, y de quales los Principes y Señores, y las Republicas se deven fiar en sus enfermedades."

41 *Ibid.*, pp. 9–10, 320–321.

42 *Ibid.*, signat. +3v.

43 *Ibid.*, p. 9.

44 *Ibid.*, signat. ++1r, pp. 9–10.

In the following pages, I will deal with Henriques' portrait of the perfect physician. Much of the content of the *Retrato* is clearly commonplace in Christian medical ethics and etiquette, and is the result of the religious and moral influence of Christianity on the underlying "Hippocratic" ideals of medical practice.[45] Henriques usually illustrated both the values he wished to promote among medical practitioners and those he denigrated with a great number of general and medical historical examples. Most of them are taken from the Bible (more from the Old Testament than from the New) and classical antiquity, with some additions from the Arab medical world. I will focus here on those features of his portrait which I see as representing the major requirements for the ideal medical practitioner in late sixteenth- and early seventeenth-century Spain. This ideal practitioner was a male, Catholic, and university trained physician.

The perfect physician should be male:
Henriques' consistent use of the Spanish masculine gender plainly shows that his *Retrato* was exclusively intended for male medical practitioners. He seems to have assumed that the exclusion of female practitioners was so "natural" that he simply ignored them, yet oblivion was not the only means of disqualification. In dealing (albeit briefly) with the "despicable old women" (*viejezuelas*), he made use of an archetypal distortion and reduced all female practitioners to a well-known locus of late medieval and early modern gynophobia, the "old women" or *vetule*,[46] to which he added the Spanish suffix *uelas* as a contemptuous intensifier. Henriques warned his readers against being treated by

45 For an overview, see D. W. Amundsen, "Medical Ethics, History of: Medieval Europe: Fourth to Sixteenth Century," in *Encyclopaedia of Bioethics*, ed. W.T. Reich, 4 vols. (New York: The Free Press, 1978), vol. III, pp. 938–951.

46 On the topic of the *vetule*, see D. Jacquart and C. Thomasset, *Sexuality and Medicine in the Middle Ages* (Cambridge: Polity Press, 1988), pp. 76, 85, 112–113, 115, 192; J. Agrimi and C. Crisciani, "Medici e 'vetule' dal duecento al quattrocento: problemi di una ricerca," in *Cultura popolare e cultura dotta nei seicento. Atti del Convegno di Studio di Genova (23–25 novembre 1982)* (Milan: Franco Angeli Editore, 1983), pp. 144–159. On the means of disqualification, see M.V. López-Cordón, "La conceptualización de las mujeres en el Antiguo Régimen: los arquetipos sexistas," *Manuscrits*, 1994, *12*: 79–117.

> garrulous, ugly, 'wise,' wandering 'despicable old women' (*viejezuelas*), brought up in the midst of an entire shamelessness, who pretend to know how to cure every disease, all of which they supposedly identify through urine; and with these deceptions they snatch money and gifts from the people.

He charged that they claim to cure everything and everybody with the same treatment and that they pride themselves on being sorceresses. He protested that "this pestilence of the Republic" could continue to live without fear of justice or the weight of the law being brought upon them. He complained that, as a result of the inroads that this "rabble" (*gentezilla*) made into other people's jobs in cities, towns and villages "we have to work hard afterwards in order to rectify their missteps and to correct their mistakes."[47]

The perfect physician should be Roman Catholic:
Henriques' *Retrato* was intended for Roman Catholic physicians.[48] Furthermore, he assumed that the first and most relevant requirement of every medical practitioner aspiring to perfection was to be a faithful Christian, and in Counter-Reformation Spain, to be a Christian was to be a Roman Catholic. Even so, Henriques claimed in a Socratic way that man had to know himself in order to know God, and he disqualified "Romans and other Gentiles" as having lost their knowledge of

47 *Retrato*, pp. 109–110: *Licenciado*: "De lo que avemos dicho y diremos se collige quan grande error y, por mejor dezir, necedad es de aquellos que se curan con unas viejezuelas, parleras, suzias, colmilludas, romeronas, criadas en el medio de toda desverguença, las quales fingen que saben curar todas las enfermedades, que todas las conocen de la orina, y con estos embaymientos sacan dineros y pieças del vulgo ¿No es esto cosa para espantar? (...) Pues, ¿como vemos que se permiten en las ciudades, villas, y lugares esta gentezilla, que usurpan el officio que no es suyo? *Arcediano*: Que me haze que aya leyes, no se executando, que me haze hablar de la justicia, si su execution se pone en olvido; y lo peor es que a vanderas desplegadas, como dizen, quieren curar a todos, a todos calan con la misma horma, dan a entender ser hechizeras, veo las vivir sin recelo de justicia, siendo la pestilencia de la Republica ¡Que harto tenemos despues de emendar sus errores, remediar sus faltas, quisiesse Dios que viniesse la gente en esta cuenta!"

48 This underlying assumption is present throughout the *Retrato*, although it is not always obvious. See, among other passages, pp. 202–203, 240–241, 240bis–241bis, 241bis–242, 243–244, 282–283, 289–290, 303–304, 312–313.

God because they did not know themselves.[49] For Henriques, a "fear of God, his Creator" was the most important prerequisite for a man who wanted to achieve perfection in medicine. Galen lacked this fear, and thus, despite having been "a very great physician, from whom we have learned the few things we know about [medicine]," he never achieved the highest degree of perfection in medicine. Henriques even alleged that Galen was ignorant of the nature of the substance of the soul, reproved "our Sainted Catholic faith" (*De differentiis pulsuum*, book iii, ch. 3), and criticized Moses (*De usu partium*, book xi, ch. 14).[50]

Being a faithful Christian had other, broader implications for medicine. Some of them illustrate the harmony which was repeatedly sought between the Hippocratic and Christian ideals of medical practice. For example, he advised that patients in a weak condition should only receive weak medicines, so as not to further debilitate their condition. Strong drugs could even cause their death.[51] He also refused to prescribe abortive drugs[52] and poisons which would help people die.[53]

At the same time, other prescriptions given by Henriques, such as those concerning fatal diseases, are mainly guided by Christian ethical values. In contrast to the views of Galen, Celsus and Guy de Chauliac ("in spite of his being a Christian"), who thought that providing medical assistance to "hopeless" patients discredited the practitioner as well as the remedies he employed, Henriques claimed that the perfect physician should always care for "hopeless" patients, as "many times they recover beyond every hope and with no explanation as to how."[54] Moreover, he added that in such circumstances the doctor

49 *Ibid.*, p. 163.

50 *Ibid.*, pp. 30, 282–283, 305. For Galen's quotations, see C.G. Kühn ed., *Claudii Galeni Opera Omnia* (Leipzig, 1821–1833), vol. VIII, p. 657, and vol. III, pp. 905–907, respectively.

51 *Ibid.*, pp. 202–203.

52 *Ibid.*, pp. 305–306.

53 *Ibid.*, pp. 312–313.

54. *Ibid.*, pp. 289–290: "Mas respondiendo conforme a nuestra christiana religion, dire yo que durante la vida del que al parecer no puede vivir, nunca ha de faltar la Medicina usando de cautela, y prognosticacion para no caer en lenguas de los maldizientes, porque muchas vezes fuera de esperança, ni entender como, ni de que manera escapan los enfermos. Y este es el parecer de Avicena, con aver sido hombre barbaro y sin fe... Deste parecer fue tambien Cornelio Celso..."

should try to delay the patient's death since his spiritual salvation could depend on "one day, one hour, one instant." Finally, he maintained that even such qualified "Gentiles" as Hippocrates and Galen seem to have sought to lengthen illness or, in other words, to delay death.[55]

In line with a widespread belief among contemporary Christians, Jews and Moslems, Henriques stated that "many famines, pestilences and other things" were allowed by God to punish mankind's sins.[56] In another passage, he illustrated this point by claiming that the "French pox, its pains and the virulent gonorrhea," all of them diseases which were never seen in previous times, were constantly afflicting people "to stop the incontinence and the immoderate sensuality of mankind."[57]

Since "many scourges and diseases come from our sins," both protagonists of the *Retrato* agreed with contemporary canon law that the "medical practitioner should make his patients confess and have the last sacraments administered" before he begins to treat the patient.[58] Henriques complained that, as physicians had usually neglected to implement this canonic rule, patients who thought themselves to be dying fell into a panic whenever any "expert and wise" doctor asked them to put their souls in order.[59] Here again, he deliberately made use of the Gentile authorities, Plato and Galen, to illustrate the correctness of his argument.[60] He added that the Christian medical practitioner

55 *Ibid.*, p. 290: "A mi me parece muy sano el parecer de Avicena, porque aunque el Medico tuviesse firmissimo conocimiento de la muerte, esta obligado a dilatar lo que pudiera con los medicos humanos, pues podria ser que en un dia, o en una hora, o en un instante estuviesse la salvacion de aquel hombre; y aun en razon de gentilidad es verdadera esta sentencia, pues Hippocrates nos dexo precepto de alargar el mal, o por mejor dezir differir la muerte, quando hablando de los Cancros, dixo: *Cancros occultos melius est non curare, curati enim citius interimunt*. Esto parece que quiso significar Galeno, quando embiava los physicos a Tabias, y affirma, que nunca vio alguno de todo sanar."

56 *Ibid.*, pp. 238–239.

57 *Ibid.*, pp. 125–126: "...el mal Frances, y sus dolores, y la gonorrea virulenta, nunca se vieron en tiempos passados, los quales males son agora muy continuos para refrenar la incontinencia y sensualidad desmoderada de los hombres."

58 *Ibid.*, pp. 239–240.

59 *Ibid.*, pp. 240–241.

60 *Ibid.*, p. 240: "Una cosa me admira, y es que algunos de los Gentiles alludieron en sus escriptos a la confession affirmando, *omnia vel bona, vel mala ab animo in*

should also be able to provide the patients with spiritual consolation, and used the opportunity to impress his readers with his wide knowledge of Biblical and Patristic sources.[61]

In order to answer those who claimed that most medical practitioners had despicable habits and lived in permanent discord with each other, Henriques concluded by reminding his readers of the many Christian cultivators of medicine who are venerated as saints as a result of the highest degree of "true nobility" they achieved in their lives. At the end of this eulogistic passage, Henriques stated that even Christ and his disciples acted as medical practitioners.[62]

The perfect physician should be university-trained:

The third main requirement of the perfect physician was that he study medicine at a university. The *Retrato* indicates not only why Henriques supported university or "rational" medical practitioners as opposed to those lacking such training, but also the kind of university training which he considered to be most appropriate.

The non-university practitioners:

According to Henriques, rational (*racional*) medical practitioners were always preferable to empirics (*emperico*). The latter were only able to cure those diseases which they had previously seen, while the former could successfully tackle every disease, not only those which, though well known, they had never seen but also the entirely new ones which periodically appeared.[63]

In several places in the *Retrato*, Henriques referred in very critical terms to several groups of empiricists. I have already mentioned his scornful comments on the old-women practitioners, but he also attacked bonesetters (*algebristas*), enchanters (*ensalmadores*), necro-

corpus et hominem totum influere. Donde vino que Platon en un dialogo [*Carmides*], dixo que assi como no se pueden curar los ojos sin la cabeça, ni sin el demas cuerpo, assi ni el cuerpo se puede curar, sin curar la alma. Acuerdome aver leydo en Galeno [*De sanitate tuenda*, lib. i, cap. viii], que curò a muchos, los quales enfermavan todos los años mudandoles solos las ruynes costumbres del alma en buenas."

61 *Ibid.*, pp. 241–242.

62 *Ibid.*, pp. 303–304.

63 *Ibid.*, pp. 125–127.

mancers and others. He sneered at the *algebristas*, who "have monopolized the job of bonesetting or, to put it more precisely, of dislocating the dislocated members, since they are like incompetent roof tilers who cause more leaks in the house they are repairing [than they fix]." He praised a "decree" (*Decreto*) by Fernando Mena, medical professor at the University of Alcalá and physician to Philip II, which was intended to put an end to the *algebristas* by requiring that surgeons show a knowledge of *algebra* when they were examined by the Protomedicato.[64] Henriques claimed that *algebra* was a part of rational medicine, as Hippocrates' *De fracturis* and *De articulis* plainly show, and therefore the perfect physician should also know about it.[65] These criticisms and claims were clearly biased by the fact that he, like every university physician, had to compete with non-university practitioners in the marketplace of medical practice.

Henriques remembered the harsh condemnations of necromancy by Thomas Aquinas and that from the Pentateuch (the fortune-teller and his or her clients). He also suggested that any other fortune-tellers, such as physiognomists and palmists, who were always successful in their forecasts should be put under suspicion of practising black magic and severely punished. Only the demon "can know, because of his

64 *Ibid.*, pp. 108–109: "Vera v.m. otra canalla de gente, que han tomado para si el oficio de concertar, o por mejor dezir, desconcertar miembros desconcertados, y son como ruynes trastejadores, que mas goteras hazen en la casa que adereçan. Esta arte llamada luxatoria en vulgar se dize algebra. (...) Entendiendo el Doctor Mena medico de Camara de su Real Magestad, los daos que estos plebeos algebristas hazen, y que esta arte es tocante a la medicina, hizo un nuevo Decreto, que ninguno se admitiesse al examen de cirujano, que no diesse cuenta del algebra, para que usandola los mismos cirujanos y examinandose della, excurriessen y acabassen los concertadores, que por ay andan sin entender la anatomia de los huessos, que por lo menos avian de tener sabida. Y sin tener entendimiento para corregir los accidentes que sobrevienen a las fracturas y dislocaciones, que ellos presumen curar."

65 *Ibid.*: "Desta parte de la medicina, que ha de saber nuestro medico, compuso Hippocrates tres libros que se llaman *De fracturis* y quatro *De articulis*, los quales Vidio Florentino bolvio de Griego en Latin con mucha vigilancia. (...) Cierto que se engañan los que piensan ser mejor que la arte de algebra este usada entre gente vulgar e indocta como agora se haze, que no entre los doctos, moviendose por una authoridad de Hippocrates dellos mal interpretada... No se antepone el vulgar al sabio absolutamente, sino a aquel sabio que con falsas y depravadas razones no se amaña a lo que el hombre plebeyo."

being more astute and clever than any man, and because of his experience and some conjectures, what is to come, so that he [the demon] would say to [the palmist] something which was entirely impossible to guess from the palms."[66]

Finally, Henriques drastically opposed the use of signet rings, enchantments, spells and other similar devices to diagnose or cure diseases. He was only willing to accept inscriptions (*nominas con caracteres*) of the "*Credo, Pater Noster* and some words from the Gospels," and even in this case only if they were used "without superstition." He claimed that none of these devices had any "natural power" in themselves, but that they worked as a result of invoking "any superior cause." Even so, he suggested that those readers interested in knowing why and how these remedies sometimes worked in medicine "should consult with wise Catholic theologians."[67] Henriques' long dissertation on this topic undoubtedly reflected the doctrines of the Roman Catholic Church after the Council of Trent.

The education of a university medical practitioner:

The *Retrato* provides a comprehensive view of what Henriques saw as the basic educational requirements for the perfect medical practitioner, but it also provides some preliminary conditions which he perceived as necessary. Some of these conditions dealt with having the appropriate physical presence, personality, way of life and natural talent (*ingenio*) for medical practice. The first three conditions were, in general terms, described according to a conventional professional pattern whose origins went back to the Hippocratic tradition. However, the last condition reflected the clear influence, detectable throughout his work, of his contemporary Juan Huarte de San Juan (*c.* 1529–*c.* 1588). According to Henriques, an inclination to wisdom was not sufficient for a medical practitioner to become wise; he must also have the appropriate natural talent (*ingenio*) for this job, in addition to intensive study and hard work in his profession. Following Huarte, he stated that the specific talent for medical practice consisted mostly of having a powerful imaginative virtue (*imaginativa*). This talent was very different from that appropriate to natural philosophy and medical

66 *Ibid.*, pp. 277–278.
67 *Ibid.*, pp. 307–311.

theory, where the intellective virtue prevailed. They both thought that the lack of the appropriate virtue explained why Giovanni Argenterio, who was far better than Galen "in reducing the art of healing to a better method," was so unsuccessful in his medical practice that "no patient of his county dared to be cured by him."[68] Again following Huarte, Henriques emphasized that medical students should leave their parents' houses in order to study in a place where they lacked "paternal protection and comfort."[69]

The medical education which Henriques' perfect physician should receive seems to have fitted to a great extent the contemporary studies of arts and medicine at the universities of Salamanca and, probably, of Coimbra, where he had studied and lectured.[70] At the same time, he did make some strong criticisms of the nature of the medical education at the University of Salamanca in a number of passages of the *Retrato*.

Henriques emphasized the importance of an education in arts as a preliminary to medicine. In a Platonic way, he recommended beginning with mathematics: first arithmetic, then geometry.[71] In addition, a good training in logic, dialectic, metaphysics, and moral and natural philosophy was necessary for any medical practitioner who took his job seriously.[72]

When discussing the nature of medical education, Henriques recommended studying the books of the authorities, having good university lecturers, gaining experience, knowing languages and travelling. He thought that Hippocrates and Galen were the main medical authorities, and claimed that medical practitioners "had to keep in mind everything written by Hippocrates," who was "a true minister and follower of nature." They must then study the works of Galen in order to know the patient's temperament and to use the appropriate medicines. Finally, they should also know the doctrines of Avicenna, Paul

68 *Ibid.*, pp. 82–83, 91, 118–120.

69 *Ibid.*, p. 121.

70 On the medical syllabus in the sixteenth-century University of Salamanca, see L.S. Granjel, *Los estudios de medicina en Salamanca* (Salamanca: Real Academia de Medicina, 1989), pp. 23–44.

71 *Retrato*, pp. 278–279.

72 *Ibid.*, pp. 278–289. In these pages, Henriques explains why he thinks that all these disciplines are relevant, and illustrates his point with a wide variety of examples taken from medical and non-medical authorities.

of Aegina, Rhazes, Aetius of Amida, Alexander of Tralles, Celsus, Haly Abbas, Johannes Actuarius "and many others, both ancient and modern, who have worked hard in cultivating and embellishing this science." Any practitioner-to-be should "work hard to imitate these outstanding men in all those good and profitable things they wrote for their faculty, because by imitating them, mistakes are reduced, art increases, difficult things become easy and intellect takes over."[73]

Henriques highly praised the good lecturers who taught students with "clarity and method," avoided giving pompous lectures, and taught "a firm doctrine, neither a sophistic one nor [one] including vain considerations."[74]

Once the student had learned "the science of medicine" (*sciencia de la medicina*), he needed to acquire experience (*experiencia*). According to Henriques, "reason (*razon*) and experience are the feet by means of which medicine walks, they are the two columns on which medicine rests." After a long discussion as to whether "science" or "experience" was more important for medicine, the archdeacon and the licenciate agreed in concluding that there is no true knowledge without knowledge of the causes and that the rational practitioner is preferable to the empiric, since the empiric "only proceeds through the demonstration *quia*," while the rational physician also "proceeds through the demonstration *propter quod*," the latter being the most precise of all demonstrations, according to Aristotle.[75]

Henriques emphasized how important it was that the perfect physician should be a "great Latinist" and that he should also have "a medium knowledge of Greek." He noted that, as all the Greek authorities had been accurately translated into Latin, Greek was no longer as essential as before. However, it was still useful, as some Greek words had not been translated into Latin.[76] He also recommended that medical students learn Arabic "in order to understand perfectly such Arabic authorities as Avicenna and Averroes," and to avoid the risk of misunderstanding their teachings because of the bad translations of their works. Together with many others of the last third of the sixteenth

73 *Ibid.*, pp. 97–103.

74 *Ibid.*, pp. 115–121.

75 *Ibid.*, pp. 121–127.

76 *Ibid.*, pp. 185bis–187.

century, he was critical of the edition of Avicenna's *Canon* and other works (first edition: Venice, 1555) by Andrea Alpago (d. 1522) and Benedetto Rinio the younger (1485–*c*. 1565), who had allegedly introduced some very serious misinterpretations of Avicenna's doctrine. Henriques took advantage of this issue to display his knowledge of Hebrew, which may have given him direct access to the medieval Hebrew translations of Avicenna's *Canon*.[77]

Henriques was strongly in favor of travel (*peregrinacion*) as a source of knowledge, and illustrated this point with many historical examples.[78] He claimed that in travelling "a great many things which are not fully learned in the schools are heard of, seen and known."[79] Thus, he believed that there should be a decree which would require every new medical practitioner to practice abroad for four or five years before beginning to work at home.[80] For those practitioners unable to travel, he suggested reading books on cosmography.[81]

Henriques emphasized three disciplines as being particularly relevant to the medical knowledge of his ideal practitioner: anatomy, astrology and therapeutics. His comments on anatomy clearly reflected his enthusiasm for Vesalian anatomy.[82] He was quite pleased that the

77 *Ibid.*, pp. 187–188. These translations were widely used in the sixteenth century in order to improve the Latin editions. See N.G. Siraisi, *Avicenna in Renaissance Italy. The "Canon" and Medical Teaching in Italian Universities after 1500* (Princeton: Princeton University Press, 1987), particularly pp. 133–144.

78 *Retrato*, pp. 262–265.

79 *Ibid.*, p. 262: "Sera tambien la peregrinacion muy necessaria a nuestro Medico, porque con ella se oyen muchas cosas, y veen y saben, que en las escuelas no se acaban de deprender".

80 *Ibid.*, pp. 262–263: "*Arcediano*: ...Esto [la peregrinacion] no consideran los Medicos deste tiempo, los quales piensan que bastan tres, o quatro solecismos, o barbarismos, que deprendieron en la Universidad ḿas vezina, con otras tantas receptas ranzias, para yrse corriendo sangre, a hazer continua y capital guerra a su patria, como perros que en beviendo del rio Nilo buelven luego raviando a morder quantos encuentran. *Licenciado*: Estos son aquellos, de los quales blasphemava Plinio, diziendo que aprenden a nuestra costa, y matando. Sin se hallar una ley que castigue tan perniciosa ignorancia, cierto que seria un decreto muy util y saluberrimo a la Republica, que ningun Medico saliendo reziente y fresco de los estudios pudiesse medicar en el Reyno, sin primero averse ensayado quatro, o cinco anõs en tierras estrageras."

81 *Ibid.*, pp. 265–266.

82 *Ibid.*, pp. 208–212.

anatomy of the human body, which was "so necessary to our physician's perfection," was taught "by showing each bodily part to the eye" at many of the Spanish universities.[83] He stated that there was nothing more necessary to medicine than "the science of anatomy," since it "allows us to point out with our finger the composition of each member, its relations and shape, and the way through which it expels its excrements and superfluities." However, anatomical studies had still higher value for Henriques; they allowed the students to contemplate this wonderful object made by God and, by admiring His infinite wisdom, they could easily find inside themselves the path to their salvation. Unfortunately, he complained, "many want to become physicians but very few are well prepared to work in the job they have chosen, and they do not take into account how much Galen has commended the knowledge of anatomy to medical practitioners."[84]

83 *Ibid.*, p. 208: "Una cosa veo agora en España, que me agrada mucho, y es que ay Cathedras en las quales se enseña la Anatomia del cuerpo humano tan necessaria a la perfection de nuestro Medico, y cada parte se muestra al ojo, lo qual no se hazia en los siglos passados." On anatomical studies in sixteenth-century Spain, see J.M. López-Piñero, "La disección y el saber anatómico en la España de la primera mitad del siglo XVI," *Cuadernos de Historia de la Medicina Española*, 1974, *13*:55–110; idem, *Ciencia y técnica en la sociedad española de los siglos XVI y XVII* (Barcelona: Labor, 1979), pp. 308–332.

84 *Retrato*, pp. 208–209: "...no se yo como podran los Medicos antiguos ser medicos faltandole la sciencia de la Anatomia, la qual muestra con el dedo cada miembro de que se compone, y la vecindad que tiene, y la figura, y por donde expelle sus excrementos y superfluidades, lo qual deve de ser tan importante saberlo el Medico, que pienso no aver en toda la Medicina cosa mas necessaria. Y dexando la utilidad, la qual obliga al Medico saberla, ¿que dize v.m. de la suavidad tan grande como de la composicion del cuerpo humano se puede recebir, andando todo con el entendimiento escudriando, ¿que Reyno mas concertado, me dara v.m. que el cuerpo del hombre? ¿que republica mas bien ornada de todo lo que importa para el buen regimiento, y sossiego y tranquilidad de los hombres? Obra hecha por manos del altissimo Dios, que dispuso todas las cosas suavemente. Dezia David rey sancto contemplando la composicion tan subida y excellente del cuerpo del hombre: *Mirabilis facta est scientia tua ex me.* Como si dixera: Considerando Señor yo el artificio de mi cuerpo, su substancia, sus actiones, su orden, sus caminos, su figura, sus cavidades, y sus sitios, sus ataduras, quedo admirado de contemplar vuestra infinita sabiduria. (...) Si quisiessemos bien considerar esto, dentro de nos mismos hallariamos el remedio de nuestra salvacion, mas todos quieren ser Medicos, y muy pocos quieren trabajar en el officio que han escogido, y no miran quanto encomienda Galeno a los que professan la medicina

Henriques dealt more with astrology than with any other discipline in the *Retrato*.[85] In several places, he defended the usefulness of astrology for medical diagnosis, prognosis and treatment. The perfect medical practitioner had to assume that the movements of inferior bodies were subordinate to those of superior ones and therefore to learn astrology in order to behave rationally in medical practice. He also claimed that neither Galen in *De crisibus* and *De diebus decretoriis*, nor Hippocrates in many passages of his works (mainly in his *Aphorismi*) could be understood without a knowledge of astrology. He felt that astrology was also a useful and necessary complement of natural philosophy, and even to some extent of moral philosophy. Nevertheless, he clearly rejected judiciary astrology whenever it opposed the Christian doctrine of free will, not only because it was condemned by the Roman Catholic Church, but also because it was completely nonsensical from a rational viewpoint. The stars could not influence human souls, as, according to Thomas Aquinas, the latter were superior to heavens, planets, stars and constellations. He made similar assumptions as to causal determinism in the case of physiognomy, which he otherwise saw as a useful tool for any medical practitioner.[86]

Henriques claimed that every medical practitioner should know the medicinal simples, since Galen stated that "only he who knows the virtues of simples can know how to use composed medicines." He illustrated this point by making use of the authority of Galen and many other ancient (Greek and Latin), Arab and contemporary physicians who were deeply concerned with herbs and their therapeutic properties. Moreover, he recommended that every medical practitioner take up the same hobby which many outstanding physicians had allegedly enjoyed in Italy, taking care of a "private garden, plenty of plants and herbs, where he looked at their birth and death," in order to devote himself to the "true knowledge of simples."[87] His claims as to the importance of gardens did not stop here. Henriques called to mind that

el conocimiento de la Anatomia de la qual compuso Galeno obras sapientissimas, como son los libros *De usu partium, De anatomicis administrationibus*. ¿Si uno quisiesse caminar sin lo saber, ni pescudar, no seria desatino?"

85 *Ibid.*, pp. 188–192, 212–224, 240–241, 243–248, 293–295.

86 *Ibid.*, pp. 272–278.

87 *Ibid.*, pp. 224–227.

God had our First Parents live in the countryside, instead of giving them "cities, palaces, castles or fortresses."[88] He also noted that in the past "many illustrious princes [had] cultivated the herbal discipline no less than the art of war," and that at present "many Italian princes and universities boast of having in their lands many and very excellent gardens which are embellished with all the plants available in the universe." At this stage, he also mentioned the royal garden which Philip II had just set up in Aranjuez, near Madrid.[89] Finally, Henriques stated that the "ancient philosophers" had gained great moral and religious wisdom from the study of plants.[90]

Henriques clearly favored attributing "occult properties" to some plants, and illustrated this issue with many examples.[91] He also dealt with the origins of human knowledge of the medicinal properties of plants and other remedies. He claimed that this knowledge was partly due to mankind, partly to animals, and partly to "demons who revealed many things to the Gentiles by means of dreams, in order to deceive them." In this respect, among others, Henriques seems to have been strongly influenced by the Neoplatonist philosophers (Iamblichus, Porphyry, Synesios and others).[92] Finally, he took into account the remedies which medical practitioners should employ and those which they should abjure, and the ways of preparing and applying the former.[93]

88 *Ibid.*, p. 261: "Y conosciendo el omnipotente Dios, quan deleytosas y llanas de recreacion fuessen las plantas que avia criado, en formando aquellos primeros hombres los puso en huertas, jardines, en praderias, en que para siempre habitassen, quiso que estuviessen entre jaxmines, violetas y olorosos narcisos, y no les dio ciudades, no palacios, no castillos, o fortalezas."

89 *Ibid.*, pp. 261–262. For the setting up of this garden by Philip II, see López-Piñero, *Ciencia y técnica* (cit. n. 83), pp. 109–111; Goodman, *Power and penury* (cit. n. 8), pp. 264–265.

90 *Retrato*, p. 262.

91 *Ibid.*, pp. 227–232.

92 *Ibid.*, pp. 224–227.

93 *Ibid.*, pp. 304–317: "*Arcediano*: No avemos dicho de las medicinas de que ha de usar, quales deven ser. *Licenciado*: Essas es menester que sean buenas, no anejas, y las compuestas que sean hechas con toda fidelidad y artificio requisito, y que no se den unas por otras, como suelen hazer algunos Boticarios poco christianos poco zelosos de la salud del proximo, de lo qual se siguen muy grandes detrimentos. Siendo cosa evidente, ser en las Medicinas el medio por donde se alcança

5. Conclusions

Up to this point, the portrait of the perfect physician which Henriques drew complied exactly with the dominant set of values in Counter-Reformation Spain. However, to a great extent every such portrait may be considered as the reverse image of an unsatisfactory reality. Henriques not only made some serious criticisms of the state of medical practice in late sixteenth-century Castile, but also put forward a number of political and moral proposals to improve it. Thus, I have already suggested that he could be considered an *arbitrista avant la lettre*, since he assumed that the implementation of his proposals would contribute to solving the problems of the "republic." Among all the topics he discussed, his strongest criticisms and alternative proposals were addressed to the following issues:

(1) *A weak arts training* — According to Henriques, many contemporary universities (including Salamanca) allowed students to complete their baccalaureate in arts in no more than six months to a year. They were then allowed to begin their medical studies. He complained that, as a result of a lack of "the foundations upon which medicine is built and the pillar around which it turns," Castile and Portugal were full of incompetent and ignorant practitioners who put their patients' lives at risk instead of curing them.[94]

(2) *Low educational standards in the medical faculties* — In his *Oratio*, which Henriques addressed to the staff of the medical faculty of Salamanca, he allegedly asked them not to treat the good and bad students in the same way. He insisted that university lecturers should promote the good students instead of indiscriminately awarding the medical bachelor degree to whoever had studied medicine for four half-years. However, he complained that his proposal had fallen into oblivion.[95]

(3) *Lack of travel experience* — Henriques was in favor of having

salud, y si esse medio es malo, no podra ser el fin bueno, una de las intenciones, y propositos que ha de tener el Medico es, que siempre en sus curas proceda seguramente" (p. 304).

94 *Ibid.*, p. 280.

95 *Ibid.*, p. 110: "Si no se remedia esto, para que nos damos a la Philosophia y Medicina con tanto estudio, con tanto gasto; y para que con tanto dispendio de nuestra salud andamos perdiendo el tiempo, y en ello nos envejecemos. Esta en la

medical students travel abroad for some years after they took their degrees. He openly claimed that it would be highly useful for the "republic" to promulgate a decree which would require every newly graduated physician to practice medicine in other countries for four or five years before he began to work in Castile. This view should probably be related to the assumption, presumably as widespread then as now, that the flesh of one's neighbors is less sensitive than one's own. Nevertheless, he complained that his views were not shared by contemporary, absolutely ignorant, physicians, who were not prepared to move beyond "the closest university" where they had studied.[96]

(4) *Lack of professional control* — Henriques denounced the fact that in contemporary Castile the *Protomédicos* were disposed to confer a license for medical practice on any ignorant practitioner who asked for it, and did nothing to punish the intrusion of non-professionals into contemporary Spain.[97]

mano del Medico la vida, y muerte, y a cada qual que se haga Medico, le dan credito, y a cada qual que curse quatro medios años en Medicina hazen las Universidades Bachilleres. Acuerdome que quando estuve en Salamanca hize una oracion en lengua latina al Claustro de los Medicos, encargandole que no lo hiziessen assi, y que no premiassen al ruyn estudiante, tanto como al bueno que siempre estudiava, mas veo que no aprovecha nada, y deve de ser porque se mete de por medio un poco del triste interes."

96 *Ibid.*, pp. 262–263. For the textual quotation, see footnote 80.

97 *Ibid.*, pp. 109–110: "La costumbre que v.m. dixo de la Universidad de Mompelier en castigar a los idiotas, que toman officio ageno, es muy galana. Pluguiera a Dios que otro tanto se hiziera en España, porque no vieramos a cada passo tantos daños, y si esta osadia y maldad se fuera con rigor castigando, oviera hombres de grande ingenio que se afficionaran a la Medicina, floreciera ella mucho mas; mas todo anda muy confuso, que es lastima y dolor muy grande pensarlo. A un sillero, a un sastre, y a un çapatero, y a los demas artifices de todas las artes machanicas, no le dexan las justicias usar de sus officios, sin que sean primero examinados. Y dase libertad a qualquiera persona inhabil y grossera para curar. O tiempos, o costumbres, a tanta miseria avemos venido, a tanta corrupcion de buenas costumbres avemos llegado, que un sayo, una capa, y las demas obrezillas, que son solo provechosas para defender el cuerpo, se tienen en mas que el mismo cuerpo, y que la misma sanidad. Bien nos pone delante los ojos el divinissimo Galeno quanto importa tenerse cuenta con este negocio, y dize que considere el Medico que quando cura el hombre, que es un subjecto tan noble y principal, no tracta con las piedras, ladrillos, palos, cueros, como los demas artifices. Y con todo veo los Illustres señores Protomedicos dar muy facilmente licencia a dos mil idiotas que ay en este Reyno para curar, y tractar cosas tocantes a esta arte tan excellente."

(5) *Exclusion of competent practitioners and the promotion of the inefficient* — At the end of the *Retrato*, Henriques openly criticized the public authorities for excluding "learned, wise and experienced practitioners" (*Medicos letrados, doctos, exercitados*) from public offices, and for preferring "illiterates" and "idiots" (*Medico indocto, Medicos idiotas*) to them, against the views of Aristotle and Plato.[98]

This item leads me to the last issue with which I would like to deal (albeit briefly) in this paper: the question of lineage. Whether or not Henriques was in his heart more radically critical of the high appreciation which a good lineage received in Castile at the time, in the *Retrato* he did not dare to openly challenge this dominant social value. Rather, he chose to emphasize that in order to actually become a virtuous man, the nobility of virtue should always accompany the nobility of blood.[99] Despite Henriques' tactfulness, I think that the relevance of his criticisms is obvious. It was precisely during the last two decades of the sixteenth century, the beginning of the decline of the Spanish empire, that criticisms of the ideal of nobility of blood grew stronger, although they only became generalized after 1650.[100]

98 *Ibid.*, pp. 319–320: "No tienen ellos la culpa, que cosa es muy usada por nuestros peccados, el interes cegar a los hombres, sino los que le dan oydos, y las justicias, y Consistorios, a los quales conviene el proveer de los officios, y artes a la Republica necessarias. Tengo cierto lastima no solo de lo dezir, sino aun de imaginarlo, que a los Medicos letrados, doctos, exercitados, que por su valor merecen honras estos quedanse por los rincones, por faltarles quien les de la mano para ser conocidos, no teniendose ya cuenta con lo que merecen, sino con lo que tienen, y pueden. Esto quiso significar Aristoteles quando en su Politica encomienda que para los cargos y officios publicos se escojan siempre los mejores de los mejores, y estos no han de ser mejores por ser mas ricos, sino por ser mas letrados y mas virtuosos. Entendia muy bien esto su maestro Platon ... Fue este parecer digno de tal varon, porque cierto, que assi como los ojos careciendo de su propia virtud, tienen corta la vista, y no conocen, ni divisan bien lo que miran; assi los entendimientos de los que tienen officios publicos careciendo de la sciencia, no pueden ver bien la verdad."

99 *Ibid.*, pp. 206–207: "*Licenciado*.... y assi querria yo que nuestro Medico fuesse de buen linaje, porque segun dezia Ciceron, los nobles favorecen la nobleza, y los que tienen cargos publicos en las Republicas, bueno es que desciendan de hombres nobles". *Arcediano*. Nascer de buenos, y por su propio valor merecer que los tengan por tales. Esta es la verdadera y perfecta nobleza. (...) Engañoso el vulgo en juzgar y tener aquel por noble, que hereda la nobleza de sus antepassados, pues es mas honrosa y mejor la que alcançan otros con sus propias virtudes. (...) [De todas formas] no se puede negar que si nuestro Medico fuere juntamente de nobles parientes, seran las letras en el mas lustrosas."

100 Kamen, *Inquisition and society* (cit. n. 2), pp. 173–181.

THE CONVERSO PHYSICIAN IN THE ANTI-JEWISH CONTROVERSY IN FOURTEENTH-FIFTEENTH CENTURY CASTILE

MARCELINO V. AMASUNO

Despite the continuous dialogue among scholars over the nature and dynamics of medieval Spanish society, we still remain quite uninformed about the specific ways in which the constituent parts of that society — Jews, Moslems, and Christians — viewed each other. Nevertheless, the peculiar way in which Spanish Christians perceived their neighbors makes it seem that Judaism and Islam were on trial.[1]

One of the most significant consequences of this attitude is that, from the thirteenth century onward, a strong and constant effort to convert Jews and Moslems to Christianity took root on the Iberian Peninsula. Christian authorities embraced the hope that all the Jews would eventually adopt the Christian faith. With this goal in mind, the Iberian Peninsula joined the rest of Christian Europe in attempting to prove that Christianity was the only true religion. This attempt led to

1 The bibliography on this topic is exhaustive to say the least; for the most recent works, see, *inter alios*, T. F. Glick, *Islamic and Christian Spain in the Early Middle Ages: Comparative Perspectives on Social and Cultural Formation* (Princeton: Princeton University Press, 1979); L. Suárez Fernández, *Judíos españoles en la Edad Media* (Madrid: Rialp, 1980); J. M. Monsalvo Antón, *Teoría y evolución de un conflicto social. El antisemitismo en la Corona de Castilla en la Baja Edad Media* (Madrid: Siglo XXI, 1985); H. Beinart, *Los judíos en España* (Madrid: Editorial MAPFRE, 1992). In the last four years, three important meetings dealing with this subject have taken place: *Las tres culturas en la corona de Castilla y los Sefardíes. Actas de las Jornadas Sefardíes y del Seminario de las Tres Culturas* (Valladolid: Junta de Castilla y León, 1990); *Proyección histórica de España en sus tres culturas* (Medina del Campo, April 1991); *Diálogo filosófico-religioso entre cristianismo, judaísmo e islamismo durante la Edad Media en la Península Ibérica* (San Lorenzo de El Escorial, June 1992).

the revival of a broad movement of conversionism directed against religious minorities. Although this movement called for amicable and low-key discussions between Christians and Jews, the goal was systematic conversion and, ultimately, the elimination of the Jewish community. Judaism had no place in the Christian world.[2]

The intensive proselytization program developed by the Christians was based on a system of missionizing in the form of anti-Jewish polemical literature. The exploitation of authoritative Jewish texts by the Christians undoubtedly had an adverse psychological impact upon the Jews, and was at least partly responsible for the conversion of an unknown number of members of the Jewish élite. The conversionist atmosphere thus created was mainly the result of the orchestration of anti-Jewish sentiment among the Christian population in Iberia by the secular religious authorities and the contributions of a number of

2 Raymond Llull, for instance, placed the Jews in the same class of infidels as the Moslems because of their blasphemous rejection of Christian beliefs. He considered them a dangerous threat to Christendom. *Liber praedicationis contra ivdaeos* in *Raimundi Lulli Opera Latina*, ed. A. Madre (Turnhout: Brepols, 1984), vol. XII, pp. 144–178. Llull took upon himself the task previously initiated by Nicolas Donin, Paulus Christiani, Raymond of Penyafort, third Master-general of the Dominican Order (the Friars Preachers), Raymond Martini, and others. His example would later be followed in Castile. The following is a selected list of the numerous studies devoted to medieval Jewish-Christian polemics in recent years: D. J. Lasker, *Jewish Philosophical Polemics Against Christianity in the Middle Ages* (New York: Ktav, 1977); idem, "Averroistic Trends in Jewish-Christian Polemics in the Late Middle Ages," *Speculum*, 1980, *55*/2:294–304; M. L. Arduini, *Ruperto di Deutz e la controversia tra Cristiani ed Ebrei nel secolo XII* (Rome: Istituto Storico Italiano per il Medio Evo, 1979). On the situation in Spain, see M.A. Cohen, "Reflections on the Text and Context of the Disputation of Barcelona," *Hebrew Union College Annual*, 1964, *35*:157–192; R. Chazan, "The Barcelona Disputation of 1263: Christian Missionizing and Jewish Response," *Speculum*, 1977, *52*:824–842; idem, "From Friar Paul to Friar Raymond: The Development of Innovative Missionizing Argumentation," *Harvard Theological Review*, 1983, *76*:289–306; idem, "The Condemnation of the Talmud Reconsidered (1239–1248)," *American Academy for Jewish Research. Proceedings*, 1988, *55*:11–30; J.M. Monsalvo Antón, *Teoría y evolución* (cit. n. 1), pp. 45–48; Jeremy Cohen, *The Friars and the Jews. The Evolution of Medieval Antijudaism* (Ithaca: Cornell University Press, 1982); H. MacCoby, *Judaism on Trial. Jewish-Christian Disputations in the Middle Ages*, ed. and trans. by Hyam MacCoby (London/Toronto: Associated University Presses, 1982), where the appropriate bibliography can be found.

converts who led this process. The polemical tracts presented by some of these converts are a legacy of this significant phenomenon in the history of medieval Spain.[3]

The collapse of the economy, the Black Death, civil war, and finally a series of anti-Jewish riots contributed to the propagation of the spirit of conversion among Spanish Jewry. As a result of these factors, the religious and social situation of the Jews became untenable. Even those who occupied positions of prestige and power in the courts of the kings and of the ecclesiastical and civil magnates lived in fear. These Jews, because of their personal power and authority, were despised by the Christian lower classes, who thought them the direct cause of their poverty and calamities.[4]

The preparations for the conversionist movement started around the second decade of the thirteenth century and reached their peak in the massacres of June 1391, when the Jewish population suffered a blow from which it never recovered. The catastrophe of 1391 acceler-

3 See, for example, Y. Shamir, *Rabbi Moses ha-Kohen of Tordesillas and his Book 'Ezer Ha-Emunah.' A Chapter in the History of the Judeo-Christian Controversy* (Leiden: Brill, 1975), pp. 40–71; A. Ravitzky, "Crescas' Theory on Human Will: Development and Sources," *Tarbiz*, 1982, *51*:445–470 (in Hebrew, abstract in English, VIII–IX); C. Sirat, *La philosophie juive au Moyen Âge selon les textes manuscrits et imprimés* (Paris: CNRS, 1983), pp. 346–347, 351–352, 407–411; S. Feldman, "A Debate Concerning Determinism in Late Medieval Jewish Philosophy," *Proceedings of the American Academy for Jewish Research*, 1984, *51*:15–54; W. Mettmann, *Die volkssprachliche apologetische Literatur auf der Iberischen Halbinsel im Mittelalter* (Düsseldorf: Westdeutscher Verlag, 1984), especially pp. 32–75. D. Carpenter, "The Language of Polemic: Abner de Burgos' Quadrilingual Defense of Christianity," in *Circa 1492. Proceedings of the Jerusalem Colloquium: Litterae Judaeorum in Terra Hispanica*, ed. I. Benabu (Jerusalem: Hebrew University of Jerusalem, Institute for Research on Sephardi and Oriental Jewish Heritage, 1992), pp. 49–57.

4 This sentiment was prevalent not only among the Christians but also among certain members of the medieval Jewish *intelligentsia*. The phenomenon of the Court-Jew as an important element of Hispano-Jewish history has been studied by contemporary historians. See, for example, H. Beinart, *Judíos en las cortes reales de España* (Buenos Aires: Biblioteca Popular Judía, 1975); B. Safran, "Bahya ibn Paquda's Attitude toward the Courtier Class," in *Studies in Medieval Jewish History and Literature*, ed. I. Twersky. (Cambridge, Mass./London: Harvard University Press, 1979), pp. 154–196; D. Romano, "Cortesanos judíos en la Corona de Aragón," in *Destierros Aragoneses. Judíos y Moriscos* (Zaragoza: Institución Fernando el Católico, 1988), vol. I, pp. 25–37.

ated the stream of conversions; the Spanish kings and nobility no longer needed the Jews, and the enviable positions held by a small minority were to be taken over by the new Christians.[5]

The role played by Vicent Ferrer was the most important factor in the next crisis, which took place between approximately 1411 and 1420. The Aragonese and Castilian Jewish communities had survived violence and conversion until that time. However, when the Dominican friar Ferrer visited the important *aljamas*, most of the upper-class members converted. Devoted to his missionary work, Ferrer believed that he was hastening the second coming of Christ and God's victory over evil.[6]

5 The bibliography on this subject is exhaustive. The social contacts between Christians and Jews during the Middle Ages have been the subject of numerous studies. See especially D. E. Carpenter, "Jewish-Christian Social Relations in Alphonsine Spain: A Commentary on Book VII, Title xxiv, Law 8 of the *Siete Partidas*," in *Florilegium Hispanicum. Medieval and Golden Age Studies Presented to Dorothy Clotelle Clarke*, ed. J. S. Geary (Madison: Seminary of Hispanic Medieval Studies, 1983), pp. 60–70; idem, *Alfonso X and the Jews: An Edition of and Commentary on ... 7.24 "De los judíos"* (Berkeley/Los Angeles/London: University of California Press, 1986). A rich bibliography is found in both works. In the final portion of VII.24.8, Alfonso forbade Christians to take medicines and cathartics manufactured by a Jew. However, a knowledgeable Jewish physician could prescribe them as long as they were prepared by a Christian fully aware of their contents. A curious example of religious disputation, common in medieval Europe, is the *Disputa entre un cristiano y un judío* [Américo Castro, ed., *Revista de Filología Española*, 1914, *1*:173–180], a fragment of about forty lines dating from the first half of the thirteenth century. The matters treated are the same as those of the Latin disputations and anti-Jewish treatises of the Middle Ages. Although Alfonso X's Castile remained for some time isolated from the fanaticism which agitated the rest of Christendom, its Jewish population soon started to feel a change of mood among their Christian neighbors. In fact, despite a certain atmosphere of laxity and toleration fostered by the king and totally unknown beyond the Pyrenees, Castilian Judaism was not free from the effects of fanaticism. Even the monarch was influenced by the teachings of the Church, and accepted the canonical doctrine that the Jews had to live in captivity among the Christians. Although not put into effect until 1348, Alfonso's systematic legal code, *Las Siete Partidas*, was permeated by the desire to punish the contumacy shown by the Jews in refusing to accept the verities of the Christian faith. For a discussion of the number of forced converts in 1391, see B. Netanyahu, *The Marranos of Spain* (New York: The American Academy for Jewish Research, 1966), pp. 235–245.

6 Y. F. Baer, *Die Juden im christlichen Spanien* (Berlin, 1929–33; facs. repr.: Farnborough, 1970), vol. I, pp. 681, 696. Another critical moment occurred

The election of Martin V in 1417 worked to the advantage of the persecuted minority. On February 20, 1422, he issued the bull *Sicut Judeis*, which was addressed to all Christians and applied to all Jews. This bull prohibited, among other things, the injury of their persons and property, and forbade preachers to preach against them. Furthermore, Jews were to be treated with kindness, and were to be allowed to enjoy the privileges granted or to be granted to them. By that time, the Castilian Jews already enjoyed such rights. After the end of King John II's minority in September 1418, the royal council had suspended the severe laws of 1412 and decided that, in practice, only one of the restrictions on Jews should be retained: the requirement that they wear special signs of identification.[7]

For almost a century (1321–1419), the Church implemented its plan, which consisted of removing the Jews from their high positions and reducing them to the servile one which, according to its traditional stance, they deserved. The Jewish-Christian disputations played a

during the Tortosa Disputation (1413–14), which lasted for twenty-one months with a total of sixty-nine sessions. Its goal was nothing less than the complete conversion of the Jews of Catalonia and Aragon. This Disputation took place under conditions of terror; the Jewish delegates were in constant fear for their lives despite the fact that the debates were presided over by the anti-pope, Benedict XIII. Even so, this deplorable affair provoked the conversion of many Jews, who succumbed and accepted baptism. Some of them were even brought into the hall of assembly at Tortosa to declare their acceptance of Christianity. Despite all his efforts, Benedict, who no doubt saw the Disputation as a means toward his recognition as the only legitimate pope of the Church, failed to achieve his goal.

7 For the popes' formal statements about the position of the Jews and the practice of Judaism in the midst of Christian society, see S. Grayzel, "The Papal Bull *Sicut Judeis*," in *Studies and Essays in Honor of Abraham A. Neuman, M. Ben-Horin*, eds. B. D. Weinryb, and S. Zeitlin (Leiden: Brill, 1962), pp. 43–80. For King John II's decree against the Castilian Jews, see *Crónica de Juan II* in *Crónicas de los reyes de Castilla* (Madrid: Biblioteca de Autores Espanñoles, 1987), p. 340a-b; F. Cantera Burgos, *Alvar García de Santa María y su familia de conversos* (Madrid: C.S.I.C., 1952), p. 238; J. Torres Fontes, "Moros, judíos y conversos bajo Fernando de Antequera," in *Cuadernos de Historia de España* (Buenos Aires: Instituto de Historia de España, 1960) pp. 60–97. For the period between 1418 and 1437, see Y. Baer, *A History of the Jews in Christian Spain*, 2 vols. (Philadelphia: Jewish Publication Society of America, 1961–1966), vol. II, pp. 244–270.

crucial role in this policy, and Church authorities sought to foster them. This activity was left in the hands of a knowledgeable few, including some of the new converts, who were among the strongest defenders of Christian theology in these disputes because of their zeal and fanaticism against Judaism.

The following addresses the topic of the disputations. This paper will not delve into all of the famous — or infamous — apostate-proselytizers who became leaders of the conversionist movement. My scope is much more limited; I will deal with the few who belonged to a very special group, the Converso physicians of Castile.

The Converso physician has rarely been seen as an important element of Hispano-Jewish history. This view persists despite the fact that contemporary historians, from Y. Baer to Américo Castro, do not deny their presence in Iberian Christian society. In clear contrast, the importance given by the former to the Court-Jew, who occupied a crucial position in his view of Hispano-Jewish history, is well known. For Baer, the Court-Jew was a recognizable social type, imbued with an Averroistic outlook. This outlook was a central issue in the tensions between the Court-Jew and the Converso physician.

There is no specific study of the effects of the polemical debates which arose between Jewish and Converso physicians during the crucial period between 1321, when Alfonso de Valladolid wrote his *Milḥamot ha-Shem (The Wars of the Lord)*, and 1419, when the Castilian king Juan II and Pope Martin V abolished the whole series of anti-Jewish edicts which had been promulgated during the previous generation. The purpose of this paper is therefore to bring to light some specific data on a few Converso physicians and some of their little-known polemical writings. Special attention will be given to Alfonso de Valladolid (ca. 1270–1346), Juan de Aviñón (? –1382?), and Alfonso Chirino (ca. 1365–1429).

The position which Jewish medicine had in Castilian society, as well as the great esteem in which the Jewish physician was generally held, are well known. Castilian kings and queens, and many of the more powerful noblemen in the realm, had in their courts and houses one or more Jewish physicians. As a result, these individuals also wielded great influence over princes and civil and ecclesiastical dignitaries. Moreover, the popularity of the Jewish physicians was not limited to the upper classes. Their high esteem among the populace is best seen in the fact that quite a number of municipalities relied on their services for the protection of public health.[8]

A well-known example of the great repute enjoyed by Jewish physicians is that of the *infante* Don Juan Manuel, who, as a regent in 1319 after the death of the *infantes* D. Pedro and D. Juan, showed great favor toward the king's Jewish vassals. One of his Jewish physicians, Isaac ibn Waqar, played a decisive role in developing the *infante's* enlightened behavior toward this persecuted minority. When the *infante* abandoned the reins of government, however, there was an eruption of anti-Jewish agitation which created an oppresive and terrifying atmosphere for the Jewish population.[9]

8 A general view of the Court-Jew is presented by H. Beinart, *Judíos en las cortes* (cit. n. 4), especially pp. 6–8, 18, 27–31. A sharp critique of the Jewish courtier is delivered by Baḥya ibn Paquda in *Ḥobot ha-Lebabot*, which, although it refers to eleventh-century Moslem Spain, is applicable to both fourteenth- and fifteenth-century Castile. See B. Safran, "Bahya ibn Paquda's Attitude" (cit. n. 4), pp. 154–196. Certain Jewish families, such as the ibn Waqars, produced a number of physicians. Nathan Koren lists several members of this famous family as doctors in the service of rulers and noblemen in Castile (*Jewish Physicians. A Biographical Index* [Jerusalem: Israel Universities Press, 1973], p. 137a). The physician Joseph b. Isaac b. Moses Waqar of Seville, who composed a calendar in 1357, might have been a member of this family. Moses ibn Waqar, who lived in the first half of the fourteenth century and whose remedy for diarrhea was quoted in a fourteenth-century manuscript, seems to belong to the same family. See B. Richler, "Medical Treatises by Moses b. Isaac Ibn Waqar," *Koroth*, 1989, *9*/9–10:700*–707*, p. 702*. Samuel ibn Waqar, to whom M. Steinschneider attributed the famous *Kitāb al-ṭibb al-qašṭąlī al-malūkī* (Book of Royal Castilian Medicine), was a physician in the service of kings Ferdinand IV (1295–1312) and his son Alfonso XI (1312–1350), and most likely a member of this illustrious family (*Die arabische Literatur der Juden. Ein Beitrag zur Literaturgeschichte der Araber, grossenteils aus handschriftlichen Quellen* [Frankfurt a. M., 1902], p. 165). See L. García-Ballester, and C. Vázquez de Benito, "Los médicos judíos castellanos del siglo XIV y el galenismo árabe: el *Kitāb al-ṭibb al-qašṭālī al-malūkī (Libro de medicina castellana regia)*, c. 1312," *Asclepio*, 1990/1: 119–147. Jewish physicians occupied municipal posts during the fourteenth century, as is the case with the Çemerro family in Seville; some of its members were municipal physicians who engaged in tax-farming and money-lending activities. See Y. Baer, *Die Juden* (cit. n. 6), vol. II, doc. 163, p. 162; doc. 249, p. 235; idem, *A History* (cit. n. 7), vol. I, p. 312.

9 Isaac's son, Judah, would later obtain important social and political advantages from his royal masters, enhancing in this way Castilian Jewry's status. When Alfonso, who was not yet fourteen, took over the reins of government in 1322, he

Rabbi Abner de Burgos emerged in this atmosphere. He subsequently became known as Maestre Alfonso de Valladolid. As Yitzhak Baer pointed out more than six decades ago, "Abner wrestled in spirit for some twenty-five years, until (shortly before the year 1321) he announced his profession of the Christian faith in a book in Hebrew entitled *The Wars of the Lord*."[10] Little is known about him after he was baptized and changed his name to include the name of the Castilian city where he spent his later years, other than that he was assigned to the newly founded collegiate church of Santa María la Real as a sacristan.

In 1336, Alfonso, holding an order granted by the Castilian king, summoned the Jews of Valladolid to a public disputation over the *birkat ha-minim*. The charge that the "prayer against heretics" referred to Christians is a commonplace of medieval anti-Judaism. Declared the winner in this debate, he succeeded in convincing the Castilian king to order the deletion of that passage from the prayer books of the Jews. This triumph ended a phase of spiritual transformation which had been initiated with the writing of the *Milḥamot*. From then until his death in 1346, he wrote many books and pamphlets in which he recommended, among other restrictive measures, that Christians refrain from eating with Jews as Jews avoided food made by Christians.

extended his personal favor to another Jewish courtier, Samuel ibn Waqar (Semuel aben Huacar), his physician and astrologer. Samuel's political clashes with the *almojarife mayor* of the kingdom, Yuaf de Ecija, created violent reactions on the part of some Christian courtiers. The fortunes of the unscrupulous royal major-domo, Gonzalo Martínez de Oviedo, were favored by the king. A crypto-enemy of the Jews, he succeeded in throwing both Yuaf and Samuel into jail, where they died; their wealth and properties were confiscated by the crown in 1336. By this time an overt enemy of the Jews, Martínez de Oviedo, presented the king with a proposal to expel the Jews from the kingdom. In spite of his success in the war against the Moroccans in the Andalusian campaign, he was charged with high treason, imprisoned, and finally executed by the king's order: "And the Lord saved His people in the twelfth month, that is the first Adar" (Y. Baer, *A History* [cit. n. 7], vol. I, pp. 325–327, 354–359). Baer follows the account given by Solomon ibn Verga's chronicle *Shebet Yehuda*, from which this quotation comes (p. 359). On December 8, 1340, Alfonso XI revoked his decree for the imprisonment of all the Jews. See F. Cantera Burgos, "*De Hispania judaica*. La judería de Miranda de Ebro (1099–1350)," *Sefarad*, 1941, *1*:89–140, pp. 132–133.

He advised the latter to shun Jewish doctors, and finally, to the Christian authorities, he strongly advised the outright persecution of the Jews in order to effect their conversion.[11]

Abner/Alfonso drew the title *Milḥamot ha-Shem* from a work written in 1170 by Jacob ben Ruben, who resided in either Catalonia or Provence, in which the latter undertook to refute Christian dogma. Unfortunately, Abner's work has not been preserved, except for some passages quoted by such fifteenth-century Spanish authors as Pablo de Santa María and Alonso de Espina, and during the sixteenth century by Ambrosio de Morales. Very little of its content is known, and what remains is only available through the quotations of such anti-Jewish

10 Alfonso XI granted important privileges to all the Jewish communities of his realms in Valladolid on August 20, 1320. This event and Gonzalo Martínez de Oviedo's rise to power might have been the direct reasons for the ex-rabbi's behavior (Baer, *A History* [cit. n. 7], vol. I, p. 329). Baer provides a very convincing historical portrait of Abner/Alfonso on pp. 327–354. He had previously focused on the former rabbi in "Abner von Burgos" in *Korrespondenzblatt des Vereins zur Gründung und Erhaltung einer Akademie für die Wissenschaft des Judentums*, 1929, *10*:20–37. See also H. Graetz, *Geschichte der Juden von den ältesten Zeiten bis auf den Gegenwart* (Leipzig: O. Leiner, 1863), vol. VII, pp. 337–341 and 485–513; I. Loeb, "Polémistes chrétiens et juifs en France et en Espagne," *Revue des Études Juives*, 1889, *18*:43–69. The interest aroused by Abner/Alfonso's writings among Hispanists has increased considerably after a long period of silence. See, for instance, the studies by C. Sainz de la Maza Vicioso, "Aristóteles, Alejandro y la polémica antijudaica en el siglo XIV," *El Olivo*, 1986, *10*/24:145–154; idem, "Alfonso de Valladolid y los caraítas: sobre el aprovechamiento de los textos históricos en la literatura antijudía del siglo XIV," *El Olivo*, 1990, *14*/31:15–32; idem, "El converso y judío Alfonso de Valladolid y su *Libro del zelo de Dios*," in *Las tres culturas* (cit. n. 1), pp. 71–85; idem, *Alfonso de Valladolid: Edición y estudio del Mss. Lat. 6423 de la Biblioteca Apostólica Vaticana* (Madrid: Universidad Complutense, 1990). See also the articles written by D. E. Carpenter and W. Mettmann in *Litterae Judaeorum in Terra Hispanica* (cit. n. 3).

11 This proposal is spelled out in his most important work, *Moreh Ẓedek* (Teacher of Righteousness), which is only extant in a Spanish translation (*Mostrador de Justicia*) in the Bibliothque Nationale de Paris (Ms. espagnol 43, fourteenth century, 338 ff.). This article cannot deal with Abner/Alfonso's theological and polemical *opus*. A very useful and short synthesis of the subject is offered by Carlos Sainz de la Maza in "El converso y judío" (cit. n. 10), where some other biographical and bibliographical data can also be found.

writers. Some authors have assumed that the *Milḥamot* contained an attack on the polemics of Jacob ben Reuben.[12]

According to its *incipit*, which is preserved in Ambrosio de Morales' *Viage... por orden del rey D. Phelipe II, a los reynos de Leon, y Galicia, y Principado de Asturias* [1572], the book was translated into Spanish by order of Alfonso's patroness the *infanta* Doña Blanca, a bastard granddaughter of Alfonso the Learned and mother superior of the convent of Las Huelgas near Burgos. The relationship between this Castilian princess and the ex-rabbi is not clear. It is most likely that Abner was attached to the monastery as its physician, as monasteries like Las Huelgas had to rely on their Jewish vassals for medical care. As Américo Castro has pointed out, "the truth is that, from the king down, Spanish Christians consulted with them [the Jewish physicians] regarding their most private difficulties," trying to find a solution for their pain and sufferings.[13]

Given the interest of the Church in the spiritual well-being of its people, as illustrated by the canon of the Council of Letran IV, it is not surprising that Church authorities sought to impose and enforce a

12 See I. Loeb, "La controverse religieuse entre les chrétiens et les juifs au Moyen Âge en France et en Espagne," *Revue de l'Histoire des Religions*, 1888, *18*, Part 2, p. 142. Jacob ben Ruben's tract is perhaps the first Jewish polemic writing against the articles of Christian belief, and it became the principal guide for similar works in the following centuries [*Milḥamot HaShem*, ed. J. M. Rosenthal (Jerusalem, 1963)]. The Castilian *Milḥamot ha-Shem*, known in Spanish as the *Libro de las batallas de Dios*, is the first work written by Abner after his conversion to Christianity. As Alfonso de Valladolid, he himself mentions it in his *Mostrador de justicia* in these words: "Entróme en voluntad de conponer un libro en razón de la fe, el qual pus' nonbre *Libro de batallas de Dios*; sino que era puridat encubierta entre mí, porque me lo non sopiessen los diçiplos et que me nasçiesse algún danno d'ellos" [Ms. espagnol 43, fol. 12v. See C. Sainz de la Maza, "El converso y judío" (cit. n. 10), p. 74, note 15].

13 Ambrosio de Morales' book, edited by Enrique Flórez (Madrid, 1765), gives the details of Doña Blanca's orders to Maestre Alfonso (p. 9). A. Castro's quotation is my own translation from his *España en su Historia. Cristianos, moros y judíos* (Buenos Aires: Editorial Losada, 1948, p. 508), where an extremely short section is devoted to the Spanish (mainly Castilian) Jewish physicians (pp. 504–509). Carlos Sainz de la Maza also suspects that this kind of medical connection existed between Maestre Alfonso and the famous monastery. As for the date assigned to the *Milḥamot* (between 1320 and April 1321, the date of the *infanta*'s death), see "El converso y judío" (cit. n. 10), p. 74.

policy which restricted the use of non-Christian physicians by Christian patients. Particularly during the thirteenth century, Church councils strictly forbade Christians to obtain medical or surgical services from Jewish or Moslem physicians under pain of excommunication. The Church could — and did — exhort, threaten, and plead, but it could not effectively control the attitudes of the sick, who continued to employ Jewish doctors despite such prohibitions. Castilian royalty and also civil and religious leaders were the first to break Church law in this respect; they never ever felt bound by such laws. The *infanta* Doña Blanca is not an exception to this rule.[14]

It should therefore not be surprising that, because of their conversion to Christianity, certain apostate Jews warned against the alleged duplicity of Jewish physicians. Thus, Alfonso de Valladolid launched his "holy war" against the Castilian rabbinate. His attack was a direct attempt to prove that Jewish morality had a double standard, a different system of values, which was most obvious in the practice of medicine by *all* of the Jewish physicians. The immorality of the Jewish healer stems, according to Abner/Alfonso, from his oral tradition. This tradition shows that Jewish society has two different yardsticks of moral behavior, one for its members and another for outsiders, the infidels and gentiles. Abner/Alfonso goes on to say that the paramount goal of Jewish physicians in their contacts with Christian patients is to destroy them. This goal is the final conclusion which can be drawn from a chapter of the *Milḥamot*, according to the Franciscan friar Alonso de Espina, in his *Fortalitium Fidei (Fortress of the Faith).*[15]

14 On the Church and its attitudes toward the sick, see D. W. Amundsen, "The Medieval Catholic Tradition," in *Caring and Curing. Health and Medicine in the Western Religious Traditions* (New York/London: MacMillan Publishing Co., 1986), pp. 65–107, especially pp. 92–94.

15 This famous work by Alonso or Alfonso de Espina, a real "cathecism of Jew-hatred" in Prof. H. Beinart's words, was written between 1458–59 and published in 1460 "in the cause of his zealous fidelity to the Catholic faith, and concerning the evil and injury caused to it by Jews, Muslims, and demons." It is divided into four books, and its special character derives from the fact that it does not just discuss the issue, but puts forward specific solutions to get rid of those evils, including Conversos. It was edited several times during the third quarter of the fifteenth century. I have only been able to use the 1525 edition (Lyon: Stephan Gueynard), from which I have drawn all the quotations. For Alfonso de Espina and his vitriolic polemical tract, see Y. Baer, *A History* (cit. n. 7), vol. II, pp.

In fact, according to de Espina, confessor to the Castilian King Henry IV, "the thirteenth cruel deed perpetrated by the Jews upon the Christians *commonly* takes place in the administration of medicines." Numerous Jews, seeing that Christians despise the learning of medicine, try hard to become knowledgeable in this art in order to curry favor with both the civil and ecclesiastical ruling classes. If, as very often happens, the Jewish physicians find a competent Christian practitioner, he is smeared and publicly proclaimed an ignoramus. De Espina, after describing the sad circumstances surrounding the death of a patient in Sigüenza at the hands of a Jewish physician, declares that

> there are many of these physicians, who if they cure one patient, they kill fifty. As has been found out, in their religious gatherings the Jewish physicians themselves praise the one who has managed to kill the most Christian patients.[16]

It seems very reasonable to assume that in this segment of his work, Alonso de Espina is directly quoting from Abner/Alfonso, for immediately afterward, he refers to the ex-rabbi from Burgos in these terms:

> And if you want to find out why Christians should not receive medicines from Jews, listen to a witness, the most famous of their progeny, maestre Alfonso Converso, in his book, *The Wars of the Lord*, chapter xliiij, where he says: 'Every Christian should avoid taking medicines from a Jew for three reasons: first, because the Jew knows by hearsay and not by experiment (*experientia*) which he ought to carry out himself the nature and temperament (*complexio*) of all the foods he prescribes. For instance, the Jewish physician knows neither through experience nor through books the nature of the hare, the rabbit, small fish, and the conger eel and other meats, as he knows the meat of beef, lamb, goat, and other foods which he usually eats. And wise

283–299; B. Netanyahu, "Alonso de Espina: Was He a New Christian?" *PAAJR*, 1976, *43*:107–165; H. Beinart, *Conversos on Trial. The Inquisition in Ciudad Real* (Jerusalem: The Magnes Press, 1981), pp. 9–20.

16 "De similibus autem non est numerus intantum quod si vnum curant quinquaginta occidunt. Sicut repertum est iudeos medicos se ipsos in suis solemnitatibus laudare conferentes ad inuicem quis eorum plures occideret xristianos" (*Fortalitium*, fol. 191a-b).

> physicians have said many times that book knowledge is not enough; what the good and true physician does — beside reading in books — is to carry out experiments and tests (*probationes*) on medicines, foods, and illnesses, and to visit the sick.[17]

Alfonso de Valladolid presents here one of the most common charges against Jewish physicians. In the first place, he claims that the Jewish physician's ignorance of foods capable of preserving the patient's health or curing his illness endangers the Christian patient's well-being. Alfonso explains that the Jewish healer is unable to determine the specific qualities of the foods to be used in the treatment of his patient. In addition, the Jewish physician is not aware of the qualities which define the somatic characteristics (*complexio*) of a particular patient, therefore putting his health and ultimately his life at risk. The good physician must know how to determine the nature and character of foods and nutritional substances, and he can only do so if he is acquainted with the doctrinal basis for preserving health and curing illnesses. This basis is obtained through a) texts, which are the medium for the transmission of medical knowledge, and b) tests (*experimenta*), which allow the physician to determine the *forma specifica*, which are the qualities and effects (*operationes*) peculiar to a particular medicine. The latter can only be achieved through the personal experience of experimental verification (*probatio*). The good doctor should therefore test his medicines before he actually applies them. A medicine must be verified for two reasons: to see what forces (*virtutes*) it possesses, and

17 "Et si vis scire causas quare xristiani non debent recipere medicinam a iudeis. Audi testem famossum ex eorum genere, s[cilicet] magistrum Alfonsum conuersum in libro bellorum dei. ca. xliiij. vbi dicit. Non expedit xristiano alicui medicinam recipere a iudeo triplici ratione. Prima est quia iudeus secundum veritatem non cognoscit naturas et complexiones omnium ciborum qui eis deferuntur nisi ex auditu; non tamen ex experientia quam ipse per se facere posset. Verbi gratia, non cognoscit medicus iudeus naturam carnis leproris (sic) et cirogriti (i.e. cyrogrilli) et fiscedule (i.e. pisciculi) et piscis congri et sic de alijs carnibus per libros sicut cognoscit carnem bouis: arietis: et hyrci et alios cibos quos habuerit in vsu comedendi. Et iam dixerunt sapientes medici: quod non sufficit alicui ad hoc quod fit bonus et verus medicus. Legere in libris quo usque vtatus experimentis et probationibus medicinarum et ciborum et infirmitatum et infirmos visitando" (*Fortalitium*, fol. 191b). For the forbidden and allowed meats, fowl, and fish among the Jews, see *Deuteronomy*, 14:3–19.

to find out whether it is harmful or not. The Jewish physician fails to verify his medicines, and is carried away by his own ignorance (*parva sapientia*).[18]

Maestre Alfonso continues that:

> The second reason [for avoiding Jewish physicians] is that such a physician (the Jew) is either afraid of sinning according to his law or is not afraid. It is clear that he is [not] because the Jewish wisemen said that the best of the physicians will go to Hell. And the reason is that the physicians' intentions are generally to acquire wealth and renown and not to serve God. And this is why they sometimes either prolong the illness or make it worse or precipitate the patient's death. And if such is the nature of healers in general, it is even more so in the case of the Jews, for, by and large, they are not afraid of sinning, as has been said.[19]

Maestre Alfonso's second argument clearly displays his hatred for Judaism by alluding to the common Christian belief in the "Judaica iniquitas." His attitude here follows that of those who, having abandoned the religion of their fathers, show profound contempt for their former co-religionists. He makes use of the grossest falsehoods in portraying the Jewish physician as inimical to Christianity and again attempts to show that Christian morality and customs are superior to talmudic law and ethics. In doing so, he is willing to denigrate the medical profession by presenting a very distorted view of it. His sharp

18 "Medicus autem non potest experire naturam ciborum sibi vetitorum nisi in corpore alieno. Sicut probant et experiuntur venena in alieno corpore parua sapientia sufficit ad discernendum cibos: vel ea que semper sunt nociua: qui sufficit quod sciat de illis solummodo quod sunt nociua. Secundum non sufficit parua sapientia ad vetandum ea que non sunt semper nociua: nec semper vtilia. Et ideo qui caret magna sapientia in similibus adducit infirmum ad periculum vel ad mortem" (*Fortalitium*, fol. 191b-c).

19 "Secunda ratio est: quod talis medicus vel timet facere peccatum secundum legem suam vel non. Et constat quod [non] timet facere peccatum: qui sapientes iudeorum dixerunt quod melior medicorum ibit ad infernum. Et causa huius est, quod intention modicorum (sic) vt plurimum est vt acquirant diuitias: vet (sic) acquirant magnum nomen sibi non vt serviant deo. Et hoc est eis aliquando causa, ad elongandum aliquando infirmitates: vel ad peiorandum eas: vel vt infirmos perimant. Et si talis est natura medicorum magis hoc erit de medicis iudeis cum vt communiter non fit in eis timor peccandi: vt dictum est" (*Fortalitium*, fol. 191c).

attack on Jewish physicians is based on the well-known maxim, "The best of physicians is fit for Gehenna."[20]

According to a generally accepted explanation, medieval commentators to the Mishna censure physicians for two reasons. They are blamed for overconfidence in their craft, which leads them to place their trust in it, instead of in God. They are further blamed for their greed and for the commercialization of the profession to the extent that they sometimes refuse to take care of the poor. The death of an untreated poor person is tantamount to a homicide committed by the physician and both sins are rightly punished with the sufferings of Gehenna. It is not surprising, then, that some Jewish theologians also condemned the medical profession.[21]

The third argument in Maestre Alfonso's disputation is based on the statement that religious differences can lead the Jewish physician to commit contemptible acts against his Christian patients. The very essence of his religion causes the Jewish healer to perform criminal acts as an enemy of the Christians, for his intentions are always prone to evil and predisposed against the pious. Alfonso claims that even in the Talmud, the sages prohibited Jews from receiving medicines made by Christians or other gentiles; Jews were to refrain from having any social contact with the former. Therefore, the farther the Christian keeps from the Jewish practitioner, the more he will be rewarded by God, for he will save not only his soul, but also his body. In doing so,

20 *Mishna Kiddushin*, IV, 14.

21 For a short review of this topic, see H. Friedenwald, *The Jews and Medicine. Essays* (Baltimore: The Johns Hopkins University Press, 1967), vol. I, pp. 11–13. An explanation of this sentence is found in Rabbi Solomon ibn Verga's *Shebet Yehuda* (chap. 41). In a discussion held in Rome in 1418 between Pope Martin V and Samuel Abrabalia and Solomon ha-Levi, ambassadors of the Castilian Jews, Solomon, a physician from Seville, said to the Pope: "*The best physician is fit for Gehenna* signifies that he should always see Gehenna open before him, should he cause the death of anyone whose health has been entrusted to him. As a consequence, he must carefully consider (the treatment) and apply all his thought to it. It is well, therefore, that he should be mindful that he is destined for Gehenna if he does not give sufficient thought to his patients." Solomon ibn Verga's work has been translated into Spanish by Francisco Cantera Burgos with the title *La Vara de Judá* (Granada, 1927).

Alfonso believed that Christians would render a service to both God and to Jesus Christ, his son.[22]

There is nothing surprising in Alfonso's condemnation of the Jewish healers, who were widely esteemed for their skill and competence. Some of them, as has been seen, ranked among the most powerful aristocrats of Castilian Jewry. Since medicine was sanctioned by biblical and talmudic law, its practice was regarded as something sacred. The rabbinate played a crucial role in developing and strengthening this belief among all members of medieval society due to its dedication to this craft. It is therefore obvious that Alfonso, by advocating restrictive measures against Jewish physicians, was attacking the rabbinate on a different front, broadening his campaign against the Jews, and making their religious leaders the special target of his diatribes.[23]

Here Alfonso was following the path previously established by ecclesiastical and secular decrees, which sought to forbid Christians

22 This is the longest of the three reasons (*rationes*) adduced by Alfonso de Valladolid. In this particular section of the *Fortalitium fidei*, it is somewhat difficult to determine where he stops and where Alonso de Espina, the Franciscan friar, starts. The quotation here is intentionally limited: "Tertia ratio est: quod licet medicus iudeus [non] esset timidus in peccando secundum legem suam, expedit multum vt unusquisque se custodiat ab eo; quia lex sua percipit ei occidere xristianos et eorum bona accipere. Defenditur etiam iudeus a reddendo xristiano ea que prodiderit et oblitus fuerit [...] et quare christianus confidet de fide iudeorum cum ipsi non confidant de christianis, quia intentio eorum ad malum prona est et ad suspitiones habendas de bonis [...] et sic dixerunt sapientes eorum in thalmuth: quod non debent recipere medicinam a christianis: nec ab alijs gentilibus nec debent eorum capilli ab illis circinari vel radi: nec habere societatem cum illis in via nec soli cum [eis] in vno loco. Sed si christianus catholicus elongauerit se a iudeo in dando et recipendo specialiter si elongauerit se ab eo in facto medicine recipiet magnam remunerationem a deo: quia in hoc implet magna dei precepta cum custodiat animam et corpus suum [...] si christiani in his se custodierint a iudeis facient in hoc seruitium deo et iesu christo filio eius..." (*Fortalitium*, fol. 191c-d).

23 Alfonso's words in the last chapter of one of his books, *Teacher of Righteousness*: "...until the Jews possess no authority, not even such petty authority as is exercised over them by their rabbis and communal wardens, those coarse creatures who lord it over the people like kings. The rabbis hold out vain promises to their people in order to keep them under their constant control. Only with the elimination of these dignitaries and judges and officers will salvation come to the masses." See Y. Baer, *A History* (cit. n. 7), vol. I, p. 350.

from seeking the assistance of Jewish doctors. The Christian authorities used charges similar to those spelled out by the *maestre* in order to try to instill a sense of fear and distrust in the lower classes.

Thus, a series of restrictive and punitive measures were dictated against the Castilian Jews at the Council of Zamora in 1313. The Council enacted a successful ban against Jewish physicians, prohibiting them from visiting Christian patients. At the Cortes of Valladolid of 1322, some months after Alfonso's conversion to Christianity, the representatives of the cities demanded that all Jews be removed from all offices connected with the royal chancellory and that they be banned from collecting taxes. Some months later, the Council of Valladolid reflected this attitude when it decreed that "the Church of God, in which the divine offices are celebrated and the sacrament of the Eucharist is consecrated, ought to be purged, in order that it not be profaned by contact between infidels and the faithful." In May 1335, the Council of Salamanca tried to enact similar measures. All of these measures failed to eradicate the widely held opinion that the Jewish physician had superior medical knowledge and competence.[24]

24 For the Council of Zamora, see Y. Baer, *Die Juden* (cit. n. 6), vol. II, pp. 118–120. The eighth decree deals with the restrictions affecting Jewish physicians: "El otavo es que non usen de fiseca con los christianos, por letrados nin provados que sean" (p. 120). For the Cortes and Council of Valladolid, see pp. 140–141. Here is the text of the latter: "(declaratio 74): Adversus Judaeorum & Sarracenorum induratam malitiam, qui sub velamine medicinae, chirurgiae & apothecariae, callid insidiantur & nocent populo Christiano, dum eis medicinas propinant, ex quibus nonnunquam pericula mortis incurrunt, sanctorum Patrum Canones salubriter, providere, prohibentes ne Christiani ni infirmitatibus suis vocent, aut ab eis recipiant medicinam" [Josef Saenz de Aguirre, *Collectio maxima conciliorum omnium Hispaniae, et novi orbis*, III (Rome, 1694), p. 567]. The council of Salamanca used the same terms in its declaration number 34 (*Ibid.*, p. 589). During this period, Isidoro of Seville's polemic, *De fide catholica ex veteri et novo testamento contra judaeos ad Florentinam sororem suam* [in I.P. Migne, *Patrologia Latina*, 83, pp. 449–538A (Faustino Arévalo, ed.)], enjoyed enormous popularity among the Spanish clergy. The number of extant manuscripts as well as the numerous quotations drawn from it by anti-Jewish polemicists during the Middle Ages demonstrate the great popularity of this Christian writer's ideas and position toward the Jews. [See, for instance, Bat-Sheva Albert, "The sixty fifth Canon of the Fourth Council of Toledo (633) in Medieval legislation and its interpretation in the 'Converso' Polemics in fifteenth-century Spain," in *Proceedings of the Eighth World Congress of Jewish Studies* (Jerusalem, 1982), pp. 43–48].

The Black Death brought mournful days to the Jewish people. They were victims not only of the plague itself but also of attacks by the European Christian population, who thought that the Jews were the originators of the dreadful pestilence. They were accused of poisoning brooks and wells in Germany and Southern France, where the plague was widespread as early as the beginning of 1348. From there, the Black Death reached Aragon and Castile, along with the massacres of Jews. So far as I have been able to ascertain, in the Andalusian city of Arjona there was one case of pillage and slaughter of the local Jewish population; this does not mean that there were no other cases.[25]

When Pedro I ascended the throne of Castile in April 1350 after his father's death, the Jews had a prosperous future ahead of them. Around this time, though, another would-be renegade from Southern France entered the controversy in Castile.

Moses ben Samuel de Roquemaure was born in the small town in Provence whose name he bore and studied in Avignon, where he lived until approximately 1348. The persecutions suffered by the Jews in this region as a result of the outbreak of the Black Death drove Moses to Toledo at an unknown date. There he may have met Shemariah ben

25 For the poisoning of brooks and wells, see E. Wickersheimer, "Les accusations d'empoisonnement, portées pendant la première moitié du XIVe siècle contre les lépreux et les Juifs; leurs relations avec les épidémies de peste," in *Comptes-rendus du quatrième congrès international d'histoire de la médicine*, eds. Tricot-Royer & Laignel-Lavastine (Antwerp/Anvers, 1927), pp. 76–83; S. Guerchberg, "La controverse sur les prétendus semeurs de la 'Peste Noire' d'après les traités de peste de l'époque," *Revue des Études Juives*, Nouvelle série, 1948, *8*:3–40. For Arjona, see S. Morales Talero, *Anales de la ciudad de Arjona* (Madrid: Ayuntamiento de Arjona, 1965), doc. XVIII, p. 268; J. Rodríguez Molina, *El reino de Jaén en la baja Edad Media. Aspectos demográficos y económicos* (Granada: Universidad de Granada, 1978), p. 139; A. Collantes de Terán, *Historia de Andalucía* (Barcelona: Planeta, 1980), vol. III, p. 78; and C.E. Dufourcq and J. Gautier-Dalché, *Historia económica y social de la España cristiana en la Edad Media* (Barcelona: El Albir, 1983), p. 280. For the effects of the Plague in Aragon, see Y. Baer, *A History* (cit. n. 7), vol. II, pp. 24–34. He remains silent in relation to Castile. The lack of documentation does not justify Heinrich Graetz's statement that "in Castile also the Black Death held its gruesome revelries; but here the population, more intelligent than elsewhere, did not dream of holding the Jews responsible for its ravages" [*History of the Jews* (Philadelphia: The Jewish Publication Society of America, 1891), IV, p. 113].

Elija ben Jacob Ikriti (of Negroponte), a philosopher and biblical commentator who had lived at the court of Robert, King of Naples, until 1328. This Roman rabbi was chiefly known for his efforts to reconcile the Karaites and the Rabbanites in Southern France, where he had taken part in religious disputations with Christian visionaries. Sometime before 1350, King Alfonso XI invited Shemariah to the Castilian court as royal physician and astrologer.[26]

It is not farfetched to assume that after Alfonso XI's death in 1350, Shemariah was trying to reconcile the theological differences between the Castilian Rabbanites and Karaites and to repeat his previous success in Provence. During this time, Moses wrote a poem against Shemariah, who had proclaimed himself a prophet and the Messiah. The ex-royal physician had apparently announced publicly in 1352 that the Day of Deliverance would come six years later. There had been certain messianic speculations about the year 5118 (1358) that Shemariah would most probably have been very aware of. For instance, Moses ben Naḥman (d. ca. 1270), a noted mystic and biblical exegete, mentions this date in his commentary on Genesis 2:3. Since Moses ben Naḥman's commentary on the Pentateuch was widely studied, his discussion of this date was unlikely to have been overlooked by Shemariah.[27]

26 The persecutions inflicted on the Jewish population by the flagellants moved both Clement VI (bull of October 1349) and the King of France, Philip VI (February 1350), to condemn the excesses of these Christian zealots. For the royal decree, see A. Colnat, *Les épidemies et l'histoire* (Paris, 1937), p. 56; for the papal bull, S. Simonsohn, *The Apostolic See*, doc. 375, pp. 399–401. See also Y. Baer, *A History* (cit. n. 7), vol. I, pp. 359–360, and for a bibliography on Shemariah, pp. 447–348 note 43a. According to a report by Rabbi Jacob ben David Provençal, "he stayed in Spain and was highly esteemed by the king, Don Alfonso, as a great astronomer and expert physician. The king rewarded him with many gifts and with fine garments on the day he disputed mystic lore with the scholars of Salamanca" [*Divrei Ḥakhamim*, ed. E. Ashkenazi (Metz, 1849), p. 69]. In Baer's opinion, this report, except for the statement concerning the disputation, seems credible (p. 448). Additional information on this famous rabbi can be found in H. Graetz, *History* (cit. n. 25), vol. IV, pp. 69–70.

27. According to Abraham Bar Ḥiyya, Levi ben Abraham ben Ḥayyim, and Moses ben Naḥman, 1358 was a date with messianic significance. A Christian astrologer, Johannes de Muris, reports that based on astrological considerations the Jews expected the coming of the Messiah between 1345 and 1355. See B. R. Goldstein

Moses' poetic composition, *Shir La'ag* (A poem of scorn) may have been written between 1352 and 1353, when he was staying in Toledo. The copyists of the still extant manuscript where this poem is found state that it is the work of "Moshe Druka — Mi-Bara, in the city of *Toletol*, on Shemariah the Greek, who claimed to be prophet and angel." In its short introduction, Moses himself explains why he decided to write these verses:

> Because that extravagant Shemariah the Greek boasts that he is connected to the separated intellects, he, who, nevertheless, finds himself so far away from any intelligence whatsoever [...] I have written the following few verses, in which I will describe his manners, dreams, and words. I, the most insignificant one in the society (of the studies), whose name is Moses, son of Samuel of Roquemaure, living in Avignon, although, for the moment I reside in *Toletol*.[28]

As I have previously suggested, Moses was in Toledo after fleeing the persecutions which the Provençal Jews were suffering at the time. Toledo was his first Castilian refuge, and by 1353 he was living in Seville, where it has been suggested he converted to Christianity between 1358 and 1360. It is therefore most likely that Shemariah and Moses met either in Avignon or in one of the Castilian cities mentioned above. Shemariah died in prison after certain accusations were leveled against him, including the charge that he regarded himself as the Messiah. Moses gives some information about his adversary's fate:

> ...Our neighbors (i. e., the Christians) will say: truth is / lies, our ancestors inherited / vanity and bequeathed it. / They captured and put him (i.e., Shemariah) in the / jail house and bound his / feet in chains.[29]

It is not clear whether Moses/Juan de Aviñón contributed to the old rabbi's (1275–1355) fate, but only that from 1353 until his death (ca.

& D. Pingree, "Levi ben Gerson's Prognostication for the Conjunction of 1345," *Transactions of the American Philosophical Society*, 1990, *80*, Part 6:1–60, p. 5.

28 A. Neubauer, "Documents inédits," *Revue des Études Juives*, 1885, *10*:79–107, mentions this poem. Neubauer draws all his data from Ms. 166 in the Library of Horace von Zünzburg.

29 *Ibid.*, pp. 90–91.

1382), Moses/Maestre Juan de Aviñón lived in Seville, where he devoted himself to the medical profession. He also translated Bernard of Gordon's *Lilium medicine* into Hebrew and, above all, he wrote one of the most remarkable medical treatises of medieval Spain, the *Sevillana medicina*.[30]

Only this early poetical composition shows a clear connection with the anti-Jewish controversy. Written before his conversion, it is another of the many satirical diatribes which the Jewish intellectuals of the day wrote on each other. Moses may have had in mind Kalonymos ben Kalonymos' famous *Eben Boḥan* (The Touchstone), an ethical treatise written in 1322, where he undertook the task of condemning Shemariah as an arrogant and false scholar. By rebuking him, Moses presented the old rabbi with his messianic fervor as an extravagant zealot. Shemariah's prophecy of the liberation of Israel could only deserve Moses' ridicule and contempt.

Among the many consequences of the disaster of 1391 was that many Jews were killed and many others converted to Christianity to escape death or slavery. Synagogues were transformed into churches and most of the still prosperous Jewish communities were ruined or disappeared. This new wave of conversions continued through the fifteenth century until the final expulsion of 1492.[31]

30 Nicolás Monardes, the first editor of this work (Seville, 1545), explains in his prologue that its author went to the Andalusian capital in 1353, during the reign of Pedro I the Cruel. He served as personal physician to Pedro Gómez Barroso, archbishop of Seville (*Sevillana medicina*, p. 4ra). Maestre Juan's translation of the *Lilium medicine (Peraḥ ha-Refu'ot)* anticipates by several years the one done by Jekuthiel ben Solomon (Bonsenyor Salamon) of Narbonne, who gave it the following title: *Šošan ha-Refu'ah* [See M. Steinschneider, *Die hebräischen Übersetzungen des Mittelalters und die Juden als Dolmetscher* (Berlin, 1893), vol. II, p. 785]. George Sarton states that Moses' conversion, as well as his change of name, took place around 1358. I do not know the sources he used to choose such a precise date [*Introduction to the History of Science* (Baltimore, 1947), vol. III, p. 1378]. Henri Gross follows him [*Gallia Judaica. Dictionnaire géographique de la France... après les sources rabbiniques* (Amsterdam: Philo Press, 1969), pp. 629–630].

31 See Y. Baer, *A History* (cit. n. 7), vol. II, pp. 96–110. The enormity of the massacres of 1391 is described by Hasdai Crescas in his chronicle composed for the Jewish community of Avignon and written on 20 Marḥeshvan 5152 (19 October 1391): "Were I to tell you many adversities that have befallen us, your

The important contributions of some figures to the so-called conversionist movement, such as Vicent Ferrer, Jerónimo de Santa Fe (the ex-rabbi and physician from Alcañiz Joshua Ha-Lorqui), and Pablo de Santa María, has been well established. An ex-rabbi from Burgos, Solomon Ha-Levi, converted to Christianity and became a theologian. Driven by a profound desire to convert his former coreligionists, he decided to champion Christianity by initiating another round of anti-Jewish polemics. This new phase, which developed between 1391 and 1415, was, in Y. Baer's words, "unparalleled for its splendid literary talent, its passionate impetuosity, and the use of every weapon in the armory of scholasticism."[32]

Hidden by the splendid intellectual luminaries who shone during this period, the royal physician to the Castilian kings, Alfonso Chirino, is practically an unknown figure. His deep belief in the superiority of Christianity over Judaism was strengthened by his academic Aristotelianism, where the criterion of truth is human reason, and religion is a political law in accordance with them both. His venomous diatribes against his Jewish colleagues were mainly designed as a vivid illustration of the errors and vices of Judaism which they represented in his eyes. Thus, by showing his hatred against his former brethren, he sought to disguise his own Jewish origins. His main work, *Espejo de medicina (Mirror of medicine)*, depicts in a biased fashion the moral depravation, the sheer jealousy, and the despicable pride of the Jewish physician in general, and of the courtly doctor in particular.[33]

minds would be devastated. [...] On the bitter and impetuous day of the New Moon of Tammuz 5151, the Lord bent the bows of the enemy against the (Jewish) community of Seville, full of people, in which were some six or seven thousand householders. They set its gates afire and killed there many people, but most of them converted and others — from among the children and women — they sold to the Ismaelites. Thus, in the streets of the Jews they sit solitary, many having died in sanctification of the (divine) Name and many having desecrated the holy covenant..." See W. Harvey, *Hasdai Crescas's Critique of the Theory of the Acquired Intellect* (Columbia University, Ph. D. dissertation, 1973), p. 15.

32 Y. Baer, *A History* (cit. n. 7), vol. II, p. 139.

33 I deal with this important Castilian author in my book, *Alfonso Chirino, un médico de monarcas castellanos* (Valladolid: Junta de Castilla-León Press, 1993). There, I address in greater depth the topic of this paper, see pp. 72–81. *The Mirror of medicine* is one of two works first published by A. González Palencia and L.

Although the *Espejo*, written between 1414 and 1418, is a passionate defense of the idea that medical knowledge is a skill rather than a science, its author also denounces his colleagues' morals and professional *modus operandi.* His vitriolic accusations are even applied to the official institutions which allowed the practice of medicine in the realm, the *examinadores* and *alcaldes mayores* on the one side, and the universities (mainly Salamanca) on the other. Chirino was not satisfied with the procedure used by the schools of medicine to grant the *licentia practicandi* to medical students who did not deserve it, as may be seen from these words:

> ...And one has to notice and marvel at how the Schools indiscriminately grant their degrees to all those who study there and consider them sufficiently prepared and fit for the practice of medicine.[34]

This irresponsible behavior on the part of the academic authorities must have been widespread, for Chirino denounces many instances of scandalous intrusiveness which such an attitude must have produced. He singles out one of the main consequences of this practice:

> Many call themselves physicians and doctors (*maestros*) and they are not. They have become used to this name because not only they themselves but also others continuously bestow it upon them. And this produces in their souls such a strong and powerful

Contreras Poza, *Menor daño de la medicina. Espejo de medicina por Alonso Chirino. Con un estudio preliminar acerca del autor* (Madrid: Imp. Cosano, 1945), pp. 359–609. It desperately needs a suitable critical edition. As far as the moral depravity of the Jewish courtiers is concerned, Solomon ben Lahmish, author of *Iggereth Musar* (Epistle on Morality), denounces their social degeneracy in these words: "...these great men of the community who stand before kings in their castles and courts and whom God has caused to be favored by their captors [...] so that the kings exalted and elevated them, appointing them to administer the kingdom and placing the keys to their treasures in their hands [...] And they despised religion and humility and all work and handicraft [...] And each man of them envied his fellow, and spoke ill of him to the king and his deputies..." [See Y. Baer, *History* (cit. n. 7), vol. II, pp. 241–242]. Chirino makes the same accusations in his writings as does the severe Jewish social critic.

34 "E conviene notar e marauillar qu'en los Estudios onde dan grados en el arte de medeçina, cómo fallan dignos e sufiçientes en este dicho examen a todos los que allá aprenden" (*Espejo de medicina*, p. 606).

> illness that they themselves would swear that it is true that they are wise. And they repeat it over and over again everywhere, especially in front of people who do not know them.[35]

Although Chirino's accusations are addressed against the dishonest physician and his quackery in general, his darts are particularly aimed at Jewish healers. They, through their guile and false humility, obtain the favor of powerful magnates:

> ...By means of their malevolent tricks they build their reputation among the ignorant. They sow the seeds of lies and harvest vanity, thus becoming the physicians of powerful noble men and women. Through these notables, some of these physicians are introduced to the kings and queens and the grandees; and once they have their favor, they exert their power to hurt whatever they wish.[36]

In this oblique manner, Chirino slanders the Jewish practitioners, especially those close to the Castilian monarch. The continuous pres-

35 "Que muchos se llaman físicos e maestros non seyéndolo, e tienen tan habituado este nonbre porque muy de continuo se lo llaman ellos e los llaman asy otros muchos. Qu'esto les engendra en el ánima enfermedad tan rezia e entensa qu'esos mesmos jurarían qu'es verdad que son sabios, e porfíanlo en toda plaça, e mayormente çerca de los que non lo pueden conosçer" (*Espejo de medicina*, p. 578).

36 "Con estas maliçiosas artes cresçen fama entre los non sabios, e de vnos en otros sienbran mentira e cojen vanidat, e llegan a ser fisicos de grandes caualleros e dueñas. E ellos allegan a muchos d'estos a los reyes e reynas e a otros grandes señores, e desende tienen actoridat para dañar quanto quieren" (*Espejo de medicina*, pp. 418–419). For a succint and panoramic view of the intellectual background and academic education of the medieval Jewish physician in Western Europe, see C. Roth, "The qualification of Jewish physicians in the Middle Ages," *Speculum*, 1953, *28*:834–843, especially pp. 837–839; see also J. Shatzmiller, "On Becoming a Jewish Doctor in the High Middle Ages," *Sefarad*, 1983, *43*/2:239–250; L. García-Ballester, "Los médicos judíos castellanos del siglo XIV y el galenismo árabe" (cit. n.8); idem, "Dietetic and Pharmacological Therapy: A Dilemma Among Fourteenth-Century Jewish Practitioners in the Montpellier Area," *Clio Medica*, 1991, *22*:23–37; L. García-Ballester, L. Ferre, and E. Feliu, "Jewish Appreciation of Fourteenth-Century Scholastic Medicine," *Osiris*, 1990, *6*:85–117.

ence and influence of cultivated Jewish physicians and advisers in royal circles and their unrestricted interaction with the highest social ranks infuriated the Converso royal physician. His malign attacks are intended for Enrique III's personal physicians, Moses ibn Çarçal and, later on, Meir Alguadex, both of whom enjoyed the king's unconditional confidence.[37]

Alfonso Chirino declares that the wicked and faithless Jews who claim to be physicians try to injure their patients severely and even to bring about their deaths. He adds that such wickedness and faithlessness are much more obvious among the royal practitioners. Chirino does not hesitate to back up his words with the authority of the Holy Bible (*Psalms*, 58:3):

> The malicious doctor can do harm in many different ways; therefore, neither the unfaithful or heretic doctor nor the sorcerer, witch doctor, diviner, liar, greedy, handicapped-from-birth physician should use his profession, especially with kings and grandees. On these the psalmist says: *The wicked are estranged from the womb; they go astray as soon as they be born.* From which it follows: *speaking lies*. Therefore, these are the worst of all men.[38]

37 Moses ibn Çarçal was a gifted poet who wrote in 1405 a poem in Castilian to celebrate the newly born heir of King Enrique ("Este desir fiso Don Mosse, çurgiano (sic) del rey don Enrique [III], quando nasçio el rrey nuestro sseñor en la çibdat de Toro." *Cancionero de Juan Alfonso de Baena*, ed. J.M. Azáceta (Madrid: CSIC, 1966), vol. II, 230, pp. 453–454). Moses was personal doctor to King Juan I and had taken care of the future Enrique III since his early years. Moses' father was Abraham ibn Çarçal, former personal physician to Muhammad V of Granada. In 1359, he took refuge in Castile, becoming personal physician to King Pedro and a royal tax collector. Pero López de Ayala, chancellor and royal chronicler, might have referred to him in his *Rimado de Palacio* ["*Libro de poemas" o "Rimado de palacio"*. Edición crítica, introducción y notas de Michel García (Madrid: Gredos, 1978), v. 254a, p. 154]. Meir Alguadez assisted Enrique until his death in 1406. He was an astronomer, philosopher, and translator, and is a very well-known figure in the history of Spanish Judaism.

38 "En otras muchas maneras puede dañar el malicioso médico, e non debe vsar d'este ofiçio, mayormente con los reyes e grandes señores, médico de poca fe nin herege, nin fechizero encantado[r], nin adevino, nin mucho mintroso, nin mucho cobdiçioso, nin menguado o sobrado de mienbros, nin otro defecto de natura a natividat. Por los quales dize el salmista: *alienati sunt pecatores, a vulua erraverunt*

Alfonso Chirino's writing illustrates once again the hostility which was part of the difficult relationship between Jewish and Converso physicians. This hostility reaches a turning point during the period between 1391 and 1412. It was fostered by the Conversos in the Castilian court and especially by Pablo de Santa María, and was enhanced by the influence and prestige of Vicent Ferrer, who stirred up hatred and fanaticism in his sermons. After Enrique III's death in 1406, the edicts of 1412 and 1415 put Castilian Jewry on the verge of extinction, and represent the culmination of a political campaign designed to complete the ruin of the *aljamas*. The *Espejo de medicina*, written sometime between 1414 and 1418, is a faithful witness of the goal of this policy. Its purpose is obviously to cause the eventual exclusion of Jewish physicians from the practice of medicine in Castile. The nature of the problematic coexistence of Jewish and Converso practitioners in the royal court is not different from that in other echelons of late medieval Castilian society. After all, baptism bestowed on the Converso identification as a full-fledged member of the Christian majority; he therefore received the everlasting right to establish his power over his former co-religionists.[39]

A logical corollary of this historical picture is that the Conversos in power tried hard to remove the courtier Jews from their *milieu*, the private chambers of the kings and magnates. Their behavior was consequently oriented to implement any measures which would rid them of this hated caste. In the medical field, this attitude was reflected in a series of punitive measures which called for the complete annihilation of the Jewish professional healer. The success of such a program relied on at least two factors: the University and the royal "examiners."[40]

ab vtero. De lo qual se sigue: *et locuti sunt falsa*, porque éstos de tal defecto son peores omnes que otros" (*Espejo de medicina*, pp. 534–535).

39 The converted Jew was eligible for any position in the Church or the State for which his abilities or training had prepared him. Up to 1391, conversions, although not uncommon, had been rare, and the Conversos, for the most part, were too humble to play a distinctive role in the Castilian social network. After this date, the Conversos found all doors open to their ambitions. Having embraced Christianity, they played an important social role in Castile. In this sense, Chirino clearly reflects the pragmatic ideology of the new ruling class.

40 On this topic in the medical field, see, for Catalonia and Aragon, the synthetic view given by L. García-Ballester, *Historia social de la medicina en la España de*

This complex undertaking, which started with Alfonso de Valladolid, reached its climax with the writings of Alfonso Chirino. It had to be initiated from the very summit of the Castilian political pyramid, the royal chamber. Obtaining the favor of the monarch was the first step necessary in order to fulfill the Conversos' ambitions. If it was to be successful, the Converso physician must use every weapon at his disposal, including slander. In his criticism of his Jewish colleagues, the Converso physician reflected not only a distorted vision of his former brethren but also an accurate perspective of himself. Both are the result of the deep and strong religious radicalism found in the spirit of the neophyte who had embraced the faith of the powerful and wanted to be one of them.

los siglos XIII al XVI (Madrid: Akal editor, 1976), pp. 59–75; L. García-Ballester, M.R. McVaugh, and A. Rubio-Vela, *Licencing, Learning and Medical Practice in Fourteenth-Century Valencia* (Philadelphia: The American Philosophical Society, 1989); M.R. McVaugh, *Medicine before the Plague. Practitioners and Their Patients in the Crown of Aragon, 1285–1345* (Cambridge: Cambridge University Press, 1993). For Castile, see — cautiously — the article signed by Valentina Gómez Mampaso, "Los alcaldes examinadores mayores. Origen y competencia," *Boletín de la Real Academia de la Historia*, 1983, *180*, cuad. III:551–560. For the intentions of the Castilian Monarchy to control the medical profession, see my *La Escuela de medicina del Estudio salmantino. Epoca medieval (siglos XIII–XV)* (Salamanca: Publicaciones de la Universidad de Salamanca, 1990), pp. 19–23.

Minorities and Medicine in Sixteenth-Century Spain: Judaizers, 'Moriscos' and the Inquisition

Luis Garcia-Ballester

During the fourteenth and fifteenth centuries, the Christian-controlled areas of Spain contained two substantial minority groups: the Jews and those Moslems who had not departed for the lands still held by their co-religionists. The members of both minorities were persecuted by the members of the Christian majority, especially from the late fourteenth century (1391) onwards. Many Jews converted to Christianity as a result of these persecutions.[1] In contrast, Moslems did not often convert during this period. They were, however, forced to adopt Christianity at the beginning of the sixteenth century, and were then called *Moriscos*.[2]

On several occasions I have discussed the study of medicine among the Morisco minority in Spain in the sixteenth century and the first decade of the seventeenth century. I have studied the disintegration of

1 Y. Baer, *A History of the Jews in Christian Spain*, 2 vols. (Philadelphia: The Jewish Publication Society of America, 1978).

2 L. Cardaillac, *Morisques et chrétiens. Un affrontement polémique (1492–1640)* (Paris: Klincksieck, 1977); A. Domínguez Ortíz, B. Vincent, *Historia de los moriscos. Vida y tragedia de una minoría* (Madrid: Revista de Occidente, 1978). With respect to the relationship between the Jewish minority and the Christians, at least in its intellectual aspect, the reality was more complex, see L. García-Ballester, L. Ferre, E. Feliu, "Jewish Appreciation of Fourteenth-Century Scholastic Medicine," *Osiris*, 1990, *6*:85–117; E. Gutwirth, "Actitudes judías hacia los cristianos en la España del siglo XV: Ideario de los traductores del latín," *Actas del II Congreso Internacional 'Encuentro de las Tres Culturas,'* 3–6 Octubre 1983 (Toledo, 1985), pp. 189–196; and L. García-Ballester, "A Marginal Learned Medical World: Jewish, Muslim, and Christian Medical Practitioners Faced with Arabic Medical Sources in Late Medieval Spain," in *Practical Medicine from Salerno to the Black Death*, ed. L. García-Ballester, R. French, J. Arrizabalaga, A. Cunningham (Cambridge: Cambridge University Press, 1994), pp. 353–394.

their medical system and the characteristics of their form of medicine and their medical practice.[3] I have recently undertaken a comparative study of the differing relationships which the Inquisition had with Morisco physicians and with those suspected of being of Jewish descent. The different social circumstances of the two groups led to widely different consequences and also to the use of different methods of action by the Inquisition. In this paper, I shall discuss some of the ideas used in this comparative approach, with special emphasis on the so-called Judaizers. The dictionary defines a Judaizer as "a person who conforms to the spirit, character, principles, or practices of Judaism." I will concentrate on the period between 1560 and 1610, which was the peak period of the Counter-Reformation, and also the period just before the Moriscos were expelled from the lands of the Spanish monarchy between 1609 and 1612.[4]

I

Many of the converted Jews were sincere Christians, while others thought that they could lead a double life and maintain their old religious beliefs. The latter became a new social category, and were called in legal and theological language 'Judaizers' and in popular terms *Marranos*.[5] From the fifteenth century onward, converted Jews were suspected of judaizing, or returning to their original faith. This

3 See my *Los moriscos y la medicina* (Barcelona: Editorial Labor, 1984); idem, "Academicism versus Empiricism in Practical Medicine in Sixteenth-Century Spain with Regard to Morisco Practitioners," in *The Medical Renaissance of the Sixteenth Century*, eds. A. Wear, R.K. French, I.M. Lonie (Cambridge: Cambridge University Press, 1985), pp. 246–270, 338–342.

4 L. García-Ballester, "The Inquisition and Minority Medical Practitioners in Counter-Reformation Spain: Judaizing and Morisco Practitioners, 1560–1610," in *Medicine and the Reformation*, eds. O.P. Grell and A. Cunningham (London: Routledge, 1993), pp. 156–191.

5 C. Roth, *A History of the Marranos* (Philadelphia, 1947; repr. New York: Sepher-Hermon Press, 1974); H. Beinart, *Conversos on Trial. The Inquisition in Ciudad Real* (Jerusalem: The Magnes Press, 1981). This work, although it focuses on fifteenth-century New Castile, is a very good survey of the relationship between the Conversos and the Inquisition.

suspicion was based on forms of ritual behavior related to the Jewish religion (among them cleansing of the hands, washing of meat, rejection of bacon, and death rituals) and also on forms of religious behavior which were suspect from the point of view of what was subsequently defined as Catholic orthodoxy (for example, anti-clericalism, particularly in the case of religious orders; reticence toward the cult of the saints; the role of the Virgin Mary and certain forms of messianic hopes).[6]

In 1478, the new monarchy created by the marriage of the so-called Catholic Monarchs (Isabella, Queen of Castile, and Ferdinand, King of the Crown of Aragon) introduced the Inquisition.[7] The same monarchs signed the decree expelling the Jews from Spain in 1492. The Jews thus disappeared from Spain, although there remained the suspicion of the *Converso* as a possible Judaizer. One of the purposes of the Inquisition was to control the religious life of the *Conversos*.[8] In 1492, many of the Jews left for Portugal, where many methods were used to force them to convert. This point is important since, in addition to the long frontier between the two countries, Portugal was united to the Spanish crown from 1580 to 1640.[9] During this period, there was a flow of Portuguese Conversos to Spain, in addition to ties between Portuguese and Spanish families and mixed marriages. It is thus

6 J. Caro Baroja, *Los judíos en la España moderna y contemporánea*, 3 vols., 2nd ed. (Madrid: Editorial Istmo, 1978), II, pp. 289–510. See Beinart, *Conversos on trial* (cit. n. 5), pp. 237ff. Interesting evidence on these topics may be found in the Archivo Histórico Nacional (hereafter AHN), Inquisition of Toledo, leg. 168, 1, fols. 291v–292v, 334v–336v.

7 A good brief survey is H. Kamen, *The Spanish Inquisition* (London: Weidenfeld & Nicholson, 1965). See also H. Ch. Lea, *A History of the Inquisition of Spain*, 4 vols. (Philadelphia, 1906; repr. New York: AMS Press, 1966). Two recent approaches are A. Alcalá, ed., *The Spanish Inquisition and the Inquisitorial Mind* (New York: Columbia University Press, 1987); and G. Henningsen, J. Tedeschi, eds., *The Inquisition in Early Modern Europe. Studies on Sources and Methods* (DeKalb, Ill.: Northern Illinois University Press, 1986).

8 Lea, *A History of the Inquisition* (cit. n. 7), I, p. 149; see Alcalá, ed., *The Spanish Inquisition* (cit. n. 7).

9 Good surveys are H. Kamen, *Spain 1469–1714. A society in conflict* (London: Weidenfeld & Nicholson, 1983); and J. Casey, "Spain: a failed transition," in *The European crisis of 1590*, ed. P. Clark (London: George Allen and Unwin, 1985), pp. 209–231.

somewhat artificial to separate Portuguese Judaizers (or suspect Conversos) from Spanish ones during the Counter-Reformation period.[10]

For the Jews, conversion was more than a personal or collective religious issue. It also affected their ability to practice medicine. Conversion to the Christian faith, together with a certain economic status and a high regard for learned culture, opened the universities to members of Converso families. As a result, they gained the prestige and social mobility characteristic of university-trained individuals. Their Jewish ancestors had not been able to do the same, as only Christians had access to the faculties of medicine. These families were still under suspicion, however, as all the trials of Converso physicians held in the various Spanish Inquisitorial courts between 1560 and 1610 were on the charge of judaizing. They were never accused, at least not during that half century, of deviant practices rejected by academic medicine, such as the invocation of devils, witchcraft, the use of charms and spells, and similar practices. In addition, almost all the Converso physicians who appeared before the Inquisition had studied at a university (see Table 2).

Throughout the sixteenth century, but especially during its first and last thirds, the so-called "condition of purity of blood" was imposed against the new Christians, especially the Conversos, probably because of the greater social prestige of the posts which they occupied. This measure was designed to prevent anyone who might be 'stained' with Jewish blood from holding any position in society (civil or ecclesiastic). It was contrary to the principle of the social unity of all those who had been baptized. This principle was not accepted by Spanish Catholicism. It became the cause of great social unrest.[11] These measures also spread to the universities, as can be seen in the constitution of the University College of San Ildefonso (1519), which belonged to the prestigious new University of Alcalá:

10 Caro Baroja, *Los judíos en la España moderna* (cit. n. 6), I, pp. 207–226.

11 A. Domínguez Ortíz, *La clase social de los conversos en Castilla en la Edad Moderna* (Madrid: CSIC, 1955), pp. 36–73; a revised edition of the book with the title *Los judeoconversos en España y América* (Madrid: Istmo, 1971) has been published; Caro Baroja, *Los judíos en la España moderna* (cit. n. 6), vol. II, pp. 285ff.

> It is ordained that no-one shall be admitted or elected as a member of the college... without it first being ascertained that he is neither the son of, nor a descendant of, a Jew, or Moor, or Converso..., and if on any occasion, whether by error, or by fraud or negligence, any such person should be elected, he shall be expelled from the College... The information should be drawn up on his parents and four grandparents.[12]

Despite the measures taken to prevent the descendants of the new Christians from entering the faculties of medicine, they found ways to get around these prohibitions.[13] The Converso physician, and the Converso population in general, intermingled with the old Christian population. They did not represent an identifiable social grouping. There remained, however, a certain amount of suspicion about them. The strength of these suspicions varied during the sixteenth century, but they became particularly strong during the Counter-Reformation. At that time, the Inquisition developed an obsession about particular communities or institutions, both civil and ecclesiastic, where accusations of judaizing had accumulated against families or individuals.[14]

Unlike the Converso, who might be poor but who was never a serf, the Morisco was generally a serf. With few exceptions, becoming a new Christian did not make it possible for young Moriscos to enter the medical faculties of the universities. On the other hand, members of reasonably wealthy Converso families, such as the sons of physicians, artisans, or merchants, did gain entrance to the universities. Moslem healers and the whole system of medical care for the Morisco population were more affected by the general disintegration of their cultural life.[15]

The growing tension which the New Christians (both Conversos and

12 *Constitutiones insignis Collegii Sancti Ildefonsi...* (Alcalá, 1716), p. 10.

13 J. T. Lanning, *The Royal Protomedicato. The regulation of the medical profession in the Spanish Empire*, ed. J. J. TePaske (Durham: The University of North Carolina Press, 1985), pp. 175–200.

14 A. A. Sicroff, *Les controverses des statuts de "pureté de sang" en Espagne du XVe au XVIIe siècle* (Paris: Didier, 1960); Domínguez Ortíz, *La clase social de los conversos* (cit. n. 11); and Caro Baroja, *Los judíos en la España moderna* (cit. n. 6).

15 García-Ballester, "Academicism versus Empiricism" (cit. n. 3), p. 246.

Moriscos) experienced from the last third of the sixteenth century onward was the most serious social problem in Spanish society. The expulsion of the Moriscos, just over a hundred years after the expulsion of the other great minority, the Jews who had refused to accept baptism (1492), was the greatest social upheaval in Spain during the Counter-Reformation. The realms of the Spanish crown (Portugal, Castile, Aragon, other European territories and the extensive overseas territories) may have gained in uniformity, but they lost in freedom and openness. During this period, the Spanish monarchy not only made use of every political means available in secular society to control the life of its subjects, but also reinforced its position using the authority of the Church. The ecclesiastical institution which played a pre-eminent role in this process was the Inquisition.[16]

II

The Inquisition played a decisive role in the twofold process of destroying the Islamic culture of the Moriscos and of attempting to assimilate the converted members of both minorities into the orthodox form of Catholic Christianity imposed in Spain by the Counter-Reformation. It delved into even the most intimate parts of the everyday life of the Moriscos and Conversos. The Inquisition made use of every available means, especially anonymous accusations. One of the most negative consequences of these accusations was the introduction of fear and mistrust into human relationships and between social groups.[17] For example, the wife of Enrique Leiton (*fl.* 1588), a graduate in medicine, confessed that her husband was ignorant of her Jewish

16 The Royal decrees were published by P. Boronat, *Los moriscos españoles y su expulsión*, 2 vols. (Valencia, 1901; repr. Granada: Universidad de Granada, 1992), vol. II, pp. 190–285. A good brief survey is Kamen, *The Spanish Inquisition* (cit. n. 7). See also the books by Cardaillac, Domínguez Ortíz and Vincent (cit. n. 2).

17 See R. García Carcel, *Orígenes de la Inquisición española. El Tribunal de Valencia, 1478–1530* (Barcelona: Editorial Península, 1976); and idem, *Herejía y sexo en el siglo XVI. La Inquisición en Valencia, 1530–1609* (Barcelona: Editorial Ariel, 1979). The more recent Alcalá, ed., *The Spanish Inquisition* (cit. n. 7), is also useful.

practices, lest he be put on trial. Despite his wife's efforts, he was arrested and subjected to torture.[18] On other occasions, the wife accused her own husband, as in the case of Luis Castro (*fl.* 1606), doctor of medicine, who was sentenced *in absentia* (he had managed to flee to France), abandoning his wife and family to their fate.[19] Two prolonged sessions of torture, which were noted down in detail with dispassionate detachment by the scribe of the Inquisition, led to the collapse of Felipe de Nájera (1560–*ca.* 1610), bachelor in medicine, "full of fear and bewildered... with his arms and body destroyed," as the Inquisition's own physician recognized.[20] Still, fear did not completely eliminate solidarity. One of the accusations made against the physicians Mateo Nuñez (*fl.* 1595) and Felipe de Nájera was "having received in their houses fugitives from Portugal fleeing the Holy Office."[21] The mere possession of the medical works of Isaac Israeli came to be a cause for suspicion on the part of the Inquisition "because the author was Jewish."[22] It is thus not at all surprising that the Inquisition was perceived by the Moriscos as the very symbol of repression, especially from 1570 onward, and that the Converso accused of being a Judaizer should consider it worse than "the devil himself."[23]

The Inquisition's near obsession with those of Jewish and Moslem descent is immediately apparent from the tables of cases recorded by the court of the Inquisition in Toledo between 1575 and 1610, the period in which the Counter-Reformation was fully implemented in Spain (see Table 1).

There were 364 trials of Judaizers and Moriscos (45% of the total); trials of Moriscos alone made up almost a quarter of the total.

The Inquisition rarely applied the death sentence to Moriscos. The ratio of death sentences to total sentences in the courts of Zaragoza (Aragon), Cuenca (Castile), Granada, and Murcia in the late sixteenth century was in the region of 1 in 40.[24] While no hard data is available for Conversos, it is clear that the Inquisition was much stricter with

18 AHN, leg. 1988, case record 23, fols. 22r–23v.
19 AHN, leg. 2106, 4, fol. 10r-v.
20 AHN, Inquisition of Toledo, leg. 160, 1, fol. 230r, marginal note.
21 AHN, leg. 1988, 49, fol. 16r; leg. 168, 1, fols. 283v–284r.
22 AHN, Inquisition of Toledo, leg. 168, 1, fol. 124r-v.
23 AHN, Inquisition of Toledo, leg. 2106, 9, fol. 41r.
24 García Carcel, *Herejía y sexo en el siglo XVI* (cit. n. 17), pp. 187ff.

TABLE 1
Offences recorded in the sentences of the Court of the Inquisition at Toledo (1575–1610)

Offence	*Number of cases*
Judaizer	174
Morisco	190
Did not consider fornication a crime	264
Blasphemy	46
Witchcraft	18
Heresy	62
Soliciting in confession (priests)	52
Total	806

Source: H. Kamen, *The Spanish Inquisition* (London, 1965).

them and that they were often condemned to death.[25] About one-fifth of the physicians tried for judaizing between 1560–1610 were sentenced to death. However, the Inquisition usually preferred to impose fines, as it needed ever increasing amounts of money to cover the costs of its bureaucracy. To meet this need, the Inquisition and Morisco communities agreed on the amount of special contributions, and Conversos were sentenced to confiscation of their worldly possessions. For example, of 36 Converso physicians or members of their families who were tried, 26 had their property confiscated (seven of them were condemned to death), two were heavily fined and seven were acquitted. The Inquisition's greed was so infamous that one of the physicians on trial, Felipe de Nájera (1609), said to the inquisitors at one stage of the interrogation, after undergoing torture:[26] "if you do this because of my estate, take it."[27] Physicians and healers also lost their right to practice for life as part of the sentences.[28]

All of these measures together reduced those who were tried and their families to poverty. The Moriscos, who were the more numerous

25 Caro Baroja, *Los judíos en la España moderna* (cit. n. 6), II, pp. 209ff.
26 On the use of torture, see F. Tomás y Valiente, *La tortura en España* (Barcelona: Editorial Ariel, 1973).
27 AHN, Inquisition of Toledo, leg. 2106, 9, fol. 46r.
28 AHN, Inquisition of Valencia, leg. 549.

and the better organized social group, were deliberately fined in order to prevent any improvement in their social status. The Archbishop of Valencia, Juan de Ribera (1532–1611), a typical representative of the Spanish church during the Counter-Reformation, made the point very clearly:

> There is also a great advantage to this method [punishing the Moriscos with fines and imposing special taxes on them], for it makes them poor.[29]

The Dominican Friar Bleda, also from Valencia, maintained that:

> These dogs should not be given the best of our [Christian] culture, but they must be expelled from colleges and assigned to low trades or to the galleys, never to [study] the liberal arts [the step prior to the study of medicine].[30]

The Inquisition wished to make the Moriscos disappear as a cultural group by means of judicial persecution. The magical forms used by Morisco healers in their practice of medicine were attacked by the Inquisition. The confrontation between the Inquisition and Morisco healers was a confrontation between academic medicine and the popular forms of medical practice which were steeped in magic and empiricism. The system of medical care which was gradually created among the Moriscos (by their own healers), the physician-patient relationship when a Morisco was one of the parties involved, and the body of medical doctrine used by Morisco healers, which was considered effective by Morisco and non-Morisco patients, were all carefully monitored and consciously undermined by the Inquisition.[31]

Converso physicians were fully integrated into the 'establishment' medical system and practiced an orthodox variety of medicine acceptable to the Christian majority (I leave aside the popular forms of

29 "Ay también en este medio una gran conveniencia que es hacerlos pobres," Archivo del Colegio del Patriarca. Valencia, I, 7, 8, 275. The letter was written *ca.* 1590. See Boronat, *Los moriscos españoles y su expulsión* (cit. n. 16), I, pp. 24ff.

30 "Non igitur est dandus panis filiorum his cannibus, sed abigendi sunt ab illis seminariis et ad sordidas artes, aut ad triremes destinandi, non ad studia literarum," see I. Bleda, *Defensio fidei in causa neophitorum sive morischorum Regni Valentiae* (Valentiae, 1610), p. 374.

31 García-Ballester, "Academicism versus empiricism" (cit. n. 3), pp. 251ff.

medicine, which historians have not yet studied). Thus Converso physicians were tried for being Judaizers, but not for medical practices deviating from what was considered 'normal' neo-Scholastic Galenism, which prospered in the Spanish faculties of medicine of the period.[32] In 1559, Spanish universities and their staff and students were forbidden by royal decree from maintaining intellectual contact with any other university in Europe. Strict control over intellectual publications, from theology to natural philosophy and medicine, had also been introduced by royal decree in 1558; a censor's office was established which had negative repercussions on Spanish intellectual life. These measures were another result of the Counter-Reformation in the Spanish realms.[33]

The Conversos did not have their own form of medicine, nor did they organize a separate system of medical care for their own community. They did not in fact form a separate community. The 36 Converso medical practitioners (physicians and surgeons) who were tried for judaizing between 1560 and 1610 belonged to the medical establishment. Their medical training is shown in Table 2.

TABLE 2

Medical training of practitioners prosecuted by the Inquisition for judaizing (1560–1610)

University training:		
Doctor:	4	
Licenciate:	16	
Bachelor:	7	
Student of medicine:	1	
Total	28	
Physicians (medical training unrecorded):	6	
Without university training:	2	(barber-surgeons)

Sources: AHN, Inquisitorial records. J. Contreras, *Database* (personal information). Additional data provided by the author.

32 For neo-Scholastic medicine in the Spanish faculties of medicine, especially that of Valladolid, in the period under discussion, see J. Riera, *Vida y obra de Luis Mercado* (Salamanca: Universidad de Salamanca, 1968).

33 J. M. López Piñero, *Ciencia y técnica en la sociedad española de los siglos XVI y XVII* (Barcelona: Editorial Labor, 1979), pp. 126–128 and 140–148.

III

Any Morisco or Converso was liable to be prosecuted by the Holy Office simply because of his origin and therefore distrusted all of those around him. The Spanish civil courts intervened under the same circumstances as did civil courts in the rest of contemporary civilized European society, but the Inquisition poked into the most remote corners of society without respecting the norms of the other courts. Although it was not equally strict in all regions, it was omnipresent, and its power and methods left the Moriscos and Conversos perpetually worried and afraid. The Inquisition even prosecuted Moriscos and Judaizers in the Americas and in India after Goa became Portuguese and finally a Spanish crown territory between 1580 and 1640.[34]

Paradoxically, the strictness and efficiency of the Inquisition help further a knowledge of the medical sociology of the Moriscos, Conversos, and Judaizers, providing material on their methods of healing which would otherwise be very difficult, if not impossible, to reconstruct.[35] The zeal of the Inquisition provides evidence for the existence of a not inconsiderable number of general practitioners (most of them university-trained physicians) who were Conversos, many of them Judaizers. They served as town physicians throughout Spain, and were the protagonists of a situation which led many of them into exile. They searched for a place where "they might be well received" and where they could live "with freedom to be Jews," as a Judaizer confessed,[36] or where they could "be able to renounce our Holy Catholic faith and apostatize and live in greater freedom in the sect of Mohammed," according to the words of a Morisco healer.[37] According to the evidence of Conversos (directly from those on trial or indirectly from those who fled), these places were: Italy, and especially Rome (the Popes were more tolerant within their own territories), France (Bordeaux, Paris,

34 Caro Baroja, *Los judíos en la España moderna* (cit. n. 6), II, pp. 175ff.

35 H. Beinart, "The records of the Inquisition. A source of Jewish and Converso history," in *Proceedings of the Israel Academy of Sciences and Humanities*, 1969, *2*: 211–216.

36 AHN, Inquisition of Toledo, leg. 168, 9, fols. 42r and 44r.

37 AHN, Inquisition of Valencia, leg. 552, 9.

Rouen), the Low Countries (Amsterdam), Germany (Hamburg), North Africa (Algeria), Turkey (Constantinople), and the overseas territories (the New World and Goa).[38]

The current state of research is not sufficient to quantify the number of Converso or Morisco physicians who had to go into exile, nor to measure the effects which the emigration might have had on the medical system in sixteenth- and seventeenth-century Spain. I know of only one Morisco healer sought by the Inquisition who went into exile. More Judaizers opted for exile, such as the famous physician and naturalist Garcia d'Orta,[39] whose life story would be repeated by many Conversos. The son of Spanish Jews who had been deported to Portugal and who converted there, he studied medicine in the Castilian Universities of Salamanca and Alcalá between 1515 and 1522–23. In 1534 he left for Goa, where he died quietly in 1568, even though the Inquisition had been established there in 1560. His sisters were prosecuted by the Inquisition in Portugal; one of them (Catalina) was tried for a second time in 1568 and burned at the stake in 1569. This trial raised suspicions about Garcia d'Orta, who was tried *post mortem*. On December 4, 1580, his remains were exhumed and burned. His work as a naturalist (*Coloquios dos simples e drogas da India*, Goa, 1563) was permeated by the memory of his parents' expulsion from Spain in 1492 and by his fear of the Inquisition as a Converso.[40] Two generations later there is the case of Zacuto (born 1575). He was a descendant of the Spanish Jewish astronomer, Abraham Zacuto,[41] who had also been exiled to Portugal in 1492. The younger Zacuto also studied in Salamanca and graduated from the minor University at Sigüenza. After practicing medicine in Lisbon, he returned to Castile in 1625, but his fear later drove him into exile in Amsterdam. There he wrote his *De*

38 These places all appear in the records of the Inquisition between 1560 and 1610. See also Caro Baroja, *Los judíos en la España moderna* (cit. n. 6), I, pp. 227–288, and the references cited therein; Beinart, *Conversos on Trial* (cit. n. 5), p. 209.

39 For a brief biographic survey, see Caro Baroja, *Los judíos en la España moderna* (cit. n. 6), II, pp. 189–193; A. G. Keller, "Garcia d'Orta," in *Dictionary of Scientific Biography* (hereafter *DSB*), ed. C. C. Gillispie (New York: Charles Scribner's Sons, 1980), X, pp. 236–238.

40 It was edited by the Count of Ficcalho in 2 vols. (Lisbon, 1891–95). The passages mentioned here are in *Coloquios*, I, 24.

41 See L. de Alburquerque, in *DSB* (cit. n. 39), XIV, pp. 583–584.

medicorum principum historia (Amsterdam, 1629), which is of great interest, for his medical correspondents indicate the widespread network of Conversos which existed in the various parts of Europe (including Castile) and overseas. They came from the Low Countries, Germany and France, and as far away as Turkey and Goa. Their evidence provides some idea of the importance of this gradual but continual drain of exiled physicians, a flow that increased during the Counter-Reformation.[42] Judaizing physicians clearly thought that this emigration had negative consequences for Spain, according to their testimonies in the records of the Inquisition.

IV

The theological justification for prohibiting the practice of medicine by Morisco and Converso practitioners was based on a puristic Catholic attitude with roots in the years when primitive Christian communities asked themselves whether Christ or the pagan physician who treated them was responsible for the cure.[43] The Spanish also wondered if an old Christian could be treated by a new Christian who was suspected of being a secret Moslem or Jew.

The Moriscos and many Conversos were only officially Christians. They were constantly suspected by the Church and by society of deviating from the true path, and the Inquisition stigmatized them as *heretics*. *Heresy* was a very wide category which, according to the famous declaration of the University of Paris in 1398, included all forms of superstitious practice whose results could not be explained as proceeding reasonably either from God or from nature.[44] The Inquisition used this definition to attack Morisco practitioners.

42 J. Hernández Morejón, *Historia bibliográfica de la medicina española*, 7 vols. (Madrid, 1841–46, repr. New York-London: Johnson Reprint Co., 1967), I, pp. 104–106; M. Lemos, *Zacuto Lusitano. A sua vida e a sua obra* (Oporto, 1909); Caro Baroja, *Los judíos en la España moderna* (cit. n. 6), II, pp. 195–198.

43 P. Laín Entralgo, *Enfermedad y pecado* (Barcelona: Península, 1961); O. Temkin, *Hippocrates in a World of Pagans and Christians* (Baltimore-London: The Johns Hopkins University Press, 1991), pp. 249–256.

44 Lea, *A History of the Inquisition* (cit. n. 7), IV, p. 185.

Explicitly or implicitly, any cure produced by a Morisco physician was considered to be the work of the Devil, and thus the result of a pact between the physician and him. Torreblanca, a Spanish theologian of the end of the sixteenth century, even suggested in his *Epitome delictorum sive de magia*[45] that a pact was present in any cure which made use of recited or murmured words, or even employed the merest touch or a simple piece of clothing with no special properties. A pact was also to be suspected if verbal imprecations were used against the disease; the Church only allowed such imprecations to be used by those in holy orders. Most generally, any cure which the physicians could not explain was suspicious. All the activities of healers and charlatans therefore fell under the jurisdiction of the Inquisition, as endorsed by the Bull of Sixtus V in 1585 (*Caeli et terrae*).[46] The wide and poorly defined areas which the Inquisition investigated meant that any cure carried out by Morisco practitioners was potentially the result of a pact with the Devil if Inquisition experts (physicians in the service of the Holy Office[47]) found it difficult to explain. At the trial of the physician Gaspar Casal,[48] a Morisco physician who practiced in the town of Buñol in western Valencia, an area with a large number of Morisco inhabitants, the prosecutor concluded:

> 1. I accuse him especially of having an express pact with the Devil, with whom he communicates freely... 2...and in accordance with the contents of the preceding chapter, the said Morisco is held to be a physician who carries out extraordinary cures

45 F. Torreblanca, *Epitome delictorum*, 2 vols. (Hispali, 1618), II, p. 9.

46 "Statuimus et mandamus ut tam contra astrologos, mathematicos, et alios quoscumque dictae astrologiae artem, praeterquam circa agriculturam, navigationem et rem medicam in posterum exercentes, aut facientes iudicia et nativitates hominum..., qui supradictas damnatas, vanas, fallaces et perniciosas divinandi artes sive scientias exercent, profitentur et docent aut discunt, quive huiusmodi illicitas divinationes, sortilegia, superstitiones, beneficia, incantationes...," *Bullarum diplomatum...* (Augustae Taurinorum, 1873), vol. 8, p. 650.

47 The collaboration between physicians (including Converso doctors) and the Inquisition has been studied by D. Gracia, "Judaism, medicine, and the inquisitorial mind in sixteenth-century Spain," in *The Spanish Inquisition*, ed. A. Alcalá (cit. n. 7), pp. 375–400. He did not use the records of the Inquisition in his paper.

48 Casal's medical training is described in García-Ballester, "Academicism versus Empiricism" (cit. n. 13), pp. 267–270.

which could not be achieved by human art or by other physicians, and that many people come to him, drawn by his reputation...[49]

An additional cause of problems was the professional competition with Old Christian university-trained practitioners, which involved money and prestige. One of the Morisco physicians (without university training) made the point clearly: "And since the Morisco took both honor and money [by attending to rich patients], he was hated by the [Old Christian] physicians."[50] These reasons supported a feeling which could be called "professional anti-Semitism" against both Converso and Morisco practitioners.[51] Such "professional anti-Semitism" appears at the trial of the judaizing physician Felipe de Nájera. In this case, an Old Christian barber-surgeon felt humiliated by what he saw as arrogance on the part of the university physician in the exercise of his profession.[52]

Reasons of a religious-pastoral nature (those related to the care which the religious authorities, as shepherds of their flocks, were supposed to provide) supported the arguments against Morisco and judaizing physicians. "How could a Morisco or a judaizing physician encourage a patient to confess his sins if he himself did not consider confession a sacrament or receive Holy Communion?"[53] If Old Christian physicians were negligent with regard to the sacraments, it was much more probable that new Christian physicians would be more so. Therefore, "it is convenient for the service of God and for good government that new Christians should be prohibited from curing and using the arts of medicine on Old Christians."[54]

This last reason led the courts of the Inquisition to examine closely the knowledge of Christianity possessed by those physicians accused

49 AHN, Inquisition of Valencia, leg. 175, 1.

50 *Ibid.*, leg. 840.

51 The concept of "professional anti-Semitism" was first used in this way, but only for Converso physicians, by Caro Baroja, *Los judíos en la España moderna* (cit. n. 6), II, pp. 175ff.

52 AHN, Inquisition of Toledo, leg. 168, fol. 229v.

53 "Quomodo igitur monebit aegrotum peccata sua confiteri medicus, si Sacramentum Confessionis contemnit, et nunquam legitime confessus est, nec sacra communione refectus?" Bleda, *Defensio fidei* (cit. n. 30), p. 366.

54 Cortes de Castilla's Proceedings, Madrid, November 13, 1607, vol. 23, pp. 583–587.

of returning to Jewish practices. They were interrogated about their fulfillment of their obligation to confess and to take communion at least once a year (reinforced by the Council of Trent and the Counter-Reformation), about their knowledge of prayers such as the Lord's Prayer and the Creed (the confession of Catholic faith), and external signs of pious behavior were carefully investigated (the cult of the saints; devotion to the Virgin Mary). All of these practices were also encouraged by the Counter-Reformation, which followed the Council of Trent. Any relaxation in carrying out these practices, total or partial ignorance of these prayers, or indifference toward external signs of devotion (not to mention the reaction if these things were rejected) worsened the suspicions that a physician was a Morisco or Judaizer. The evidence from this sort of investigation is particularly abundant. One particular case is that of Felipe de Nájera, accused of judaizing by the Inquisition in Toledo in 1607, two years after having been accused of homosexuality. He was observed by his cellmates, who reported to the Inquisition judges that he did not pray in prison[55] and even made fun of those of his fellow prisoners who did:[56] he also did not know how to recite the Creed in an orderly fashion.[57] He obviously did not fulfill the precept which stated that a sick patient should be induced to make his confession with the diligence required by the Fourth Lateran Council of 1215.[58] The poorly defined frontier between the physician of the soul and the physician of the body was used by the Inquisition, which dusted off this old medieval polemic.[59]

* * * * * *

55 AHN, Inquisition of Toledo, leg. 168, 1, fol. 173r.

56 *Ibid.*, fol. 187r.

57 *Ibid.*, fol. 206r.

58 "Quod infirmi prius provideant anima quam corpori. Cum infirmitas corporalis nonnunquam ex peccato proveniat...," J.D. Mansi, *Sacrorum conciliorum nova amplissima collectio* (Repr. Graz, 1960–62), vol. 22, pp. 1010–1011.

59 L. García-Ballester, M.R. McVaugh, A. Rubio, *Medical licensing and learning in fourteenth-century Valencia* (Philadelphia: The American Philosophical Society, 1989), pp. 42–44 [Transactions of the American Philosophical Society, vol. 79, part 6].

The Spanish monarchy linked its methods of political control to the Counter-Reformation, which was concerned with the preservation of Catholic dogma. This decision created a mixture of political, religious, and legal ideas, a mixture which clouded the life of the whole of Spain.[60] The records of the Inquisition's interrogations demonstrate that members of both minorities were in an increasingly desperate situation; that fear and mistrust permeated all of Spanish society; and that Moriscos and Conversos (whether or not Judaizers) wished to live unmolested and in freedom. Old Christian society in Counter-Reformation Spain was unable to integrate Morisco culture on illness and medicine and to endow them with social and intellectual legitimacy. Sixteenth-century Spanish society was unable to accept religions and cultures other than Catholic Christianity as reinterpreted according to the principles of the Counter-Reformation. It therefore opted for the easiest, but most traumatic, solution to the problem: to make the Moriscos and Judaizers disappear.[61] This solution was an attack on human dignity and covered the Spanish past with shame.

ACKNOWLEDGEMENT

I am indebted to Jaime Contreras, who has allowed me to use his database of inquisitorial records. Funding for this research was provided by CICYT grant no. PB/89–0066, from the Spanish Ministry of Education and Science.

60 Domínguez Ortíz and Vincent, *Historia de los moriscos* (cit. n. 2), pp. 129ff.

61 García-Ballester, *Los moriscos y la medicina* (cit. n. 3), pp. 211–212.

ACADEMIC DISCOURSE AND PAIN IN MEDICAL SCHOLASTICISM (THIRTEENTH–FOURTEENTH CENTURIES)

FERNANDO SALMÓN

Nowadays, the medicalization of the experience of pain in Western societies has reduced pain to the need for quick relief from it.[1] This approach, which does not allow pain to be seen as an experience worth having, whether pleasurable as in some sexual practices or transcendental like a religious experience,[2] also makes it very difficult to understand pain in different cultural or historical contexts.

The period that I will deal with here provides the most bizarre representations of human pain. The medieval iconography of saints' tortures, which depict a sharp contrast between the painful nature of the tortures and the ecstatic faces of the sufferers, can hardly leave us indifferent.[3] However, the celebration of pain was not the only Christian approach to it during the Middle Ages. Pain was handled in different ways depending on the particular aims of different groups and individuals. For example, the relation between pain and knowledge

1 The need to rediscover pain as a general human experience has recently been stressed. See D. Morris, *The culture of pain* (Berkeley: University of California Press, 1991).

2 For a comparison of social attitudes about Sadism / Masochism with other sexual practices, see G. Rubin, "Thinking sex: notes for a radical theory of the politics of sexuality," in *Pleasure and danger: Exploring female sexuality*, ed. C. Vance (London: Pandora, 1989), pp. 267–319. For an analysis of a transcendental idea of pain from a Catholic viewpoint, see P. Laín Entralgo, *Mysterium Doloris. Hacia una teología cristiana de la enfermedad* (Madrid: Publicaciones de la Universidad Internacional "Menéndez Pelayo," 1955).

3 Mystical experiences of pain as portrayed on women's bodies are analyzed in C. W. Bynum, *Fragmentation and Redemption* (New York: Zone Books, 1991), esp. ch. 6 and 7.

was understood very differently by the Franciscans and the Dominicans, two mendicant orders who were widely influential in thirteenth-century intellectual life.[4] Self-inflicted pain and the glorification of suffering were at the center of the mystical way to knowledge of some Franciscan groups.[5] On the contrary, the Dominicans, who stressed learning as the pathway to God, emphasized that pain was a cause of distraction from the study of God.[6]

The centrality of pain in the Christian definition of what was human, notably Adam's gaining the ability to suffer after the Fall and Christ's humanity as defined by his physical suffering, was also accepted by the Schools of Arts of the thirteenth century. Aristotle's *libri naturales* were used to teach the student of the Arts and/or Medicine that pain was at the very core of the definition of man as a living animal.[7] Works from a medical tradition, as the Hippocratic *De natura hominis*, were also used in the thirteenth century to show that pain was a definite human characteristic.[8]

My analysis in this paper will leave aside these theological and natural philosophical considerations to focus on some particular aspects of pain in relation to medicine. In a medical practice based on Hippocratic and Galenic sources, pain was significant as a cause of disease, as a disease itself, and as a prognostic and diagnostic symptom. Well-known medical treatises written in Latin and in vernacular gave

4 On the academic influence of Franciscans and Dominicans and their different religious programs, see R. French and A. Cunningham, *Before Science: The Friars and the Invention of Natural Philosophy* (in preparation). I am grateful to the authors for allowing me to read the typescript.

5 L. J. Bruce-Chwatt, "A Medieval Glorification of Disease and Death," *Medical History*, 1972, *16*:76–77.

6 "Et ideo dolor corporalis magis impedit contemplationem, quae requirit omnimodam quietem, quam dolor interior, si multum intendatur, ita trahit intentionem, ut non possit homo de novo aliquid addiscere." Thomas Aquinas, *Summa Theologiae*, prima secundae, quaest. XXXVII, art. 1. (Turin, 1895–98), vol. ii, p. 215.

7 *Alberti Magni Opera Omnia*, vol. xxxv: *Summa de creaturis*, ed. A. Borgnet (Paris, 1890–98), p. 305.

8 *Corpus Medicorum Graecorum*, vol. II, 3: *Hippocrates De natura hominis*, ed. J. Jouanna (Berlin: Akademie-Verlag, 1975), p. 169. By the late thirteenth century there were two different versions in circulation, an anonymous one from the fifth or sixth century and another from the mid thirteenth century. See P. Kibre, *Hippocrates Latinus* (New York: Fordham University Press, 1985), pp. 192–195.

prominence to diseases where pain was at their core and where remedies were offered to alleviate it.[9] However, I will not go into the more practical aspects of handling pain such as the procedures for alleviating it, nor will I explore the place of patients' voices in the negotiation of pain.[10] Instead, I will focus on academic discussions of pain which took place in various European *Studia* in the late thirteenth and early fourteenth centuries.[11] I will pay particular attention to Arnald of Vilanova (*c.* 1240–1311), who taught at the Montpellier *Studium* and practiced medicine in various western Mediterranean countries, especially the Crown of Aragon.

I contend that by the late thirteenth century, academic discussions of pain in the various European *Studia* were part of a wider program which stressed the Christian nature of the learned medicine which was being developed in those Schools. These discussions included three main aspects to which I will refer below. First, I will analyze the presence of references to the Fall in discussions of the causality of pain. Some medical works did incorporate the Fall in the causality of pain, but generally speaking, the medical discourse developed by the

9 See, for example, the list of pain-related diseases and pain-killers in the *Thesaurus pauperum*. See the edition and the introductory study in *Obras Médicas de Pedro Hispano*, ed. M. H. da Rocha Pereira (Coimbra: Acta Universitatis Conimbrigensis, 1973). See also the various references to pain and its alleviation in the Anglo-Norman collection of receipts edited in T. Hunt, *Popular Medicine in Thirteenth-Century England* (Suffolk: Brewer, 1990).

10 For an analysis of bloodletting as a procedure for alleviating pain, see *Arnaldi de Villanova Opera Medica Omnia*, vol. iv: *Tractatus De consideracionibus operis medicine sive de flebotomia*, ed. L. Demaitre, intr. P. Gil Sotres (Barcelona: Publicacions de la Universitat de Barcelona, 1988), pp. 77–79.

11 Little has been written on the history of pain in medical scholasticism. A brief account can be found in K. D. Keele, *Anatomies of Pain* (Oxford: Blackwell, 1957), esp. ch. 4, pp. 55–59. See also D. de Moulin, "A Historical-Phenomenological Study of Bodily Pain in Western Man," *Bulletin of the History of Medicine*, 1974, *48*:554–560; L. García-Ballester's introduction (discussion on pain on pp. 81–82) to *Arnaldi de Villanova Opera Medica Omnia*, vol. xv: *Commentum supra tractatum Galieni de malicia complexionis diverse*, eds. L. García-Ballester, E. Sánchez Salor (Barcelona: Publicacions de la Universitat de Barcelona, 1985); N. Siraisi, *Taddeo Alderotti and his pupils: Two generations of Italian medical learning* (Princeton, N.J.: Princeton University Press, 1981), pp. 222–226; P.-G. Ottosson, *Scholastic medicine and philosophy* (Naples: Bibliopolis, 1984), pp. 239–246; R. Rey, *History of Pain* (Paris: La Découverte, 1993), pp. 55–61. See also P. Gil in note 10.

university-trained practitioners in the late thirteenth century did not offer a wider analysis of this point. Second, it is interesting to notice that various medical works written by pagan authors which were used in discussing pain had been already prepared for Christian consumption by direct manipulation of the text[12] or by adding a commentary and/or introduction.[13] Galen, who wrote some of these medical works such as *De interioribus*, *De morbo et accidenti* and *De malicia complexionis diverse*, was presented without family lineage or religion and was thus ready to be converted or transformed into an author sympathetic to the Christians. Finally, academic discussions of pain will be analyzed as part of the rhetoric used by the university-trained practitioner in his attempt to establish the supremacy of the university-trained physician (male and Christian) as the ethical practitioner over other practitioners (Christian women, Jews and Moslems).[14]

1. The Fall, unbalanced complexion and solution of continuity

In 1308, Bernard of Gordon (*c.* 1258–*c.* 1320), a devoted Christian and master of the medical school at Montpellier, wrote a treatise on how to preserve human life (*De conservatione vitae humanae*).[15] After reading the preface, however, it is not clear which life the physician should

12 R. K. French, "*De Juvamentis membrorum* and the Reception of Galenic Physiological Anatomy," *Isis*, 1979, *70*:96–109.

13 C. O'Boyle, "Medicine, God, and Aristotle in the Early Universities: Prefatory Prayers in Late Medieval Medical Commentaries," *Bulletin of the History of Medicine*, 1992, *66*:185–209.

14 On the Christianizing role of the founding of the new university at Lérida see L. García-Ballester, M. McVaugh and A. Rubio Vela, *Medical Licensing and Learning in Fourteenth-Century Valencia* (Philadelphia: Transactions of the American Philosophical Society, vol. 79, no. 6, 1989), esp. pp. 41–44.

15 This treatise, which has the general title *Tractatus de conservatione vitae*, has four different parts which often circulated separately: works on bloodletting (*De flebotomia*), urine (*De urinis*), the pulse (*De pulsibus*) and lastly a regimen of health (*Regimen sanitatis*). See L. Demaitre, *Doctor Bernard de Gordon: Professor and Practitioner* (Toronto: Pontifical Institute of Mediaeval Studies, 1980), pp. 59–70; Y. O'Neill, "The History of the Publication of Bernard of Gordon's *Liber de Conservatione Vitae Humanae*," *Sudhoffs Archiv*, 1965, *49*:269–279.

preserve. Bernard wrote that, in order to somehow prolong the life of our insignificant human bodies, he began, with God's help, a regimen of health which will follow the three ages of man from the day of birth to the final hour of death. As a result, after departing, we shall, with God's help, come rejoicing before the tribunal of the Judge.[16] According to Bernard, childhood was characterized by a pursuit of pleasure and old age by reflection as the last step before death. Between the two stages was an age characterized by hard work, affliction and pain. The origin of this state of suffering was the Fall of our first parents as was promised in Genesis.[17] Bernard's *De conservatione vitae* contains little more about pain, just a short reference to the pain suffered by manual workers and a remark about the use of pain as a prognostic tool in old age.[18] However, Bernard's *Lilium medicinae*, written at Montpellier in 1303, contains more about pain. He does not refer here to the Bible or to the opinions of the Church Fathers on pain, but to Galen and Avicenna instead.[19] The entire discussion of pain was placed in the

16 "Ut igitur vitam huius corpusculi aliqualiter possimus praelongare, regimen sanitatis cum Dei auxilio inchoemus, istas tres aetates diligentissime prosequendo a die nativitatis usque ad ultimam horam mortis. Et ita post separationem cum Dei auxilio gaudentes ante tribunal iudicis veniemus". Bernard de Gordon, *Tractatus de conservatione vitae humanae* (Leipzig, 1570), p. 10. The word "vitam" is omitted in the Vatican Ms. Vat. Pal. 1174, fol. 54rb. This omission led Demaitre to misinterpret Bernard's intention. Demaitre, *Doctor Bernard de Gordon* (cit. n. 15), p. 63. The Cambridge ms. Gonville and Caius 373 (593) contains the word "vitam" (fol. 31rb), as does the Leipzig edition.

17 "Et hoc totum intelligitur auctoritate preallegata, cum dicitur nasci, et per hoc intelligitur prima etas, que durat circiter annos xiii. Et sequitur, cum dicitur per Augustinum, laborare, ubi intellexit secundam etatem, que est Adolescentia et Iuventutis. Ista enim est etas laboris, et doloris, et angustie, quoniam homines mundi huius, aut laborant in speculando, aut in operando. Si in speculando, ibi est labor et afflictio, secundum quod dicit sapiens, qui addit scientiam, addit et laborem. Si autem laboret in operabilibus, semper erit afflictio, quoniam universaliter nutrimento cum labore acquiruntur... Et hoc fuit promissum primo parenti post suam prevaricationem sicut scribitur Genesis: in sudore vultus tui vesceris pane tuo, donec revertaris in cinerem unde venisti." Bernard de Gordon, *Tractatus de conservatione* (cit. n. 16), pp. 8–9.

18 Ch. 16: "De dispositione corporis laboriosi, et de cura eius" (pp. 80–87) and Ch. 26: "De prognosticatione morbi futuri per ea quae sunt extra naturam" ("De dolore," p. 136). Bernard de Gordon, *Tractatus de conservatione* (cit. n. 16).

19 Pain is discussed by Bernard mainly in ch. 18 ("De dolore") of part I and ch. 1 ("De dolore capitis") of part II. The main authorities mentioned are Galen (*De*

general context that the best road to God was the study of the truth, which Bernard ascribed to a pious Galen, God's servant and the prince of physicians.[20]

Although not very common, references to the Fall as the prime cause of human suffering can also be found in the works of other medical authors, such as the *Tractatus contra calculum*, attributed to Arnald of Vilanova. This treatise, composed in 1301, was dedicated to Pope Boniface VIII, who suffered acute pain from bladder stones. The work opens with a reference to medicine as God's gift and to suffering as man's Fall, but there is no additional commentary on the Fall as a cause of pain.[21]

I have been unable to find any contemporary medical treatise which presents an extensive analysis of the Fall as the first cause of human suffering. The university medical discussions of the cause of pain which took place in various European *Studia* at the end of the thirteenth century focused instead on the immediate cause of pain: unbalanced complexion or solution of continuity. Numerous authors of medical works describe this set of causes in their commentaries, ignoring the biblical curse. One example of this approach is Dino del Garbo (*d.* 1327). Dino was a prolific medical author who practiced and taught medicine at various Northern Italian schools — Bologna, Siena and Padua — in the first third of the fourteenth century. One of his works is probably the only extant Latin commentary on *De natura fetus*, a work attributed to Hippocrates.[22] In this commentary, which may be the result of his academic duties, Dino asked if childbirth must be

morbo et accidenti, *De ingenio sanitatis*, commentary on Hippocrates' *Aphorismi* and *Regimine acutorum*) and Avicenna (*Canon* and *Sextus de naturalibus*). See Bernard de Gordon, *Lilium Medicinae* (Lyon, 1550), fols. 61–65 and fols. 162–181.

20 "quoniam secundum Galienum VII de ingenio nullus potest Deo melius approximare quam studendo in veritate et pro veritate." Bernard de Gordon, *Lilium Medicinae* (cit. n. 19), prohemio, fol. 4. See also Demaitre, *Doctor Bernard de Gordon* (cit. n. 15), pp. 113–115.

21 "Reor quod medicina est scientia quam divina statuit providentia fore auxiliatricem hominique contra incommoda necessitatem quam genus humanum ob praevaricationem primi parentis incurrerit delictuose." Arnau de Vilanova, *Tractatus contra calculum* (Basilea, 1585), fol. 1565.

22 On Dino's career and other activities, see Siraisi, *Taddeo Alderotti* (cit. n. 11), pp. 55–64.

accompanied by pain. This topic presented an opportunity to use the curse in order to defend the affirmative part of the *questio*. However, the Fall does not appear in Dino's analysis, and, even more, he clearly states that childbirth *per se* was not painful. However, his account of women's experiences confirmed that pain occurred in childbirth and its existence was justified in medical technical language by the solution of continuity and the strong movement caused by the expulsive virtue present in childbirth.[23]

2. Pain and a Galen of unknown origin

The absence of references to the Fall or to any religious authority in the arguments and counterarguments employed by Dino in the *questio* about childbirth may be seen as evidence for the lack of a religious bias in academic medical discourse. However, references to the Bible or to the Church Fathers are not the only way to understand the Christian nature of academic discussions about pain, but the analysis of the elements on which academic medical discourse on pain was built provide additional information.

Galen's *Tegni* with Haly Ridwan's commentary, Haly Abbas' *Pantegni*, and Avicenna's Canon were used in framing theoretical discussions about pain. However, if the elements which were part of medical discussions about pain in the mid thirteenth century are compared with those of the late thirteenth century, one of the main differences is the extensive use in the latter of at least two of Galen's works, *De morbo et accidenti*[24] and *De interioribus*.[25] This fact is highlighted

23 "Dico quod verum est quantum est de se, quia in partu non accideret dolor ut partus est quid naturale; sed quia non potest fieri apte sine disiunctione iuncturarum, ideo concurrit dolor per accidens. Item concurrit ibi dolor quia partus fit cum vehementi motu expulsive virtutis, modo vehemens motus expulsive est causa egritudinis, et per consequens accidentis huius quod est dolor que consequitur egritudinem." Dino del Garbo, *Supra librum Ypocratis de natura fetus* (Venice, 1502), fol. 58va.

24 The medical community of the late thirteenth century found in *De morbo et accidenti* an aggregation of Alexandrian origin of Galen's works on disease, its causes and its symptoms. The work was divided into six parts. The first three correspond respectively to Galen's *De morborum differentiis*, *De causis morbo-*

when the approaches to pain of two medical masters are compared: Peter of Spain (*c.* 1205–1277), who wrote in the mid thirteenth century, and Taddeo Alderotti (1223–*c.* 1295), from the late thirteenth century.

Peter of Spain wrote about pain when he commented on the whole of the *Articella* collection, probably as part of his teaching activities, in the *Studium* of Siena between 1245 and the 1250s.[26] He developed at least four questions on pleasure and pain in his commentary on Galen's *De crisi et de diebus creticis*. Although Peter stated very early on the importance of pain as a sign which allowed the physician to localize the internal organs and their disorders, he was more concerned with fitting pain into Aristotelian patterns of perception. Thus, Peter first asked if pain was an object of the senses and if so, of which senses. Second, he compared pleasure and pain and tried to explain which came first. The third question dealt with the causes of pain, which return to the problem of the perception of pain. The last question defined pleasure. The whole discussion was presented in a transformed Aristotelian framework. This perceptual scheme, by the late thirteenth century, had been expanded with important anatomical and physiological details of Galenic and Neoplatonic origin. The works used by Peter of Spain in discussing pain were Aristotle's *De anima*, Avicenna's *Sextus de naturalibus* and *Canon*, Constantine's *Pantegni* and Galen's *Tegni* and *De simplicium medicine*.[27]

rum and *De symptomatum causis*; the last three books of *De morbo et accidenti* were the Latin version of Galen's *De symptomatum differentiis*. See *C. Galeni Opera Omnia*, ed. C. G. Kühn (Leipzig, 1821, rept. Hildesheim: Georg Olms, 1964), vol. VI, pp. 386–880; vol. VII, pp. 1–41, pp. 42–84 and pp. 85–272.

25 *De interioribus* was the title given to the medieval Latin translation of Galen's *De locis affectis*, see *C. Galeni Opera Omnia* (cit. n. 24), vol. VIII, pp. 1–452. By the end of the thirteenth century, two different versions were in circulation: an anonymous Arabo-Latin translation and a Latin version translated directly from the Greek by Burgundio of Pisa (1110–1193). See R. Durling, "Corrigenda et addenda to Diel's Galenica," *Traditio*, 1981, *37*:376–377.

26 MS 1877 of the Madrid National Library contains Peter of Spain's most important medical commentaries. He commented on the following works: Iohannicius' *Isagoge*, Galen's *Tegni* and *De crist et diebus creticis*, the Hippocratic *Prognostica*, *Aphorismi* and *Regimen acutorum morborum*, Isaac's *De dietis universalibus*, *De dietis particularibus* and *De urinis*, Constantine's *Viaticum* and Philaretus' *De pulsibus*. For an up-to-date biography of Peter, see D. Jacquart, *Supplément au Dictionnaire biographique des médicines en France au moyen age* (Genève: Droz, 1979), pp. 232–236.

Thirty years later the panorama changed. In the 1280s, Taddeo Alderotti, medical master at Bologna, was dealing with various problems related to the definition and perception of pain.[28] However, the questions which he asked were derived from the clinical examples contained in Hippocrates' *Aphorismi.* For example, one question was why mentally ill people did not always perceive pain;[29] another was whether a large pain could conceal a smaller one.[30] The two questions deal with subjects such as how pain was perceived, if pain was an object of the senses and if it was possible to differentiate between the cause of pain and pain itself. If Taddeo's approach is compared with that of Peter of Spain, one of the features that differentiates between the two men is Taddeo's references to Galen's *De interioribus* and *De morbo et accidenti.* Neither of Galen's works was used by Peter. Taddeo was conscious of the novelty of his approach, and explained in his discussion of the first question that, given the novelty of his approach, his solution was a tentative one, and he would have no qualms about changing it.[31] It has been argued that the novelty to which Taddeo referred was that physicians undertook a philosophical inquiry into the nature of pain.[32] I suggest instead that what was novel in Taddeo's eyes was the use of the "new Galen" to reinterpret the old topics contained in the Articella collection.

By 1300, medicine was a well established branch of several European *Studia.* It had a well defined technical literature and shared with the

27 Petrus Hispanus, *Questiones super libro de crisi et super libro de diebus creticis*, Madrid, Bibl. Nac. 1877, fols. 248r–255r. "Hic queritur quatuor de dolore. Primo utrum dolor sit obiectum sensus et cuius sensus. Secundo de comparacione dolorem ad suum contrarium quod est delectacio quid istorum primitus sit. Tercio de causis dolorum. Quarto quid sit dolor (sic)," fol. 249ra.

28 Siraisi, *Taddeo Alderotti* (cit. n. 11), pp. 223–226.

29 Taddeo Alderotti, *Expositiones in arduum aphorismorum Ipocratis volumen, In divinum pronosticorum Ipocratis librum, In preclarum regiminis acutorum Ipocratis opus, In subtilissimum Ioannitii Isagogarum libellum* (Venice, 1527), fols. 30vb–31ra.

30 *Ibid.*, fols. 66vb–67ra.

31 "Hic tamen attende quod est in ista solutione propter novitatem questionis ego multum dubito et propter hoc si quando sentencia verior occurrerit, eam sine pudore mutarem." *Ibid.*, fol. 31ra.

32 Siraisi, *Taddeo Alderotti* (cit. n. 11), p. 223; Ottosson, *Scholastic medicine* (cit. n. 11), p. 239.

Arts a grounding in Aristotelian logic and natural philosophy. By then, the medical masters had already adopted a number of works by Galen in Latin translation, the "new Galen," to enlarge the set of works which had previously defined medical education. Among these works were Galen's main treatises on pathology, *De interioribus*, *De morbo et accidenti* and the brief *De malicia complexionis diverse*.[33] Pain was an important topic in these treatises. In *De malicia complexionis diverse* (chapters 3, 4 and 10) and in *De interioribus* (book II), pain was given prominence as a diagnostic symptom which would help in the understanding of internal problems; in *De morbo* (book IV), a wider theoretical framework was applied to the analysis of the perception of pain. These treatises were popular among the medical elite of the *Studia*, and at least seven commentaries on *De morbo et accidenti* were written between the last decade of the thirteenth century and the first third of the fourteenth century.[34] By 1309, the new academic ordinances at Montpellier made *De morbo et accidenti* and *De malicia complexionis* required texts.[35] *De malicia complexionis* was used in both Montpellier and Bologna as an introduction to Galen's major work on therapeutics (*De ingenio sanitatis*), thus emphasizing the role of the "new Galen" in daily medical practice.[36] *De interioribus*, although not part of the new curriculum in Montpellier, was used extensively by the medical masters of the late thirteenth century. Several of these masters offered their own versions of the work and some rearranged the texts circulated in the different *Studia*. Johannes of Saint-Amand, the Parisian master, provided a summary of the work in his *Revocativum memorie*.[37] Taddeo Alderotti's version resulted

33 L. García-Ballester, "Arnau de Vilanova (*c.* 1240–1311) y la reforma de los estudios médicos en Montpellier (1309): El Hipócrates latino y la introducción del nuevo Galeno," *Dynamis*, 1982, *2*:97–156.

34 Two of the commentaries were written by masters of the Montpellier *Studium*: Arnald of Vilanova (*c.* 1240–1311) and Bernard of Gordon (*c.* 1258–*c.* 1320); three in Bologna: Bartholomew of Varignana (*c.* 1260–*c.* 1321), Albert of Bologna (*c.* 1280–*p.* 1348) and Anthony of Parma (*f.* 1315); and the others were anonymous.

35 *Cartulaire de l'Université de Montpellier* (Montpellier, 1890), vol. I, p. 220.

36 *Arnaldi ... Commentum supra tractatum Galieni de malicia complexionis diverse* (cit. n. 11), pp. 73–74.

37 *Johannes de Santo Amando Abbreviationes librorum Galieni*, ed. O. Paderstein (Berlin, 1892), pp. 28–45.

from his comparison of two different Latin translations while teaching at the medical school in Bologna.[38] Finally, Arnald of Vilanova re-worked the two first books of the Arabo-Latin version, and also complained about the poor quality of the copies available at Montpellier.[39]

It is not yet clear why this new Galen shaped the activities of the medical elite of the late thirteenth century. The works were extremely complex, repetitive and offered no immediate improvement in clinical practice. Furthermore, academic physicians already had a well-defined technical *corpus* of medical literature. Why, then, were the medical masters William of Brescia, John of Alestio and Arnald of Vilanova so keen to convince Pope Clement V to furnish Montpellier's curriculum with these works of Galen?[40] I think that we are far from a satisfactory answer, but I would like to outline a hypothesis that involves both a consideration of the university physicians' claim as to the practical benefit inherent in the reading of Galen's new works and a reflection on the benefit of building an exclusive curriculum for Christians, alongside an author — Galen — of unknown origin.

Medieval praise of Galen, who emerges from the pages of the commentaries as the most clear or the most holy, is known by historians, although this praise has not yet been systematically studied. However, historians have not paid much attention to the Galen who emerges from the *accesus* which medical commentators used when introducing a medical work to their public. One of the questions which the master answered in the *accesus* was about the *causa efficiens* of the treatise, that is, about its author. In most commentaries on Galen's works, the answer to the *causa efficiens* was that Galen was the author and no additional commentary was provided. Even so, some medical

38 Siraisi, *Taddeo Alderotti* (cit. n. 11), pp. 101–102.

39 On the authorship of this treatise, see M. McVaugh, "The authorship of the Galenic compendium *De interioribus 'Quoniam diversitas ...'*," *Dynamis*, 1981, *1*:225–229. A modern critical edition of this treatise is available in *Arnaldi de Villanova Opera Medica Omnia*, vol. xv: *Doctrina Galieni de interioribus*, ed. R. Durling (Barcelona: Publicacions de la Universitat de Barcelona, 1985), pp. 305–351.

40 "de consilio et ad instanciam dilectorum filiorum magistrorum Guillermi de Brixia et Johannis de Alesto, phisicorum et capellanorum nostrorum, necnon et magistri Arnaldi de Villanova, phisici." *Cartulaire* (cit. n. 35), p. 220.

commentators of the late thirteenth and early fourteenth centuries provided additional information. In the Krakow manuscript, for example, which contains a commentary on *De morbo et accidenti* attributed to Arnald of Vilanova, the author pointed out his ignorance of Galen's life (*Galienus quis autem fuerit ignoramus*), but also stated that the works of the ancients confirm that Galen was the son of a rich family and very learned.[41] The same ignorance was expressed in the Vatican manuscript which contains a commentary on the same work attributed to Albert of Bologna. Albert stated that it was known only that Galen was a man of great activity and learning and that he was the son of a rich family.[42] If these authors had a genuine interest in Galen's life, why did they not reconstruct it from the autobiographical accounts present in several of the works which were already available to the medical community in Latin? I would like to suggest that they were not interested in clarifying Galen's biography, but rather in pointing out that Galen had no known past. This unknown Galen could then be linked to the Christian tradition. Thus, Mondino de' Liuzzi, a contemporary medical author who taught and practiced in Bologna, created a passage of Galen's life which had a definite Christian flavor. Mondino described Galen as a contemporary of Christ, who went to meet him after hearing of Christ's miraculous healings.[43] The study of the works of a man who was not only the ancients' prince of physicians, but who also had some sort of acquaintance with the miraculous healings of Jesus Christ, was no doubt a necessary step for any aspiring physician.

41 "Tercium est que sit causa efficiens huius libri, quia Galienus quis autem fuerit ignoramus, verum tamen certa penitus auctoritate antiquorum exprimitir, ipsum divitum parentum filium excesisse et eruditum fore erudicione mirabili." Arnau de Vilanova, *Commentum supra tractatum Galieni De morbo et accidenti*, Krakow, Bibliot. Jagiell. 781, fol. 131r.

42 "Primo que sit causa efficiens huius libri. Quia Galienus de quo scitur tantum quod fuit homo magne industrie et maxime sciencie, fuit eciam filius divitum parentum ut de eo narratur." Alberto da Bologna, *Commentum supra tractatum Galieni De morbo et accidenti*, Vatican, Reg. Lat. 2000, fol. 28ra.

43 "et dicitur quod ipse (Galenus) fuit coetaneus Christo; et dicitur in cronicis quod ipse audiens miracula que faciebat Christus de sanatione infirmorum venit ad ipsum." Mondino de' Liuzzi, *Comm. Tegni*, Vatican, Vat. Lat. 4466, fol. 57r. *Cf.* Siraisi, *Taddeo Alderotti* (cit. n. 11), p. 190 n. 117.

3. The discourse of practical interest

The analysis of the perception and nature of pain was contained in various commentaries on Galen's *De morbo et accidenti* and *De interioribus*. Questions such as: if pain was a kind of alteration of the sensitive action; if only the object of the sense of touch could produce pain; if it was possible that the sensitive species of an object could cause a material effect; inquiries into the painful or delightful effects of the objects of the senses were present in the medical commentaries on these works.[44] At the same time, other, more clinically oriented questions were also raised by the medical communities of Bologna and Montpellier by the end of the thirteenth century. In a medical model based on Hippocratic-Galenic principles, pain, together with inflammation and alterations of function and of bodily excretions were the signs through which internal afflictions could be known.[45] Thus, Bartholomew of Varignana, when commenting on *De interioribus* (book II), was concerned with classifying different kinds of pain — *congelativus, pulsativus, gravativus, extensivus, frangitivus, pungitivus, compressivus* — as aids in the diagnosis of internal diseases.[46] The same insistence on the practical value of discussions about pain can be found in Montpellier in the works of Arnald of Vilanova. For example, he insisted in his *Speculum medicine* that the patient's account of pain was relevant in making a good diagnosis.[47] The same practical aim

44 See, for example, some of the questions raised by Bartholomew of Varignana in his commentary on *De morbo et accidenti*: "Utrum dolor sit aliqua species accionis sensitive lexe," fol. 77ra; "Utrum dolor sit passio partis in qua est causa doloris" fol. 77ra; "Utrum humiditas et siccitas per se sint causa doloris," fol. 77ra; "Utrum in omni sensu preter quam in sensu tactus — quia de hoc non est dubium — contingat dolor et eius contrarium scilicet delicia," fol. 77rb. Bartolomeo da Varignana, *Commentum supra tractatum Galieni De morbo et accidenti*, Vatican, Vat. Lat. 4452, fols. 67r–82v.

45 On the relevance of pain in Galen's medical practice, see R. Moreno and L. García-Ballester, "El dolor en la teoría y práctica médicas de Galeno," *Dynamis*, 1982, *2*:17–24.

46 Galen, *De interioribus* in *Opera Omnia* (Venice, 1490), fols. 102r–106r; Bartolomeo da Varignana, *Comm. De interioribus*, Vatican, Vat. Lat. 4454, fols. 89v–91v. On Bartholomew's views see Siraisi, *Taddeo Alderotti* (cit. n. 11), p. 223.

47 "Propterea dicitur, quod genera signorum demonstrantium aegritudines interiorum membrorum sunt quatuor. Unum sumptum a doloribus, nam cum dolor

may be seen in Arnald's analysis in his commentary on Galen's *De morbo et accidenti*, written a few years earlier. Following Galen's statements, Arnald treated pleasure and pain in their relation to the five senses and their objects. His discussion did not follow the natural philosophical analysis of sense perception and the nature of the various sense objects, and did not even make use of Aristotelian technical language. Instead, Arnald provided an analysis which would have clinical significance. For example, he discussed the painful effect of moving from a dark place to a very bright one and the pleasant effect which grey or green could have on sight.[48] Arnald's interest in speculation only where it would have had clinical benefit was repeated in his commentary on *De malicia complexionis diverse* in the 1290s.[49] In this commentary, Arnald devoted a long discussion to the causality of pain: unbalanced complexion and/or solution of continuity.[50] He became involved in very subtle disquisitions about how humidity, dryness, heat and cold could cause pain. He referred his readers to the fourth book of Galen's *De morbo et accidenti* where, according to Arnald, Galen explained "very subtly and profoundly" the causality of pain.[51] However, Arnald strongly emphasized that his theoretical disquisitions were only worthwhile if they would produce a change in therapeutical decisions.[52]

percipiatur ab aegro et omnis dolor causetur immediate vel a malitia complexionis vel a solutione continuitatis, vel ab utroque constat quod ubi patiens apprehendat circumstantias doloris, aut differentias, poterit aliqualiter iudicari per eius confessionem genus et species aegritudinis." Arnau de Vilanova, *Speculum introductionum medicinalis* (Basel, 1585), fol. 230.

48 On the painful and pleasurable effects of some colors on sight, see F. Salmón, "La couleur dans les théories visuelles des cercles médicaux universitaires de la fin du XIIIe siècle," in *Maladies, Médecines et Sociétés*, ed. F. Touati, 2 vols. (Paris: L'Harmattan et Histoire au Présent, 1993), vol. I, pp. 159–169.

49 *Arnaldi ... Commentum supra tractatum Galieni de malicia complexionis diverse* (cit. n. 11), pp. 81–82.

50 *Ibid.*, pp. 182–195.

51 "ex verbis Galieni quarto de morbo et accidenti, ubi subtilissime et multum profunde loqutus est Galienus de causis doloris et deliciarum." *Ibid.*, p. 192.

52 "Hoc enim accidens tantum considerat Medicus in proposita materia, quoniam est principium variandi et regulandi opus curacionis, aliud vero non. Si enim humor calidus causat dolorem acutum et scit medicus quia racione caliditatis causat illum dolorem per se, ad regulandum opus curacionis non eget considerare

Arnald's anti-intellectualism or anti-Aristotelianism has already been the subject of comment, and has been linked with his sympathy with Franciscan views of intellectual life.[53] His own assertions provide support for this conclusion. However, Arnald was not the author of a handbook like the *Thesaurus pauperum* or other medical *compendia*, but rather wrote highly technical works and commented on several of Galen's more complex treatises, such as *De malicia complexionis* and *De morbo et accidenti*. At the same time, Arnald constantly emphasized that the main theme of his medical epistemology was the achievement of a better practice. He wanted to be seen as putting this aim forward by his audience: colleagues, students and illustrious patients. More generally, I would suggest that he wanted to advertise the new medicine which he was so successfully establishing at Montpellier in the same way.[54] In this sense, it is very interesting to see how Arnald manipulated certain paragraphs of Galen's *De interioribus* in his reworking of this treatise, in order to strengthen his own insistence on the uselessness of medical theory for its own sake.[55]

This was not an exclusively Arnaldian attitude. Other contemporaries used some of Galen's works on pathology to discuss pain in the same light. For example, the medical masters expounded Galen's *De morbo et accidenti* as the book which presented a general understanding of disease, its causes and its symptoms (*res praeter naturam*). Far from pursuing knowledge for its own sake, various commentators such as Bartholomew of Varignana and Albert of Bologna advised their readers that their aim in building this theoretical framework on

quia humiditas, que inest illi humori, est causa per accidens, quamquam hoc verum sit. Similiter posset dici de colore humors et sapore et odore et ceteris eciam qualitatibus eius, quia verum est quod sunt causa illius doloris per accidens; tamen non est medicinalis ista consideracio, quia inutilis est ad opus; non enim per hoc regulabitur in aliquo actus curacionis. Immo, si penitus ignoraretur hoc, non minus compleretur bene canon." *Ibid.*, pp. 193–194.

53 Ch. Crisciani, "Exemplum Christi e sapere, sull' epistemologia di Arnaldo de Villanova," *Archives Internationales d'Histoire des Sciences*, 1978, *28*:255–259.

54 García-Ballester has analyzed in great detail Arnald's role in the incorporation of this "new Galen" at Montpellier. See García-Ballester, "Arnau de Vilanova" (cit. n. 33), pp. 119–127.

55 On this point, see M. McVaugh, "The Nature and Limits of Medical Certitude at Early Fourteenth-Century Montpellier," *Osiris*, 1990, *6*:73–74.

the "contra naturals" was the attainment of a better practice.[56] Bartholomew justified the reading of Galen's *De interioribus* because of its *utilitas*.[57] Jean de Saint-Amand, when presenting his abbreviation of *De interioribus* to the Parisian academic medical community in the 1280s, had the same practical orientation. He saw this work as the tool from which the physician learned about those afflictions which were hidden from sensual knowledge.[58]

Arnald also insisted on the utility of the first two books of Galen's *De interioribus*. More significantly, he indicated to his students his distrust in the medical expertise of those physicians who were not familiar with them.[59]

Therefore, by the late thirteenth century there was a growing attempt by the medical masters at various European *Studia* to link the medicine taught and learned at the university with the best possible medicine.

56 "Res preter naturam in communi est hic subiectum... Causa finalis est duplex: scilicet propinqua et inmediata, et illa est cognicio perfecta rerum preter naturam scilicet morbi cause et accidentis; sed causa finalis remota et mediata est finis tocius medicine." Alberto da Bologna, *Comm. De morbo et accidenti* (cit. n. 42), fol. 28ra.

"Cum igitur artis medicine finis sit adepcio sanitatis, secundum Galienum in libro sectarum, habet ars medicine considerare ea que sunt ad illum finem; modo cum ea que sunt ad illum finem sint illa per quarum cognicionem adipiscere sanitas, est artis medicine considerare res preter naturam... asumpta sunt in esse communi ut hoc libro." Bartolomeo da Varignana, *Comm. De morbo et accidenti* (cit. n. 44), fol. 67ra.

57 "Causa finalis est duplex scilicet operis et hec est utilitas eorum que traduntur in isto libro," fol. 85ra; again later "In prima parte Galienus intendit talem rationem: inspicere in arte medicine quod utile est ad finem medicine; Sed cognoscere loca paciencia et passiones et earum causas et diversitates accidencium est utile ad finem medicine; Ergo (...) etcetera." Bartolomeo da Varignana, *Comm. De interioribus* (cit. n. 46), fol. 89vb.

58 "Intencio Galieni in isto libro est disputare de nocumentis membrorum... et monstratio locorum infirmorum que nec visu nec sensu cognoscuntur." Jean de Saint-Amand, *De interioribus*, Brux, Bibliot. Roy. 9905-14, fol. 13rb.

59 "et quoniam prime due particule de interioribus utilem continent doctrinam et valde necessariam medico, nec per communem translationem poterat intellectus elici propter differentiam reductionum et reducta fuerit anno preterito ad statum latinorum, ita quod omnis studens potest in eis modo proficere et notabiliter defectus est medici qui caruit scientia illarum duarum particularum." Arnau de Vilanova, *Repetitio super canonem Vita brevis* in *Opera Omnia* (Venice, 1505), fol. 321vb.

Academic medical training thus became an ethical duty for any physician-to-be who wanted to practice the Art with the best results for his patients. Arnald expressed this need with an interesting religious analogy. When commenting on his own aphorisms in one of his last works, he presented various ways of understanding the patient's affliction. The first came through divine revelation which, according to Arnald, only happened to a few people. The second and more general path to a proper understanding of the disease was, in Arnald's words, human revelation, or the observation and questioning of the patient and his or her relatives about the course and characteristics of the affliction.[60] The message of the analogy is clear: the voice of revelation, in this case human, could only be heard by those whose minds had been enlightened with the right (university) training, which alone would allow them to operate according to the light of reason and not by chance.[61]

Whatever its actual results, the attempt to equate university medical training with the practice of the best possible medicine did have repercussions, not only in controlling the product which came out of the universities, but also on the unlicensed professional. Thus, the professional product of academic training was designed to become identified with the decorous and ethical practitioner, and only Christian men could get this training.[62]

60 "I.16 *Propietas incognita, etc.* Ostensa necessitate agnoscendi propietatem individualem, iam exprimit modos quibus potest cognosci. Et primus est revelatio, que prout fit a Deo paucis conceditur, sed prout fit ab homine debet communiter a medicis observari. Nam prudens medicus debet suum patientem diligenter interrogare vel asistentes ut ei proprietas indicetur illius. Tali etiam revelatione, humana scilicet, multarum medicinarum proprietates individuales multis innotuerunt." *Arnaldi de Villanova Opera Medica Omnia*, vol. vi.2: *Commentum in quasdam parabolas et alias aphorismorum series*, eds. J. A. Paniagua and P. Gil (Barcelona: Publicacions de la Universitat de Barcelona, 1993), p. 160.

61 "Intendit ergo quod medicus qui predicta quatuor plene cognoscit medetur egris corporibus cum lumine rationis et iuvamentum procurabit eis artificialiter et non casualiter." *Ibid.*, p. 159.

62 On the attempt to control unlicensed practice by the medical masters of Paris, see P. Kibre, "The Faculty of Medicine at Paris, Charlatanism and Unlicensed Medical Practices in the Later Middle Ages," *Bulletin of the History of Medicine*, 1953, *27*:1–20. An account of the topic's complexity has been written for the case of the kingdom of Valencia and the Crown of Aragon. See García-Ballester *et al.*, *Medical licensing* (cit. n. 14).

The debates on pain which I have mentioned must be located within this context. If we look only at what the medical masters said about pain, it can easily be concluded that their statements had no religious flavor, but the social context which created the theoretical discussions of pain and used them to build up and strengthen the new medical culture which was in the making was exclusively Christian.

Fixing a Cost for Medical Care: Medical Ethics and Socio-Economic Reality in Christian Spain as Reflected in Jewish Sources

Y. Tzvi Langermann

One of the important questions debated in medical ethics concerns the financial compensation which the medical doctor may charge for his services. There are a number of reasons why this should be considered a problem in ethics. From one perspective, there is a moral imperative to relieve suffering and save life and, consequently, it is not at all self-evident that whoever engages in those acts has a right to ask for payment. If, however, it be granted that the medical practitioner may ask for remuneration, how should his fee be fixed? Can one put a price on preserving human life and alleviating suffering?

We have formulated these questions in a purely theoretical fashion. The answers given to these ethical questions will find expression in the laws or customs which regulate medical costs; and such legislation as exists will perforce take into account — though it may not be entirely in step with — economic realities and social norms. In this presentation we shall examine some responses to these questions on the part of Jewish communal leaders in Christian Spain. As historians, we shall examine closely a number of legislative pronouncements against the background of the economic and social data that are available to us. Though we shall not be able to provide a full and comprehensive picture, I trust that our investigation shall yield some insight.

My chief source will be a passage in Moses Naḥmanides' (Ramban)

* I wish to thank Professor Michael McVaugh for making available to me then unpublished materials from his new book (see note 2), and Professor Menachem Kellner for his insightful criticisms.

Torat ha-Adam,[1] where Ramban sets the parameters for the fee which the physician may charge for his services. I shall also make use of a response of Asher ben Yeḥiel and, to a lesser extent, some other rabbinic writings. I shall supplement the halakhic materials with information concerning medical practice that I have culled from two sources: *A Mediterranean Society*, Professor Goitein's exhaustive study of documents from the Cairo Genizah; and a chapter from *Medicine before the Plague: Practitioners and Their Patients in the Crown of Aragon 1285–1345*, the new book of Professor Michael McVaugh of the University of North Carolina at Durham.[2] It should be clear that the following account is far from being an exhaustive study, and many of my observations and conclusions remain tentative. All the same, it is to the best of my knowledge the first attempt to survey this important topic from the perspective of Jewish thought during the medieval period, and I trust that it shall be of use, if only as a stimulus to a more thorough undertaking.

Let us turn straightaway to the passage from Ramban which I shall translate and analyze:[3]

> As far as the fee for medical treatment is concerned: It seems to me that [the physician] may charge for his time (*baṭla*) and exertion (*ṭirḥa*). However, he may not charge for the cost of his education, because it [illness] is a case of "losing one's body," and the Torah said, *You shall return it to him* [Deut. 22:2, i.e., one must return a lost object for free]. Moreover, with regard to religious commandments, the rule is: "Just as I [the Lord] do it

1 I used the edition of C. Chavel, *Kitvei Ramban*, vol. 2 (Jerusalem, 1964), pp. 44–45.

2 Cambridge University Press, 1993 (hereafter: McVaugh).

3 For a more complete discussion of *Torat ha-Adam* and its importance for Ramban's views on medical issues, see the article of Samuel Kottek in this volume. On Ramban's attitude towards science in general, see Y. Tzvi Langermann, "Acceptance and Devaluation: Naḥmanides' attitude towards science," *Jewish Thought and Philosophy* 1 (1992), 223–245. The most recent study of Ramban is the collection of essays edited by I. Twersky: *Rabbi Moses Naḥmanides (Ramban): Explorations in His Religious and Literary Virtuosity* (Cambridge, Mass., 1983). I should add that Ramban finds legal precedents for his rulings in a number of *halakhot* that are not widely known; I shall do my best to outline Ramban's legal reasoning without, however, straying from my topic.

for free, so too shall you do it for free." Therefore, it is forbidden to charge for one's wisdom (*ḥokhma*, here perhaps a better translation would be "professional expertise") and education, because it would be like charging for sprinkling [that is, sprinkling the special fluid used in Temple purification rituals] and sanctifying [that same fluid; see *Bekhorot* 29a for that injunction]. However, he may charge for his exertion, because that is analogous to charging for transporting and filling [that is, transporting and filling the vessel which contains the purification fluid; hence, as it seems to me, "exertion" refers to incidental expenses incurred by the doctor traveling to the patient, etc.]. Likewise, he is allowed to charge for his time; for the Mishnah [*Bekhorot* 4:6] states, "If he [here the Mishnah is referring to the expert in inspecting first-born animals] is an old man, one [may pay for his] transportation on a donkey, and one pays him whatever he would have accepted not to engage in his profession during that time [that he spent inspecting the animal]."

In addition, whoever possesses drugs which his sick comrade needs may not overcharge for them [the drugs], because they were under time pressures and could find no drugs other than the ones that [that person] had, he [the man who owned the drugs] can recover only their market value . . . [that is, the patient need not pay the exorbitant price to which he had agreed, but only the market value of those drugs; Ramban here goes to some length to prove this from Talmudic sources, and I shall skip over his proofs].

Our conclusion is that whoever agrees to an exorbitant fee as the result of an exigency and time pressure, is entitled to say, "I was only fooling [when I agreed to that price]." This rule applies to someone who overpaid for drugs on account of the pressure of the illness; he is liable only for their [market] value. The same rule applies both to leasing [!?] or buying [the drugs]. However, if he agreed to a high price for the doctor's services, he must pay; for he has sold him his wisdom [or: professional expertise], and that has no price.

Ramban then cites and refutes another opinion, which maintains that under any and all circumstances, the doctor is entitled to charge only for his time. Ramban restates his own view on the matter: "But the doctor's fee is priceless, and he [the patient] must pay whatever they agreed upon."

This document, in addition to being a brilliant piece of *ḥiddush* (halakhic innovation), is a very rich source for our topic. Let me proceed directly to the most significant statements that we may make in the light of Ramban's pronouncements.

(1) Ramban's rulings appear to reflect a period of transition from a nonprofessionalized (or, perhaps, semi-professionalized) medical practice to one which is professionalized. By "professional" I mean here the fact that the medical doctor earns his livelihood primarily or solely by means of the practice of medicine. (I do not take into account the possibility that the doctor often invested his earnings in ventures which provided additional income.) "Nonprofessional" medicine, by contrast, is that which is practiced by people who earn their livelihood by means of some other craft. The importance of this distinction for our problem is evident. The ruling that a doctor may be paid for his time (the key technical term here is *baṭla*) but not for his wisdom reflects, or is most suited to, a situation wherein the medical practitioner is generally employed in some other craft, and, therefore, his fee is determined by the amount of money that he would have earned at his main occupation during whatever period of time he spent treating the patient. Of course, this regulation makes no sense when confronted with a medical professional, someone who spends all of his working hours treating patients, and is not engaged in some other craft. Ramban recognizes both professional and nonprofessional medicine. In his first statement of the rules governing medical fees, he states that the doctor may charge for his time but not for his wisdom (*ḥokhma*, which, as I suggested above, may in this case be rendered more accurately "professional expertise"). One may safely assume that that fee, i.e., the doctor's time and nothing else, would be less — considerably less — than professional medical treatment. However, at the end of his discussion he states that if the patient had contracted for a higher fee for the doctor's services, then the agreement is legally valid. The doctor may collect his fee in court. Note also that Ramban has not even fixed any upper bound for this fee. As it seems to me — and the matter requires much further investigation, and I shall have a bit more to say on this later — these two rulings reflect a changing situation. The ruling for

nonprofessional medicine has a Talmudic precedent, and may still have been the norm in Spain; in any event, other authorities dispute Ramban's ruling. On the other hand, professional medical treatment had become widespread enough that Ramban wished to give it halakhic recognition, that is, to ensure that the courts would give relief to doctors wishing to recover the higher fees demanded by professionals. (2) In demanding that only a fair market price be charged for drugs, and in denying the right of the doctor to recover in the courts any higher prices which the patient may have agreed to under duress — note that this is the opposite of the ruling regarding professional fees, where any sum agreed upon is recoverable — Ramban addressed one of the major grievances concerning the medical practice of his day. It seems to have been the case that medical doctors hid the high fees which they wished to charge for their services in the form of grossly inflated prices which they (perhaps in cahoots with apothecaries) charged for medications. We have evidence for this assertion in some of the sources which Professor McVaugh has assembled. For example, some contracts for medical services which he examined stipulate that the fee which the patient will pay shall include all medication as well. McVaugh suggests that his clause was included to guard against fee-splitting with apothecaries; but, as we have seen, it may also have been the doctor alone who charged exorbitant prices for his prescriptions. McVaugh has also called attention to the fact that Juan Manuel, son-in-law of the King of Aragon, accused physicians of inflating the costs of medicines.

The two rulings which we have just examined are, to my mind, connected to each other. Ramban knew that doctors tended to overcharge for drugs, but he also realized that, in some cases anyway, this was done because they were not allowed to charge the higher fees for professional services to which they felt they were entitled. By allowing them to do so — at least in those cases where the patient agreed — he hoped that physicians would no longer feel compelled to sneak in these costs through charges for some other facet of the patient's treatment.

These, I submit, are the chief conclusions that may be extracted from Ramban's discussion. Before moving on to some other observations, I must say something about one more issue that is raised in our text. We recall that Ramban ruled that the doctor may *not* figure into his charges the cost of his own medical education. Now Professor

Goitein has spoken of "the expensive apprenticeship of scientific medicine;"[4] however, neither he nor any other scholar whose work I consulted (and my study has been far from exhaustive) have produced any hard data concerning the cost of medical education. Another relevant factor is the cost of medical books. It is interesting, as Goitein notes, that medical doctors seem to have been quite active in the book trade. They also had some role in the drug trade; that is to say, they seem to have had financial interests in those items that had a close connection to their own profession.[5]

Let us move on. It seems a safe generalization that legislation such as that which was innovated by Ramban was aimed at protecting certain interests. But whose? Today, when the high cost of health care is a major social and political issue, it seems a commonplace that it is the consumer of health services who needs to be protected. And, indeed, during the period of concern to us as well, the sources record no few complaints of the high cost of medical care. Avraham Avigdor, a translator of Latin texts into Hebrew who flourished in the Provence in the fourteenth century, criticizes contemporary doctors who, he states, are only in it for the money.[6] Many of the economic documents studied by Professor Goitein name doctors as those who invested in various enterprises — for some reason, they seem to have had a particular interest in the sugar industry in Egypt — which indicates that they had plenty of money for investment.[7] Goitein further notes that the image of the doctor was generally one of greed and avarice.[8]

However, we have ample evidence which indicates that medical doctors stood no less in need of legal backing as far as payment was

4 *A Mediterranean Society*, vol. 1 (Berkeley and Los Angeles, 1967), p. 128 (hereafter: Goitein).

5 Concerning physicians active in the book trade, see Goitein, vol. 1, p. 379; on physicians who prepared their own prescriptions, see Goitein, vol. 2, (Berkeley and Los Angeles, 1971), p. 253; for some data on fees charged by physicians, see vol. 1, p. 259, and vol. 2, p. 256. Goitein observes that the data at hand is insufficient for us to draw any firm conclusions concerning the fees charged by physicians.

6 Ms. Escorial, G-III-9, f. 152a.

7 Goitein, vol. 1, p. 259 (physicians investing in the sugar industry), and *passim* concerning physicians figuring as partners in various business interests.

8 Goitein, vol. 2, p. 257.

concerned. For one thing, it seems often to have been the practice not to pay the doctor unless the treatment was successful; both Goitein and McVaugh note this.[9] (This may have been one of the reasons why doctors had to disguise their fees in the form of high prices for medication.) Goitein has also noted that there was keen competition among medical practitioners, something which usually serves to lower the cost to the consumer. He also found that it was common practice for a patient to apply to more than one physician; presumably only the one whose treatment was successful (if any were) would be paid.[10]

One very valuable source for this matter is the book on surgery of Henri de Mondeville (ca. 1270–1320), which McVaugh has studied closely.[11] After some pious-sounding remarks to the effect that the money which the patient pays serves as a tangible sign of the mutual commitment of the doctor-patient relationship, de Mondeville gives some practical advice to physicians. The patient will usually bargain about the fee; therefore, the doctor should start out by asking for double the fee which he hopes to collect. Moreover, the majority of the patients will pay only if they are cured, and even then they will pay only in accordance with their perception of how quick and painless the treatment was. All of this points to a medical profession which is highly unregulated. Indeed, it is not surprising that many of the documents which McVaugh has studied are court cases in which the doctor sues the estate of his former patients.

De Mondeville also gives instructions for calculating the fee which the doctor may charge. It would be of great interest to compare de Mondeville's criteria with those of Ramban, but before proceeding to such a comparison we must make this *caveat*: De Mondeville is a physician, writing for physicians, who has the physician's interest at heart. On the other hand, although Ramban too was a physician — we have solid evidence that he took money for treating one of his patients[12]

9 *Ibid.*, 257; McVaugh, pp. 177, 178, 179.

10 Goitein, vol. 2, p. 257, and p. 583, n. 30.

11 McVaugh, pp. 172–173.

12 In a responsum of Ramban's student Shelomo den Adret (*Teshuvot ha-Rashba*, part 1, no. 120), we find testimony that Ramban took a fee for treating a Christian woman for infertility. Cited by C. Henoch, *Nachmanides, Philosopher and Mystic* [Hebrew], second edition (Jerusalem 1982), p. 29, n. 55.

— nevertheless, his work is a legal treatise, not one written for physicians, and it does not reflect a narrow professional interest, but rather the concerns of a communal leader for just and comprehensive regulation.

According to de Mondeville, three factors may be included in the calculation: the physican's professional stature; the patient's economic circumstances; and the seriousness of the patient's condition. The first two factors illustrate, perhaps somewhat remotely, some of the reflections which I offered above. The physician's stature expresses the notion that, in the period of concern to us, professional reputation was an important factor in the costs which physicians felt entitled to charge; but the second factor testifies to the fact that not everyone could afford highly respected doctors. De Mondeville left it to the doctor to make the appropriate equation in each case. Ramban, it so appears, took a different approach. Those who wished, or were forced by economic circumstances, could have recourse to "nonprofessional" doctors, whose charges were strictly regulated. (They could charge only for their "time.") Those who were willing and able to pay for the most highly regarded doctors could do so, and the doctors would have legal recourse in the matter of fee collection. (My choice of words, by the way, is quite deliberate — it is, in my opinion, the physician's reputation — how highly regarded he was — that was the major factor here.)

It is very noteworthy that both Goitein and McVaugh in their entirely unrelated investigations have found that in the Middle Ages there existed a sort of health insurance. That is, we know of contracts in which the patient paid in advance a flat fee, which entitled him to full treatment on the part of the physician for a given period of time.[13] In the light of the picture which we have sketched out, we see that this was advantageous for both parties. The patient protected himself against exorbitant fees (including, perhaps, hidden fees in the form of inflated costs for medications); and the doctor protected himself in a social-economic situation where collecting fees for medical practice seems to have been a difficult and unsure task. I may add here that McVaugh

13 McVaugh, pp. 175–176. The evidence from the Genizah is less conclusive, but Goitein, vol. 2, records that a Jewish physician was held on retainer by a Muslim family for the fixed fee of one dinar per month.

has also come to the conclusion that it was generally harder for Jews to collect their fees from non-Jewish patients than it was for Christian doctors.[14]

I should like to end this essay by discussing a source which is about a generation or two later than Ramban, namely a responsum (no. 85) of Asher ben Yeḥiel ("the Rosh"), who assumed the rabbinate in Toledo in 1305. The case with which he was confronted is as follows. The relatives of the deceased had made some expenditures on behalf of medical treatment for the deceased, even though he (the deceased) had not asked them to do so. These relatives now wished to recover their expenses from the estate; presumably (this is not expressly stated), the heirs opposed that action. I now quote the Rosh's decision:

"In my opinion, that reason — that is, that he did not ask them to make those expenditures — is not sufficient [cause] for them [that is, the relatives] to forfeit. For the custom is well-known, that when a person becomes ill and cannot take care of himself, his relatives undertake to secure for him medical treatment."

From this responsum I infer that medical care — perhaps even professional medical care, as defined earlier — had become a social norm, on the order of *piqu'aḥ nefesh* (saving a life), without, however, the norm associated with that ancient rule, that is, that it be done for free. Hence the Rosh ruled that moneys which family members expended on medical care for a sick relation (may this ruling have been extended to friends as well?) are legally recoverable even if the patient did not expressly request this treatment. Now the Rosh was not a native Andalusian, and it remains an open question whether that ruling reflects norms of his native Germany or his adopted country, Spain.

In conclusion, we note that Jewish communal authorities responded to the situation — a changing situation, as it appears — with regard to the costs that were fixed for medical care. In particular, Ramban pioneered thoughtful and detailed legislation which, it so appears, was for the most part quickly accepted, and eventually incorporated into the standard Jewish law codes, the *Ṭur* and the *Shulḥan Arukh*.[15]

14 McVaugh, pp. 177, 181.

15 *Yore De'ah*, paragraphs 335–339. R. Ya'qov ba'al ha-Ṭurim plainly acknowledges Ramban's *Torat ha-Adam* as his source for the rulings in question.

MEDICAL PRACTICE AND JEWISH LAW: NAḤMANIDES' *SEFER TORAT HAADAM*

SAMUEL S. KOTTEK

Rabbi Moses ben Naḥman was born in Gerona in 1194, and is therefore often called Rabbi Moses Gerundi. In later Spanish rabbinical literature, he was also given the title *haRav haNeeman* (the trustworthy or authoritative rabbi), while non-Jewish Spanish sources referred to him as Bonastruc de Porta. He had a broad knowledge, as was not uncommon in his times, of philosophy, biblical exegesis, poetry, kabbalah and medicine. His teachers included R. Judah ben Yakar, who spent some time in Barcelona, but had been trained by the French tosafists. Naḥmanides was a cousin of the scholar and moralist R. Jonah ben Abraham Gerundi.

One event in Naḥmanides' biography is of great importance in a discussion of interfaith influences. He participated in a famous public disputation against the apostate Pablo Christiani, in the presence of King Jaime I, in 1263 in Barcelona. Even the King praised Naḥmanides' skill and scholarship, though each side claimed that he had won the contest. Naḥmanides boldly wrote down the argument of the disputation, an act which enraged the Dominicans.[1] The Pope Clement IV requested a condemnation of Naḥmanides' work, and in order to escape, he fled to France and ultimately to the Holy Land, where he died. Naḥmanides is thus a particularly appropriate choice as a person linking Spain with the Holy Land.

Sefer Torat haAdam is a legalist work which includes a comprehensive study of the laws applying to visiting the sick, to the practice of

1 *Sefer haVikkuaḥ*, also called *Milḥamot haShem* or *Milḥamot Ḥovah*, was first printed by Wagenseil in Altdorf in 1681.

medicine, to dealing with a dying patient and, ultimately, to burial and mourning. The work is divided into thirty 'gates' (*she'arim*) or chapters. The last chapter, entitled *sha'ar ha-gemul*, was printed separately in Naples as early as 1490.[2] It deals with reward and punishment after death using talmudic and mystical sources, and also discusses later authorities' statements on the resurrection of the dead.

In a brief paper published in 1983, Benjamin Richler listed twelve manuscript copies of *Sefer Torat haAdam*, the earliest dating from the end of the thirteenth century or the beginning of the fourteenth century. The first printed edition of the whole work appeared in Constantinople in 1518, and the second in Venice in 1595. The third edition, however, did not appear until 1840, and was followed by editions in 1876, 1926, 1928–29, 1955 and 1979.[3]

Did Naḥmanides actually practice medicine? Where and how did he learn medicine? The second question has no answer, but the fact that he at least occasionally practiced medicine is documented in three responsa by his pupil R. Solomon ben Abraham Adret of Barcelona (the Rashba, 1235–1310). The first responsum is of particular interest in the context of interfaith relationships. It answers the question: "Is it permissible [for a Jew] to treat a non-Jewish woman so that she will be able to conceive?" In response, R. Solomon quotes the Talmud, which says that "A Jewish woman should not help a non-Jewish woman in childbirth, as she would bring to the world a child [who will be brought up] into heathen practices (*'avodah zarah*)."[4] The text continues: "A heathen woman should not [out of distrust] help a Jewish woman in childbirth, lest she destroy the life [of the child]." This opinion is that

2 The printer was Joseph Guntzenhauser, who also printed the first Hebrew edition of the whole *Canon* of Avicenna. *Sha'ar haGemul* was printed seventeen times, seven of them before 1840.

3 Benjamin Richler, "Manuscripts of Moses ben Naḥman's Torat ha-Adam," *Koroth*, 8 (7–8), 1983 : 265*–267* (Engl.) and 216-218 (Hebr.); Samuel Ashkenasi, "The printed editions of Ramban's Sefer Torat ha-Adam," *Koroth, Ibid.*: 219–221 (Hebr.).

4 Responsum no. 120, quoting Tos. Avodah Zarah 3:3. This topic is also discussed in the Mishnah (Avodah Zarah 2:1) : "A Jewish woman should not help a heathen woman in childbirth." However, a later talmudic authority permitted this assistance if the woman was paid for her work, thus enabling professional Jewish midwives to practice among non-Jews.

of Rabbi Meir. However, the majority of the Rabbis permitted the latter, as long as the two women were not left alone.[5] Communities of differing religion clearly distrusted each other, but solutions were devised in order to allow them to live together. It is quite possible that an additional reason for not allowing a Jewish woman to deliver a non-Jewish baby was the fear that the whole Jewish community might be endangered if an accident was to occur.[6]

Rabbi Solomon's responsum permitted the treatment of a non-Jewish woman for sterility. It also stated that he had witnessed this sort of treatment performed by his teacher Rabbi Moses (Naḥmanides), and that it had been duly rewarded (*be-sakhar*); the nature of the treatment is unfortunately not indicated.

The other two responsa deal with an amulet on which was carved the image of a lion. It was used against pains in the loins (*le-ḥoli mothnaim*).[7] R. Solomon states that he heard that his teacher R. Moses ben Naḥman had used this treatment without fear that it might be sacrilegious. Such silver or golden amulets with an image of a lion were in use throughout the Mediterranean area long before Naḥmanides.[8] R. Solomon admitted that he could not see how such a device could be effective, at least according to the ways of nature, but its use was eventually permitted.

Another source which documents Naḥmanides' interest in medical matters is a dedicatory introduction to Jacob Hakatan's translation of a brief treatise on diarrhea by Ibn Roshd. The translator attests that the work was done at the request of his teacher R. Moses ben Naḥman.[9]

5 Similarly, a Jewish woman was not to nurse a heathen child (wet-nursing), but a non-Jewish nurse could give suck to a Jewish child if she was under supervision.

6 Another issue which is mentioned several times in the Tosefta in close relationship with medical practice is embryotomy. If a mother's life was in danger during birth, she was to undergo an embryotomy in order to save her life (cf. Oholot 7:6; Tos. Yevamot 9:4). If a person who was licensed to practice, performed an embryotomy and caused damage to the mother, he/she was not liable before a human court, but only before the court of Heaven (Tos. Baba Kama 7:17; Tos. Makkot 2:5).

7 Rashba, responsa nos. 167 and 825.

8 On this amulet, see my "Le symbole du lion dans la médecine de l'antiquité." *Rev. Hist. Méd. Hébr.* (1967) 78: 161–168.

9 See D. Margalith: "Ramban (Rabbi Moses ben Naḥman) the physician," citing S. Muntner, *Koroth* 1 (9–10), 1956 : 303–315, especially pp. 310–311.

On the Right to Heal and to be Healed

Since talmudic times there has been a debate over whether it is lawful to treat a sick person and whether it is appropriate to seek medical advice whenever diseased.

The Talmud offers two opinions which are presented in a discussion of bloodletting.

According to Rabbi Aḥa (4th cent.), a person who is about to submit to bloodletting should pray to the Lord that the procedure will help him. Rabbi Aḥa thought that medicine was not a human skill, although men betook themselves to it.[10] It appears that for him, and he was most probably not the only Sage to think so, the practice of medicine was a *minhag* (or *nohag*, accepted custom). The noted scholar Abbayé strongly opposed this opinion.[11] He felt that one should not use such a prayer, as the school of Rabbi Ismael established that Scripture legitimizes the practice of medicine according to the verse "And he shall be thoroughly healed" (Ex. 21:19).

This discussion of the legitimacy of medical practice did not settle the question for later generations. Two divergent opinions can also be found in the writings of Naḥmanides, one in his commentary to the Bible, the other one in *Sefer Torat haAdam*.

In the latter (*Sha'ar ha-sakana*), Naḥmanides clearly states that medical practice is lawful. He first cites the Talmud and the ruling of R. Ismael (Baba Kama 85b),[12] and then adds: "Lest the physician say 'I had better stay away from this disheartening [process], which could lead me to commit some unintentional mistake resulting in the death of the patient.' For this reason the Bible attested that medicine is lawful." Naḥmanides protests against the idea that medicine is not a human skill. He holds the contrary view that healing is clearly permitted, a permission (*reshut*) that at once qualifies into a commandment

10 Berakhot 60a. Hebr. *she-ein darkan shel benei-adam lerapeot ela she-nahagu.*

11 Abbayé (278–338 CE) was the head of the Babylonian talmudic academy at Pumbedita. According to later authorities, he was also called Naḥmani, after his grandfather. Abbayé believed that whatever was done for healing purposes and had no obvious idolatrous implications was not among the "ways of the Emorites" and was permitted (Shabbat 67a).

12 He asserts that the Bible fully endorses medical practice, according to Lev. 21:19 (See above).

(*miẓvah*) connected to the highest ordinance about saving life (*piquaḥ nefesh*). The physician is obligated to heal, for if he refuses he is like one who sheds blood (*shofekh damim*). The latter conclusions are apparently based on Naḥmanides' own authority, and were later included nearly verbatim in the Codes.

Naḥmanides' approach to the practice of medicine is clear. The physician is not interfering with, or against, the Lord's project. His practice is not only permitted, it is a duty related to saving life.[13] If he refrains from performing his duty, the physician may come close to being considered a murderer.

From the side of the patient, medical practice could also be seen as problematic. The patient could argue, writes Naḥmanides, that he brings himself into danger, as the physician could be mistaken either in his diagnosis or in his treatment. In going to the physician he might even be considered like one who commits suicide! However, Naḥmanides soothingly adds, if the physician acts according to accepted professional rules and with sane judgment, there should be no such fear, as the Lord himself would (hopefully) intrust the healing procedure.[14]

In his *Commentary on the Bible*, Naḥmanides takes a rather different approach to the practice of medicine. He comments on Lev. 26:11, which has no apparent bearing on medicine or healing. If the great majority of the Children of Israel are accomplished,[15] they will not be subject to the laws of nature, and there will be no need for medicine. If one of them would nevertheless become sick, and given that people have "betaken themselves" (*nahagu*) to taking medicines, physicians are allowed to give advice. Physicians should not worry about the patient dying while in their care as long as they are properly trained in their art, nor should they argue that the Lord alone is the healer of all flesh, as the custom of healing was firmly established.

13 Maimonides based the commandment (*miẓvah*) to heal on an interpretation of the rule according to which one has to bring a lost article back to its owner whenever he/she can be identified. Similarly, the physician should restore the health which the sick person has lost! (*Perush ha-Mishnayot* on Nedarim 4:4).

14 Hebr. *raḥmana peqida le-ripuye*.

15 Accomplished: The Hebrew *shelemim (shalem)* includes wholeness of body and soul. Such a person could not, by definition, be ill.

Naḥmanides rather curiously adds that though the Bible clearly acknowledges the right of physicians to cure, it is less evident that it allows the sick to go to the physician. Those who do so are not really part of the "Community of the Lord" for whom "life is their portion."[16]

Summing up this review of Naḥmanides' approach to the lawfulness of curing and of being cured, in an ideal society which lives completely according to the biblical ordinances, there would be no place for medicine. Disease is a state of waste, of want. An accomplished (*shalem*) man/woman would not want, either spiritually or physically. Such a situation is clearly unnatural and improbable. When disease nevertheless occurs, there is no theological problem whatsoever on the side of the physician, though there might be on the side of the patient. It seems that making use of medicine is merely tolerated, and warranted by custom.

I would like to argue that a historical shift may be delineated from some talmudic circles (cf. R. Aḥa) where medicine was effectively objected to (though 'custom' was admitted), through Naḥmanides in his biblical commentary, where healing was not problematic, though being cured could be, and finally to Naḥmanides in *Sefer Torat ha-Adam*, where medicine received full, unrestricted acceptance.[17]

On the Liability of the Physicians

Naḥmanides' discussion of the liabilities of the physicians is based on four brief talmudic statements. All of them are recorded in the Tosefta[18] Three of them read as follows:

1.- "A trained physician (*rofe uman*) who healed by permission of

16 "Life is their portion": see Psalms 17:14. The righteous are called 'living' even when they are dead (Berakhot 18a).

17 This last approach, which fully endorses the practice of medicine, was accepted by the Codes. See *Shulḥan Arukh*, Yore De'ah, ch. 336.

18 The Tosefta, meaning 'addition,' is a collection of tannaitic rules more or less parallel to the Mishnah, together with some original data that for some reason were not included in it. The edition of Zuckermandel: *Tosephta*, based on the Erfurt & Vienna codices — with supplement by S. Liebermann (Jerusalem: 1970) — is used here.

court[19]) (*bi-reshut bet-din*) and caused damage, is free (from punishment). If however he caused an injury that was greater than was adequate for the case, he is considered guilty" (Tos. Baba Kama 9:11).

2.- "A trained physician who healed by permission of court and caused damage, is free from any punishment by human law, but his case is forwarded to the court of Heaven" (Tos. Baba Kama 6:17).

3.- "A trained physician who healed by permission of court and caused damage, in case this was done unintentionally, he is free; if done intentionally, he is guilty, for the sake of social order (*mipnei tikkun ha-'olam*)"[20] (Tos. Gittin 4:6).

A preliminary question arises regarding the definition of a *rofe uman*. A *rofe* is a physician, but the word is also used sometimes to indicate a surgeon. *Uman* (as an adjective) means 'trained,' 'skillful,' 'approved,' 'reliable.' As a noun, it is often used to refer to a surgeon, sometimes even in opposition to a physician.[21] It seems clear, though, that the Tosefta is directed at both physicians and surgeons. Moreover, the concept of "for the sake of social order" suggests, as Naḥmanides comments, that if every error, even unintentional, would be sanctioned by the law, nobody would agree to enter the medical profession.

There is a fourth statement recorded by Naḥmanides which has sometimes been misunderstood. It reads: "A trained physician that healed by permission of the court and caused damage will go to the towns of refuge (*goleh*)."[22] This statement is based on Tos. Makkot 2:5, which says nothing about the kind of damage caused by the

19 Hebr. *bi-reshut bet-din*. This raises the question of medical license in talmudic times. Physicians, like judges and other officials, were protected by the law if they had been duly licensed by judicial courts, as appears in this very early reference to medical license. On this topic, see J.O. Leibowitz, "The problem of medical license in Hebrew sources," *Koroth* (1977) : 360–363 (Hebr.) & XLVII–LIII (Engl.) and *Proceedings*, 26th Internat. Congress of the History of Medicine, (Sofia: 1981), pp. 139–140.

20 In sources 2) and 3) the same rule applies to anyone performing an embryotomy by permission of court — i.e., to a certified midwife (or surgeon).

21 See for instance, Sanhedrin 17b, where it says that a scholar should not live in a place where there cannot be found ten facilities, among them a physician and a surgeon (*rofe ve-uman*).

22 This statement is not a distorted reference to Tos. Baba Kama 9:11, as Chavel apparently thought. See *The Works of R. Moses ben Naḥman*, ed. H.D. Chavel (Jerusalem: 1964), vol. 2, p. 41, n. 55 (Hebr.).

physician. However, the context clearly indicates that the physician unintentionally caused the death of his patient. The same penalty (exile) is imposed on an embryotomist who acts by license of court and unintentionally causes the death of the mother (*Ibid.*). This penalty (exile) was no longer in use in talmudic times, and the sanction merely remained on the books. Still, it is noteworthy that a trained and licensed physician who causes the death of his patient has the same legal status as a person who has unintentionally killed another.[23]

Naḥmanides adds an important point here. He says that the physician is liable to penalty only if he becomes aware that he made a mistake which resulted in injury to the patient, or in his death. Moreover, it seems that Naḥmanides restricts the physician's liability to cases in which the damage was caused by his direct intervention (*ba-yadaim*), thus excluding any kind of indirect injury.[24]

Finally, all the sources on which Naḥmanides elaborated are found in the Tosefta, and not in the talmudic corpus. The reason may be that these questions relate to a special group (physicians), and are not generally applicable. Moreover, these topics were rarely mentioned in the early rabbinic literature, and Naḥmanides may be the first scholar who discussed this topic in depth. As a result the Codes leaned heavily on *Sefer Torat haAdam* in their brief chapter on "Medicine and Law."[25]

On Treatment by Non-Jews

Naḥmanides[26] first quotes from the Talmud (Avodah Zarah 27a): "It is permitted to be treated by them [heathen doctors], only when [healing relates] to money (*mamon*), not if [it relates] to the person (*nefashoth*)." This strange statement is discussed in the Gemara. A first suggestion, immediately rejected, is that treatment for money is opposed here to treatment gratis. A second possibility is that 'money' means a disease which is not dangerous, while 'person' refers to a life-threatening

23 Num. 35:11 and Deut. 19:2–3.

24 Indirect damage (Hebr. *gerama*) is not generally speaking liable to punishment by a human court.

25 *Shulḥan Arukh*, yore De'ah, ch. 336.

26 *The Works* (1964) vol. 2, p. 37.

illness. A third opinion is that 'money' is used for animals (cattle), whereas 'person' indicates a disease of the body (or soul), including non-dangerous cases. In the long discussion that follows, an obvious distrust of heathen physicians is apparent. It is stated, however, that if the heathen doctor merely indicates "what drug would be good, what medicine would be bad" for the patient, such advice may be accepted.

The Talmud differentiates between an 'Aramaic' physician, a Samaritan (*kuthi*), and a Nazarean (*min*). Several cases are recorded involving a certain Jacob from Kfar Sakhnia.[27] Rabbi Ismael would not allow his nephew to be cured by Jacob, even though his life was in danger from a snake-bite. Rabbi Abbahu was, however, treated by him, when he applied a powerful drug (*sam*) to Rabbi Abbahu's thigh. Rabbi Ami and Rabbi Assi promptly licked it away, if not Jacob would have amputated the leg (Avodah Zarah 28a).[28] Rabbi Joḥanan was treated by a Roman matron (*matronitha*) for a severe stomatitis (*Ibid*).[29] These two cases were considered exceptional: Rabbi Joḥanan was himself a trained healer, and Rabbi Abbahu was a well-known personage (*adam ḥashuv*) and therefore particularly immune to heretics or heathen healers.

Naḥmanides mentions most of these passages with only minor changes. The story of the 'heretic' Jacob from Sakhnia is, however, portrayed as a story of magic cure (*kishuf*). All references to heresy (*minut*) are converted here to magic or witchcraft.[30] Thus, while the

27 Sakhnia has been identified with Sakhnin in Galilee. This Jacob may have been one of Jesus' disciples, either James the son of Zebedee, or James the son of Alphaeus (cf. Mark 3:17–18). The disciples were supposed "to have power to heal sickness and to cast out devils" (*Ibid.* 15). See also Avodah Zarah 17a for more on this Jacob.

28 This *sam* (or *sama*) was most probably considered to be too strong by R. Ami and R. Assi, and they therefore sucked it (or scraped it) away. It is not clear whether the drug would have caused the loss of the leg, or whether the leg would have had to be amputated as a result of the treatment.

29 This episode is recorded in two places in the Babylonian Talmud: Avodah Zarah 28a and Yoma 84a. The "matron" was most probably the wife of a Roman official.

30 The chapter on "magic" treatments is appended to the passage dealing with heathen doctors. It begins: "One should not deal in any way with sorcerers, neither should one be treated by them," echoing the talmudic warning : "One should not deal in any way with heretics (*minin*), neither should one be treated by them" (Avodah Zarah 27b).

Talmud insists that no treatment should be accepted from heretics (here, Nazareans) because they attract people (*de-moshkha*),[31] Naḥmanides instead states that magic allures people. This shift could well have been motivated by the fear that he might be accused of raising suspicions against Christian physicians.

According to the Talmud, non-Jewish doctors used the names of 'other gods' (*elohim aḥerim*) in their incantations. Thus, if the cure was successful, people would say, "there is indeed something real in this thing" (their creed). Naḥmanides, however, thought that 'magic' cures were prohibited because they included the use of 'names,' not because they might attract people to witchcraft.

To sum up this last chapter, Naḥmanides again makes use of most of the talmudic sources related to his theme. His conclusion is that diseases involving danger to the patient should not be intrusted to 'them,' except in cases where the patient is a well-known personage and/or the healer is a specialist (*mumḥeh*).[32] Moreover, as is shown above, mere consultation with such a practitioner is not objectionable. The more problematic Nazarean 'heretics' are transformed into magicians, and are viewed with disfavor for their alleged use of 'idolatrous' means of healing.

I have considered in this study three areas relevant to Jewish medical ethics, the lawfulness of medical practice, the liabilities of the physician, and the relationship to non-Jewish healers, in Naḥmanides' legalistic work *Sefer Torat haAdam*. It is clear that Naḥmanides is of the greatest importance in these areas. He may be considered the most comprehensive codifier of medical-ethical matters during the Middle Ages. The Codes (16th cent.) epitomized, and often quoted verbatim, Naḥmanides' decisions.

A thorough critical study of Naḥmanides' use of talmudic sources remains, however, to be undertaken.

31 Avodah Zarah 17a.

32 If the non-Jewish physician has a well established reputation (*mumḥe le-rabim*) and uses accepted medicines (not incantations, etc.), then a Jew may be treated by him. This was the case with 'Aramaic' doctors, even those counted among the 'sorcerers' (*mekhashefim*).

The Relationship Between the Process of Reasoning and the Legitimacy of Medical Therapy in Medieval Spanish Halakhah

Daniel Sinclair

1. Introduction

The focus of the present study is the problem of the relationship between the process of reasoning and the legitimacy of therapy, i.e., is a cure which is obtained by a non-rational method a legitimate one or not? The views of two of the most influential medieval Spanish rabbinic scholars will be analyzed in the course of the article. The first is Maimonides, who, though he left Spain at a young age, is nevertheless, both spiritually and intellectually, part of the Spanish school of Jewish law and philosophy. He flourished in the second half of the twelfth century. The second is Naḥmanides, who lived in Christian Spain in the thirteenth century, and who only left for the Land of Israel because his clash with the Church in the famous Barcelona Disputation of 1263 made it impossible for him to remain in Spain. It is significant that both of these authorities were practicing physicians. Maimonides' role as a court physician is well known, and the fact that Naḥmanides practiced medicine is recorded in the *responsa* of his disciples. The synthesis of Jewish legal scholarship and medical knowledge — Maimonides is known for his general medical expertise, as well as his knowledge of Jewish medical law — makes them ideal subjects for an analysis of this type of legal-medical issue, and it is hoped that the themes explored will also shed some light on modern aspects of this problem.

2. Maimonides

In his famous *Letter on Astrology*, Maimonides explains that there are three sources of valid knowledge:

> The first is a thing for which there is a clear proof deriving from man's reasoning — such as arithmetic, geometry and astronomy. The second is a thing that a man perceives through one of the five senses...The third is a thing that a man receives from the prophets or from the righteous...anyone who accepts as trustworthy anything that is not of these three species, of him it is said: "The simple believes everything" (*Prov.* 14:15).[1]

These three features of rational proof, logic, empirical evidence and authoritative tradition also figure in his description of the prerequisites for sound medical science:

> For you know how long and difficult this art is for a conscientious and exact man who does not want to state anything which he cannot support by argument, and without knowing where it has been said, and how it can be demonstrated.[2]

Maimonides requires the good doctor to be concerned with the process by which medical knowledge is derived, and not merely with the obtaining of a cure. It is undoubtedly with respect to this process of obtaining knowledge and applying it to the body which makes medicine, according to Maimonides, a stage along the road to "intellectual, ethical and theological excellence."[3]

Maimonides emphasizes the need for a rational approach to medicine in various aspects of Jewish law and thought involving medical matters. In explaining the opinion of the Rabbis that someone bitten by a rabid dog is not permitted to eat the lobe of its liver in order to be cured,[4] he remarks that the laws of the *Torah* (which prohibit the

1 *A Maimonides Reader*, ed. I. Twersky (N.Y.: Behrman House, 1972), p. 464.

2 *Maimonides' Letters*, ed. D. Baneth (Jerusalem: Mekizei Nirdamim, 1946), p. 69; I. Twersky, *Introduction to the Code of Maimonides* (New Haven: Yale University Press, 1980), p. 51.

3 *Eight Chapters* (Jerusalem: Mossad Harav Kook, 1961) pp. 5, 185.

4 *Yoma* 84a. The influence of the doctrine of sympathetic cures — *similia similibus curantur* — is evident in this passage. It is also manifested in the Talmudic cure for

eating of dog) may only be overriden (for therapeutic purposes) by therapies based upon "logical and empirical proof."[5] In his commentary on this passage, Rashi mentions that physicians do, in fact, use this cure, but "it is not a proper one for the purpose of overriding the prohibition on eating forbidden flesh."[6] It is arguable that Rashi's definition of a "proper cure" is one which has cured on a number of occasions, i.e., a proven cure, and is not necessarily one which is amenable to "logical and empirical proof."[7]

Maimonides is also severely critical of any attempt to substitute prayer for medical therapy. The focus for this issue is the talmudic statement that King Hezekiah "concealed the Book of Cures and the Rabbis agreed with him."[8] The general context of this statement is the efficacy of prayer for healing illness, and Rashi explains that Hezekiah concealed the Book "in order that they should entreat God (and not simply rely upon the cures in it)."[9] Maimonides, however, takes strong exception to this explanation: "it is vain and bizarre, and attributes to Hezekiah such folly as is attributable to only the most vulgar elements of society."[10] According to Maimonides, the reason for the concealment of the Book of Cures was that the "cures" it contained were irrational, and only therapies based upon scientific experiment are permitted to be used. Maimonides draws an analogy between food and medicine and argues that just as no one would accuse a hungry person who eats bread of not trusting in God, so, too, a sick person who takes medicine is not to be regarded as lacking in faith.[11]

a bone stuck in the throat, i.e., to place a similar bone on the head and to recite the appropriate formula (*Shabbat* 67a). Also see: J. Preuss, *Biblical and Talmudic Medicine*, trans. F. Rosner (N.Y.: Sanhedrin Press, 1978), p. 196, n. 90; J. D. Bleich, "Maimonides on the Distinction between Science and Pseudoscience" in *Moses Maimonides*, ed. F. Rosner and S.Kottek (Northvale: Jason Aronson, 1993), pp. 107 ff.

5 *Commentary on the Mishnah, Yoma* 8:4. For parallels in classical Islamic thought, see I. Twersky, "Halakhah and Science," *Shenaton Hamishpat Haivri*, 1988–1989, 14–15: 136, n. 54.

6 Rashi, *Yoma* 83a, *s.v. ein maakhilin.*

7 See *Responsa Aseh Lekha Rav* 5, no. 13 and section 3 below.

8 *Berakhot* 10b; *Pesaḥim* 56a.

9 *Berakhot* 10b, *s. v. sheganaz; Pesaḥim* 56b, *s.v. veganaz.*

10 *Commentary on the Mishnah, Pesaḥim* 4:10.

11 This analogy is found in a *midrash* of uncertain date cited in *Oẓar Midrashim*, ed.

Another area in which the Maimonidean emphasis on the rationality of medicine comes to the fore is that of astrological cures. In his *Letter on Astrology*, Maimonides mounts a fierce attack on astrology and argues that it lies at the root of all idolatry.[12] In the *Guide for the Perplexed*, he asserts that the talmudic prohibition on certain cures classified as the "ways of the Amorites"[13] is based upon the fact that "they are not arrived at by way of reason, but are similar to the performances of witchcraft, which is necessarily connected with the influence of the stars."[14] Rashi comments that the Amorite rubric contains cures which are not efficacious.[15] Although there is no practical difference between them, it would appear that whereas Maimonides is concerned with the process by which a therapy is obtained and insists that it be rational in order to be legitimate, Rashi is simply concerned with its curative powers. The method through which it was derived is not of great concern to him. Naḥmanides and his school certainly used astrological cures, and their approach would appear to be the normative one in the *halakhah*.[16]

Maimonides' methodology is a very sophisticated one in the sense that his rationalist agenda is subservient to the jurisprudential system of the *halakhah*, and he studiously avoids any direct clashes with normative law. In other words, Maimonides uses his rationalist ap-

J. Eisenstein (N.Y.: Hebrew Publishing Company, 1915), vol. 2, p. 580. It also provides support for R. Judah Ayash (*Shevet Yehudah, Yoreh Deah* 336) in his rejection of the idea that Divine healing ought to be preferred over going to the doctor (see n. 34 below).

12 *Letter on Astrology* (n. 1); *Commentary on the Mishnah, Avodah Zarah* 4:7; *Hilkhot Avodah Zarah* 11:8–9; *Sefer Hamiẓvot*, no. 132. Maimonides' negative view of astrology is expressed in a theological context, and in particular that of the issue of free will. There is evidence to suggest that his position is a much more positive one in relation to cosmological astrology, see Y. Langermann, "Maimonides' Repudiation of Astrology" in *Maimonidean Studies*, ed. A. Hyman (N.Y.: Yeshiva University Press, 1991) p. 123; G. Freudenthal, "Maimonides' Stance on Astrology in Context" in *Moses Maimonides* (cit. n. 4), p. 77. See also D. Schwartz, "The Debate on Astral Magic in Fourteenth Century Provence," *Zion*, 1993, 58:141, for a general discussion on this point.

13 *Shabbat* 67a.

14 *Guide for the Perplexed* 3:32.

15 *Shabbat* 67a, *s.v. sheyesh bo.*

16 See n. 43.

proach in order to explain established laws, or to fill in *lacunae* in the law. Rational medical science may not, therefore, override established *halakhah.* A good example of this is Maimonides' treatment of the *terefah* category in his *Mishneh Torah.*[17] The term *terefah* is used in the context of the Jewish dietary laws to indicate a fatal organic defect in an animal or fowl which makes its flesh unfit for consumption.[18] Typical examples of *terefah* are a pierced windpipe or gullet, and the Talmud states that the essence of the *terefah* concept is the inevitability of death within twelve months. The normative halakhic position is that the list of defects falling within the category of *terefah* given in the Talmud is a definitive one, and may not be added to or subtracted from, even in the face of medical evidence.[19] Maimonides is completely faithful to the talmudic tradition on this issue, and makes the following unequivocal statement on the matter:

> As regards the defects which the Sages have enumerated, concerning which they have said that they render the animal *terefah,* even if it should appear from our present knowledge of medicine that some of them are not fatal and that the animal cannot survive them, one must go only by what the Sages have enumerated as it is said: "According to the law which they shall teach you."[20]

Despite the evidence of medical science, Maimonides codifies the normative halakhic position with regard to the definition of animal *terefah*, and does not attempt to resolve the contradiction between the two disciplines. In the context of a human *terefah*, Maimonides' definition is a purely medical one. According to Maimonides, a human *terefah* — for the killing of whom there is no death penalty [21] — is defined as follows:

17 D. Sinclair, *Tradition and the Biological Revolution* (Edinburgh: Edinburgh University Press, 1989), pp. 19ff.; I. Twersky, (cit. n. 5), pp. 143–145.

18 *Ḥullin* 42a. Also see S. Levin and E. Boyden, *The Kosher Code* (Minneapolis: University of Minnesota Press, 1940).

19 *Ḥullin* 54a.

20 *Hilkhot Sheḥitah* 10:12–13.

21 For an analysis of this rule and its significance with regard to the relationship between positive law and morality in Jewish criminal law, see D. Sinclair (cit. n. 17), ch. 2.

> It is known for certain that he has a fatal organic disease and physicians say that his disease is incurable by human agency, and that he would have died of it even if he had not been killed in another way.[22]

In the case of the human *terefah*, there is no authoritative talmudic definition, and hence Maimonides is free to define it in accordance with medical science.[23] Rashi, on the other hand, defines the human *terefah* in the same terms as the animal form, i.e., a pierced oesophagus or windpipe.[24] The relationship between the two definitions is a matter for halakhic discussion, and has practical significance for the treatment of the fatally ill.[25] In the present context, however, it provides a good illustration of the way in which Maimonides incorporates medical science into the *halakhah* in cases in which there is no normative bar to doing so.

3. Naḥmanides

Naḥmanides' approach to the definition of valid knowledge may be derived from the following statement in a sermon given on the Sabbath following his famous disputation in Barcelona in 1263:

> First, you must know that all knowledge is fruit or sub-fruit of the *Torah*, and without the *Torah*, there is absolutely no difference between the rider and his donkey.[26]

In the same sermon, Naḥmanides expresses his disapproval of Maimonides, who "decreases the miraculous and emphasizes the natural."[27]

22 *Hilkhot Rozeaḥ* 2:8.

23 The primacy of medical evidence in Maimonides' definition of human *tarfut* is emphasized in *Responsa Iggrot Moshe*, *Ḥoshen Mishpat* 2, no. 73.

24 *Sanhedrin* 78a, *s.v. hakol modim.*

25 See A. Steinberg, "Mercy-Killing in the Light of the Halakhah," *Sefer Assia*, ed. A. Steinberg (Jerusalem: Falk-Schlesinger Institute, 1983), vol. 3, p. 431.

26 *Torat Hashem Temimah, Kitvei Ramban*, ed. H. Chavel (Jerusalem: Mossad Harav Kook, 1963) vol. 1, p. 142.

27 *Ibid.*, p. 154.

According to Naḥmanides, all natural phenomena are concealed miracles, and it is wrong to make nature into the regnant force responsible for these phenomena.[28]

One area in which Naḥmanides' supernatural approach manifests itself is the question of the legitimacy of human healing. In his *Commentary on the Torah*,[29] Naḥmanides deals with the contradiction between the passage in the *Book of Exodus* which provides that the medical expenses of an assault victim are to be paid by his attacker,[30] thereby implying that medical treatment is an acceptable course of action for the sick, and the various passages from which it would appear that healing is a Divine prerogative. Of particular concern is the verse in *Chronicles* according to which Asa, King of Judah was criticized because "in his disease he sought not the Lord but the physicians."[31]

In order to resolve this contradiction, Naḥmanides makes a distinction between the age of prophecy, during which Israel was at a very high spiritual level, and the post-prophetic period in which the level of spirituality was much lower. In the prophetic period, the sole legitimate means for curing disease was prayer. Asa lived during the era of prophecy and ought, therefore, to have entrusted his cure to Divine rather than human hands. His reliance upon the physicians was tantamount to denying God's providence and, hence, the biblical censure of his conduct. The situation is different in the post-prophetic era, when the level of spirituality is much lower, and God has withdrawn from the healing process in favor of the human physician.

Naḥmanides does not, however, draw a hard and fast line between the prophetic and post-prophetic ages with regard to recourse to Divine healing. In the course of making a distinction between the physician's obligation to heal and that of the patient to be healed, he indicates that, even in the post-prophetic period, the spiritually inclined patient will rely on Divine rather than human healing:

> This is the intent of the Rabbis' interpretation: "And he shall cause him to be thoroughly healed — from here you deduce the

28 *Commentary on the Torah, Genesis* 17:1; *Exodus* 13:16.

29 *Leviticus* 26:11.

30 *Exodus* 21:19.

31 2 *Chronicles* 16:12.

> principle that permission has been given to the physician to heal."[32] They did not say that permission was given to the sick to be healed, but instead they stated that since the person who became sick comes to the physician to be healed, because he has accustomed himself to seeking medical help and he was not of the Congregation of the Lord whose portion is in this life, the physician should not refrain from healing him.

The general tenor of this passage suggests that even in the post-prophetic age, permission to indulge in human healing is only given to the physician, not to the patient. Ideally, a sick individual ought to strive to belong to the "Congregation of the Lord" and to rely exclusively upon the Divine Healer. In practice, however, many people will fail to attain this high standard of spirituality, and in order to ensure that their diseases will not go untreated, the human physician is given a religious mandate to heal.[33]

Naḥmanides' position, in its full-blown form, was rejected by most authorities.[34] It does, however, provide the basis for the generally accepted view that when going to the doctor, sight must never be lost of the Divine role in healing. This view is succinctly expressed in the following citation from the writings of the R. Isaiah Karelitz:

> It is necessary to strike a fine balance between reliance upon Divine providence and pursuit of the appropriate medical cure.[35]

There is also a minority view which accepts Naḥmanides' argument that human therapy is not a desideratum, even in the post-biblical period, and rules that it is permissible for a dangerously ill person to decline to eat ritually forbidden foods, even when his doctor requires

32 *Berakhot* 60a; *Bava Kamma* 85a. Also see D. Sinclair, "Non-Consensual Medical Treatment of Competent Individuals," *Tel Aviv University Studies in Law*, 1992, 11, pp. 227 ff. for a full discussion of Naḥmanides' views on this issue.

33 Naḥmanides also cites various classical texts in support of the idea that righteous conduct is the ultimate form of therapy, e.g., *Horayot* 14a; *Shir Hashirim Rabbah* 6:17.

34 See *Birkhei Yosef, Yoreh Deah* 336:2; *Shevet Yehudah, Yoreh Deah* 336; *Turei Zahav, Yoreh Deah* 336:1; *Responsa Binyan Ẓion* no. 111; *Responsa Ẓiẓ Eliezer, Ramat Raḥel* no. 20; *Responsa Yehave Daat* no. 61.

35 *Koveẓ Iggrot* no. 136. See also *Teshuva Meahavah, Yoreh Deah* 336; *Responsa Ḥatam Sofer, Oraḥ Ḥayyim* no. 177.

him to do so for therapeutic purposes. The very fact that a person chooses to trust in God rather than physicians automatically makes him one of "the Congregation of the Lord," and there is no reason to reject this course of action as an inappropriate one in the present era.[36]

Naḥmanides' position also provides the basis for R. Joseph Engel's explanation of the halakhic dictum that "a physician who causes death is liable to exile."[37] According to Jewish law, inadvertant homicide carries the penalty of exile, except in those cases in which it occurs in the course of fulfilling a religious precept (*miẓvah*) as when a father chastises his son and a teacher disciplines his student.[38] The question which arises is why the physician is not also considered to be fulfilling a precept, in the same way as a parent and teacher. R. Engel observes that since Naḥmanides regards human healing as a compromise with human spiritual frailty, rather than a recommended activity, "it is not considered a *miẓvah* to the extent of exempting a doctor who is guilty of inadvertant homicide from exile."[39] It is noteworthy that R. Engel relies upon Naḥmanides' teachings in his *Commentary on the Torah* in the context of a halakhic analysis. Presumably, he does so because of Naḥmanides' great stature as a halakhist; other Bible exegetes would not receive the same deference in the course of a legal discussion.[40] Naḥmanides also deals with the normative status of the practice of medicine in a lengthy monograph on sickness and healing, and derives it from the general obligation in Jewish law to preserve human life.[41] This monograph also preserves the distinction between the obligation of the doctor to heal and the patient to seek human therapy,

36 *Responsa Avnei Nezer, Ḥoshen Mishpat* no. 193; *Responsa Haelef Lekha Shelomo, Oraḥ Ḥayyim* no. 351.

37 Naḥmanides, *Torat Haadam, Kitvei Ramban* (cit. n.26) pp. 42–43; *Tosefta Makkot* 2:5; *Tashbeẓ* 3, no. 82; *Biur Hagra, Yoreh Deah* 336:6.

38 *Makkot* 8a; *Hilkhot Roẓeaḥ* 5:6.

39 *Gilyonei Hashas, Berakhot* 60a. According to R. Maskil-Leitan (*Yad Avraham, Yoreh Deah* 336:1), the solution lies in the fact that the physician only fulfills a *miẓvah* if the patient lives, unlike the father and teacher who fulfill a precept every time they actually chastise their respective charges. See also D. Sinclair (cit. n. 32) pp. 241–242.

40 Note the comment on Abraham ibn Ezra's lack of halakhic standing in *Tashbeẓ* 1, no. 51.

41 See n. 37 and D. Sinclair (cit. n. 32) pp. 238–239.

and the two sources are readily compatible with Naḥmanides' basic approach to the lower spiritual status of the practice of medicine as outlined above.

Naḥmanides' approach to astrology in general, and astrological cures in particular, is very different from that of Maimonides. In relation to the claim by Maimonides that the biblical prohibition on divination extends to astrology, Naḥmanides states that "the actual talmudic passage does not imply that this is the case." Indeed, he marshals other sources in order to prove that, in general, astrology is accepted as a legitimate activity in the *Talmud*.[42] Naḥmanides accepts that a miracle might be performed for someone whose fate as determined by the stars is to suffer misfortune, but does not recommend relying upon such miracles:

> If a person realizes, on the basis of astrology, that a particular day is not good for his work, he should take that realization seriously, and not rely on a miracle. Indeed, I would opine that it is prohibited to ignore astrological forecasts by relying upon miracles.[43]

Naḥmanides' approach is cited with approval by various authorities, and is incorporated in the glosses of R. Moses Isserless on the *Shulḥan Arukh*.[43]

R. Solomon ibn Adret, a student of Naḥmanides, finds support for the use of astrological cures in his teacher's use of "the image of a tongueless lion on a gold or silver plate to cure a pain in the loins." The plate had to be placed in position at the time determined by astrological calculations.[44]

42 *Shabbat* 156a–b; *Gittin* 45a; Jerusalem *Talmud, Shabbat* 6:9.

43 *Responsa Ramban* no. 282.

44 See *Nimukei Yosef, Sanhedrin* ch. 7; *Beth Yosef, Yoreh Deah* 179. R. Isserless notes that if a person knows that a certain activity is not advisable on the basis of astrology, he should avoid it, but he ought not to actively seek astrological forecasts since the ideal is to trust in God and not to consult with astrologers (*Yoreh Deah* 179:1).

4. Coercive and Alternative Medical Treatment

The differing views of Maimonides and Naḥmanides are not only of theoretical significance. The question of coercive life-saving medical treatment is discussed in both classical and modern halakhic sources.[45] In a recent article, a rabbinic commentator argues, inter alia, that medical treatment ought not to be coerced, since coercion is only applicable in the case of a *miẓvah*, and in the light of the negative view of medical therapy adopted by Naḥmanides in his Commentary on the Torah, such therapy does not constitute a *miẓvah* — for the purposes of coercion at any rate.[46] Maimonides' view of medicine is, however, a very positive one, and as a result, it is unlikely that a decision based upon his approach would yield anything other than a positive conclusion regarding the use of coercion in the context of life-saving therapy.[47]

Another area in which the different approaches of Maimonides and Naḥmanides are significant is that of alternative medicine. Maimonides' insistence upon "logical and empirical proof" clearly militates against alternative medicine which does not necessarily conform to the formal testing standards of mainline medical practice. Naḥmanides' approach, on the other hand, provides a basis for a wide range of therapies, whether or not they conform to scientific methods of testing. A practical illustration of the clash between these two approaches is the divergence of rabbinic opinion regarding homeopathic medicine. The legitimacy of this type of therapy is questioned by some authorities,[48] whilst others support "any therapy — even if it is not a rational one."[49]

An interesting illustration of this debate in the nineteenth century is the discussion of the legitimacy of hypnosis and magnetism in the halakhic tradition.[50]

45 *Responsa Rashba* 1, nos. 167, 413, 652; *Derashot Haran* no. 8.

46 S. Rafael, "Coercive Medical Treatment," *Torah Shebal Peh*, 1992, 33:74.

47 See M. Raziel, "Forcing a Patient to Accept Medical Treatment,", *Teḥumin*, 1981, 2:325; D. Sinclair (cit. n. 32) p.237.

48 G. Rabinowitz, "A Responsum Concerning Homeopathic Medicine in Jewish Law," in *Halakhah Urefuah, Vol.* 3 ed. M. Herschler (Jerusalem: 1973) p. 249.

49 See n. 7.

50 *Responsa Binyan Ẓion* no. 67.

5. Legal Reasoning in the Writings of Maimonides and Naḥmanides

An interesting parallel to the divergence of views between Maimonides and Naḥmanides in the area of medicine is provided by their different approaches to the nature of legal reasoning in Jewish law. The focus of their respective analyses is the status of laws derived by the Rabbis by virtue of the canons of juristic interpretation of the biblical text. According to Maimonides, such laws do not possess biblical status unless there is a specific talmudic tradition to that effect.[51] A major factor in Maimonides' decision to exclude laws derived by the Rabbis on this basis, would appear to be the fact that such laws are almost invariably the subject of controversy.[52] Maimonides describes the process of legal interpretation as follows:

> And of the laws which the Rabbis derived, some... became the subject of a dispute, with each side merely seeking to fortify its own position. This is often the case when interpretation by analogy is involved.[53]

The non-apodictic nature of results derived from the interpretation of legal texts figures in an early work of Maimonides on logical terms. In this work, Maimonides classifies the various forms of syllogism and specifically excludes "the legal analogy" from the proper scope of his study. For Maimonides the establishment of the logical status of any conclusion drawn in a particular reasoning process is of primary importance. Having established that the results of legal interpretation are non-apodictic and therefore inherently controversial, Maimonides excludes them from the category of biblical law, presumably on philosophical grounds.[54]

51 *Sefer Hamiẓvot*, ed. H. Chavel (Jerusalem: 1981), Second Principle.

52 *Introduction to the Mishnah* (Jerusalem: Mossad Harav Kook, 1964) p. 3; *Sefer Hamiẓvot, ibid.*

53 *Introduction to the Mishnah, ibid.*

54 "Maimonides' Treatise on Logic," *Proceedings of the American Academy for Jewish Research*, 1937–1938, 8:19; D. Sinclair, "Legal Reasoning in Maimonidean Jurisprudence," *L'Eylah*, 1990, 29:32.

Maimonides was a pioneer in the field of the jurisprudential analysis of *halakhah*, and his approach to the phenomenon of controversy in Jewish law is a good illustration of his original scholarship in this area. Maimonides' predecessors, the Gaonim, suggested that controversies arose as a result of part of the tradition having been forgotten, and were, therefore, mere exercises in its reconstruction.[55] Maimonides approaches the problem from the perspective of legal reasoning, an issue which was widely debated in classical Islamic law,[56] and reached a conclusion which was analytically sound but religiously awkward, i.e, laws derived by rabbinic exegesis did not enjoy biblical status. Maimonides does find support for his position in talmudic sources, but as he himself would be the first to admit, these could be interpreted quite differently, and his position is certainly not accepted by the majority of rabbinic thinkers.[57] The reasons for its rejection, however, may very well be polemical, since, in the words of a seventeenth century halakhic authority, "Maimonides' theory was more dangerous than it was beneficial for it leads to the conclusion that only a fraction of talmudic law originates from Sinai."[58]

Naḥmanides takes a very different position with regard to the status of the derived laws. According to Naḥmanides, all such laws are biblical, unless there is a clear talmudic statement to the effect that their status is merely rabbinic.[59] In addition to gathering support for this position from all over the *Talmud*, Naḥmanides criticizes Maimonides' view on polemical lines:

> Maimonides' position uproots great mountains in the *Talmud* and destroys mighty walls in the *gemara* (Talmudic discussion of

55 A. Halkin, "R. Saadyah Gaon's Introduction to the Torah" in *Levi Ginzberg Memorial Volume* (N.Y., 1956) p. 153; S. Abramson, "From the Fifth Chapter of R. Samuel b. Ḥofni's Introduction to the *Talmud*," *Sinai*, 1981, 88:214; G. Blidstein, "Transmission and Institutional Authority in the Oral Law," *Daat*, 1986, 16:15.

56 J. Schacht, *Introduction to Islamic Law* (Oxford: Oxford University Press, 1984) p. 21; R. Brunschvig, "Logic and Law in Classical Islam" in *Logic and Classical Islamic Culture*, ed.G. von Grunebaum (Wiesbaden: Otto Harrassowitz, 1970) p. 15; J. van Ess, *ibid.* p. 49.

57 I. Herzog, *The Main Institutions of Jewish Law* (London:1965) pp. 2–3.

58 *Responsa Ḥavat Yair* no. 162.

59 *Hassagot Haramban, Sefer Hamiẓvot*, Second Principle.

> the Mishnah). It is evil and bitter for the students of *gemara* and may it be erased from memory.[60]

It is arguable that not only does Naḥmanides differ from Maimonides with regard to the status of derived laws, but that these two talmudic Titans also disagree in relation to the status of reasoning in the context of the *halakhah*. In his glosses on the *Sefer Halakhot* of R. Isaac Alfasi, Naḥmanides makes the following statement concerning the type of reasoning required for bringing a halakhic debate to a definitive conclusion:

> There is no such thing as absolute proof in this wisdom (i.e. *gemara*) as there is in mathematics or astronomy...therefore, we devote all our energies to the rejection of one of the opinions in a dispute...and strengthen the case for adopting the other one. This is the best we can hope to achieve.[61]

Clearly, Naḥmanides does not share Maimonides' rigorous approach to legal reasoning, and accepts that the type of argument employed in halakhic debates is rhetorical rather than apodictic. The process described by Naḥmanides of strengthening one of two positions rather than looking for the logically definitive answer corresponds both to the classical Aristotelian definition of rhetorics [62] and to the modern form, which, in the context of legal reasoning, has been championed by Ch. Perelman and the New Rhetorics school of philosophy.[63]

Further analysis of the jurisprudential implications of this debate and its ramifications for Jewish law is clearly beyond the scope of the present article.[64] The short point is that legal philosophy is another area in which Maimonides and Naḥmanides disagree over the concept of rationality and its significance in the practical application of the *halakhah*.

60 *Ibid.*

61 *Milḥamot Hashem, Introduction.*

62 *Rhetorica*, Book 1, ch. 2.

63 Ch. Perelman, *The Idea of Justice and the Problem of Argumentation*, trans. J. Petrie (London: Routledge and Kegan Paul, 1963); Ch. Perelman and L. Olbrechts-Tyteca, *The New Rhetoric*, trans. J. Wilkinson and P. Weaver (South Bend: Notre Dame University Press, 1969); P. Goodrich, *Reading the Law* (Oxford: Oxford University Press, 1986) ch. 6.

64 See D. Sinclair (cit. n. 54).

6. Conclusion

The focus of the present study is the relationship between methodology and healing in the writings of two of the most influential representatives of medieval Spanish rabbinic scholarship — Maimonides and Naḥmanides. This relationship was never a simple one, and in the context of modern bioethics, it is more complex than it has been in the past. Issues such as non-consensual medical treatment and alternative medicine are just two of the areas in which it poses pressing contemporary problems. Experimental therapy and non-certified treatments are two other issues in this general rubric which have come before legal tribunals and have provoked much discussion in both popular and academic circles. Hopefully, the above outline of the problem will, notwithstanding its mainly medieval context, prove to be illuminating in a modern context as well.

Ethical Perspectives in the Care of Infants in Sixteenth to Eighteenth Century Spain

Rosa Ballester

This paper discusses specific aspects of the doctor-patient relationship in pediatrics. A historical analysis of this subject from an ethical point of view must take into account two different aspects: the first is the prevailing ideas about the biological nature of the child's body in Spanish medical books between the sixteenth and eighteenth centuries. This question is crucial in understanding diagnostic and therapeutic practice, especially the different ways of dealing with pediatric illnesses and the strategies used. In addition, it is necessary to consider social attitudes about the health and welfare of children, including modern and traditional ideologies of childhood, the principles of Christian ethics relevant to them; and the development of modern conceptions of childhood.

The historical sources used in this paper are the medical works printed in Spain between the sixteenth and eighteenth centuries which deal with the study of infancy. At that time, pediatrics did not yet exist as a specialty, and the main body of work is made up of texts on childhood illnesses and children's health and welfare. Together, these works make up a coherent and homogeneous doctrine.[1] I have also studied other medical texts which offer additional information, such

1 J.M. López Piñero, F. Bujosa, *Los tratados de enfermedades infantiles en la España del Renacimiento* (Valencia: Cátedra de Historia de la Medicina, Universidad de Valencia, 1982). This book provides both a selection of pediatric sources and a critical historical analysis of Spanish Renaissance works on pediatrics. A brief history of Spanish pediatrics is L.S. Granjel, *Historia de la Pediatría Española* (Salamanca: Universidad de Salamanca, 1965). See also R. Ballester, "Factores biológicos y actitudes vigentes frente a la infancia en la sociedad española del Antiguo Régimen," *Asclepio*, 1984, *35*:343–357.

as books on obstetrics or general medicine. The chronological distribution of these publications shows a substantial albeit variable rate of increase of publication. The first systematic texts date from the first half of the sixteenth century, but the main body of work was published between the last decades of that century and the first decades of the following one. The works of Pérez Cascales[2] and Luís Mercado[3] are the most learned of this period, and Mercado's was undoubtedly the most influential and the most often quoted. However, during the course of the eighteenth century, systematic monographic pediatric texts did not appear, although there are references to the topic in works on general medicine.[4] At the same time, there are numerous texts on hygiene and breastfeeding in which their physical and moral role in the life of the child is of primary importance. Medical texts appeared in both Latin and Spanish, with an increasing proportion of the latter in the more modern books. Moreover, Spanish was used in the practical texts, which offered simple therapeutic rules and basic advice on hygiene, and was the language used to spread knowledge beyond the medical profession.

2 F. Pérez Cascales de Guadalajara (*fl.* 1611), *Liber de affectionibus puerorum, una cum tractata de morbo illo vulgariter Garrotillo apellato, cum duabus Quaestionibus...* (Madrid, 1611). See the bibliography of works by this author in A. Carreras Panchón, "Pérez Cascales y la clínica del garrotillo," *Asclepio* 1978–79, *30–31*:319–322.

3 L. Mercado (1525–1611), *De Puerorum educatione, custodia et providentia; atque de morborum qui ipsis accidunt, curatione* (Valladolid, 1611). For Mercado's ideas on the health and diseases of children, see also *De mulierum affectionibus. Libri Quatuor... Quartus, puerperarum & nutricum accedentia, ad unquem exequitur liber quartus* (Valladolid, 1579) especially chapters XV to XIX; idem, "De recta victus administrationem," in *Institutiones Medicae iussu Regio factae pro Medicis in praxi examinandi* (Madrid, 1594). For a bibliography of Mercado's works, see J. Riera, *Vida y obra de Luís Mercado* (Salamanca: Seminario de Historia de la Medicina, 1968); R. Ballester, "La utilización de los clásicos en la obra pediátrica de Luís Mercado (1525–1611)," *Asclepio*, 1978, *30–31*:307–318.

4 Cf. F. Rubio, *Arte de conocer y curar las enfermedades por reglas de observación y experiencias para la juventud médica* (Madrid, 1761). G. Casal (1680–1759), *Historia Natural y Médica del Principado de Asturias* (Madrid, 1762).

The image of the body and the moral qualities of the child in medical works

This collection of basic sources makes it possible to speak of a biological model with clearly defined characteristics for the stages of life. This model, which was widely accepted, was influential beyond the purely medical sphere, and affected other areas of intellectual and social life. It was originally a scholastic model, but it was modified throughout the period under study. The model includes a series of *loci communes* such as the ages of man, the nature of the child in sickness and health, means for the preservation of health, and the attitude of the doctor when faced with dilemmas resulting from the doctor-patient relationship.

The ages of man.[5] The authors of the works analyzed outline the contents of their works according to the principles of the ancient world. In the Greek concept of human nature,[6] infancy is the phase of development which comes before man realizes his full potential in what Plato calls "youth" and Socrates "maturity." In this second phase, the growth process is complete and the diminution or decrease has not yet started. Therefore, in this age human nature reaches maximum perfection and man is really a 'natural' being.

From this point of view, human beings cannot be considered either healthy, beautiful or good until they reach maturity and their nature achieves perfection. Children are not healthy because their constitution lacks temperance, they are not beautiful because they have not fully developed, and they are not good, as according to the humoral theory, there cannot be a good soul in an intemperate body. The child is thus inherently lacking in virtue.

5 For the connotations of the term "edades de la vida" ("ages of life"), see D. Gracia, J.L. Vidal, "La *Isagoge* de Ioannitius: introducción, edición, traducción y notas," *Asclepio*, 1974–75, *26–27*:267–382.

6 Hippocrates, *De la génération. De la nature de l'enfant*, ed. and trans. R. Joly (Paris: Societé d'Edition "Les Belles Lettres," 1970); Plato, *Obras completas* (Madrid: Aguilar, 1972); Aristotle, *Retórica. Etica a Nicomaco* (Madrid: Aguilar, 1964); T. Linacre, *Claudi Galeni Pergameni De sanitate tuenda libri sex...* (Lyon, 1559); P. Laín Entralgo, *La medicina hipocrática* (Madrid: Revista de Occidente, 1970); L. García-Ballester, *Galeno* (Madrid: Guadarrama, 1972).

The life cycle is understood as a continuous path from the formation of the embryo until death. The course of life is ordered into different ages, each of them with its own different virtue. These works frequently make use of the Aristotelian image of childhood as covering the period between birth and the seventh year. At this point, the child has a warm and humid constitution similar to that of the seeds from which he was created. Between the seventh and fourteenth years, the warmth continues, although the humidity decreases. As a result of Stoic influence, the childhood phase is occasionally extended to the fourteenth year, when the procreative capacity begins. The names used for the different phases of growth are varied. In ordinary language, newly-born and breastfed children are "niños," those who cannot speak are "infantes," and those who have learned to speak are "parvulos."[7] These differences are, however, more of form than of content, and most of the literature is dedicated to newly-born children and to small children below the age of seven. There are very few references to older children, who are grouped with the adults.

Concepts relating to the nature of children

The Aristotelian-Galenic tradition considers the child to be intemperate in constitution because its body is warm and humid, properties which make it corruptible.[8] In contrast to women, who are also imperfect because of their coldness and humidity, the child is perfectible. Although the warmth persists as it grows, the humidity, an excess of which is harmful above all to the brain, disappears.

When treating children, the great problem confronting the doctor is the weakness which stems from the child's imperfect nature. This weakness is constantly demonstrated and causes "nervios molificados"[9] (softened nerves) and "débiles osezillos" (weak little bones). In addi-

7 S. de Covarrubias (1611), *Tesoro de la lengua castellana o española* (Madrid: Turner, 1979).

8 Mercado, *De Puerorum educatione* (cit. n. 3), pp. 23–24.

9 Luis Lobera de Avila (*fl.* 1530), *Libro del regimiento de salud y de la esterilidad de hombres y mujeres y de las enfermedades de los niños* (Valladolid, 1551), ch. XXIII.

tion, the bones of the skull are so soft that hydrocephalus[10] may easily appear and the eyelids are so soft that the eyes, as is shown below, are liable to 'fascination' and bewitchment.[11] Most of the problems are due to the excess of humidity, which makes the tissues as soft as wax.

In etymological and conceptual terms, to be a child is to be ill. The natural faculties and vegetative functions dominate the corporal side, while the rational functions of imagination, thought and memory are barely developed at birth. Children have a strong natural virtue[12] which is necessary for growth, and the process of growth makes them voracious.[13] Nevertheless, as Diego Gracia has pointed out,[14] a detailed study of the ancient texts changes the statement that, although the child is ill, weak, and has an intemperate constitution, he is totally natural. The child belongs instead to the poorly defined area of neutrality,[15] and is a "neutral thing" heading almost infallibly for illness and vice unless directed, by means of a strict *paideia*[16] of body and soul, to corporal health and moral goodness.

What properties define the condition of the soul in infancy? The most widely-read work is Aristotle's *Rhetoric*, which states that greed dominates the souls of children and leads to the most significant characteristics of their behavior. They avoid pain and search for anything which provides pleasure; they are determined to do only those things which appeal to them. They are moody and care only for those who allow them to follow their whims. Their souls also tend to overexcitement and irritability and as a result, they cry, laugh and

10 C. Pérez de Herrera (1558–ca. 1618), *Defensa de las criaturas de tierna edad y algunas dudas y advertencias cerca de la curación y conservación de su salud... Traduzido por el mesmo Autor de otro que escribio en la lengua latina* (Valladolid, 1604), pp. 8–9.

11 Pérez Cascales, "Quaestio de fascinatione" (cit. n. 2), pp. 120–129.

12 Lobera de Avila, *Libro del regimiento* (cit. n. 9), ch. XXIII.

13 Pérez Cascales, *Liber de affectionibus puerorum* (cit. n. 2), ch. XXXV; G. Soriano (*fl.* 1598), *Methodo y orden de curar las enfermedades de los niños* (Zaragoza, 1600), ch. IV; C. Carles, *Glosario médico de la obra de Gerónimo Soriano* (Valencia: Tesis de Licenciatura, 1977).

14 D. Gracia, "¿Es el niño un ser enfermo?," *Jano*, 1985, *662-H*: 801–814.

15 For a theoretical discussion of this "neutrality," see Mercado, "De morbis puerorum ac de eorum curatione," in *De Puerorum educatione* (cit. n. 3), Lib. II, p. 23.

16 W. Jaeger, *Paideia. Los ideales de la cultura griega* (México: Fondo de Cultura Económica, 1957).

chatter and are neither prudent nor constant. Their spiritual constitution prevents them from understanding or distinguishing good from bad until the age of seven, nor can they accept rational arguments. They have a great capacity for learning, but find it difficult to remember the acquired knowledge, as their minds are busy with games and superfluous things. Their positive characteristics are generosity and innocence, which make them easily manageable. In the case of young girls, the pleasant and affectionate aspect is emphasized, though they are frivolous and envious and their hearts fickle and deceitful.[17] Although this description might suggest the intrinsic "immorality" of infancy, a more appropriate term would be "moral neutrality." Infants have a natural tendency to intemperance which may be redirected through the use of an intelligent *paideia.*

In summary, the foundations of the physical and moral concepts of infancy in the works of Spanish writers of the modern era may be found in the works of ancient and orthodox science. However, it is also necessary to consider the introduction of a series of innovations throughout the period under review and particularly in the eighteenth century.

Profile of the ideal doctor

A constant theme in these sources is the image of the doctor responsible for the health of children. There are two aspects to this theme: the qualities essential to a perfect doctor and the doctor as defender and protector of infancy and his role in the moral upbringing of the child.

The conditions which a good doctor must fulfill

There are several conditions or qualities required in order to achieve perfection in the difficult art of providing medical care for the youngest members of society. Some of these conditions are the same as those required in the care of adults,[18] but must be adapted to the relations between doctor and child.

17 Mercado, *De Puerorum educatione* (cit. n. 3), p. 22; D. Carbón (*fl.* 1541), *Libro del arte de las comadres o madrinas y del regimiento de las preñadas y paridas y de los niños* (Palma de Mallorca, 1541), fol. LXXXVIII.

18 P. Laín Entralgo, *La relación médico-enfermo. Historia y teoría* (Madrid: Revista

The doctor must be learned (docto), or, in other words, *erudite* and *wise*;[19] he must be erudite because he needs to know the relevant works of the ancient and modern authors, and wise because the diagnosis and treatment of children involves greater difficulties than that of adults. With children, the doctor must guess or use his intuition to decide things about the nature of the illness which cannot be determined through the signs.[20] Wisdom consists mainly of reaching knowledge through causes, foreseeing developments, and acting accordingly. Nevertheless, these qualities are of no use if the doctor is not *experienced* and *practical*,[21] so that he will have greater self-confidence in his decisions and better results in his actions. In addition, he also needs *clear judgment* and to take special care in his prognosis if he wishes to avoid problems as a result of his errors and misjudgments, as "it is dangerous to seek by obscure and dubious conjectures to cure such feeble patients, whose tenderness and weakness does not permit any error of treatment without it costing their lives."[22] It is also stressed that the doctor must have a complete and substantial knowledge of the religious truths. Apart from being learned, experienced and prudent, the doctor must be a *good Christian*,[23] and must have two virtues: charity, the fundamental norm of behavior toward those in need,[24] and, above all, compassion.[25] The ill child appears as the most defenceless of the defenceless and as the poorest of the poor. As a pious

de Occidente, 1964); I. David Peyré, *Le personnage du médecin et la relation médecin-malade dans la littérature ibérique, XVI et XVII siècle* (Paris: Ed. Hispanoamericana, 1971). L.S. Granjel, *El ejercicio medico y otros capítulos de la medicina española* (Salamanca: Universidad, 1974); J.M. López Piñero, *Ciencia y técnica en la sociedad española de los siglos XVI y XVII* (Barcelona: Labor, 1979); L. García-Ballester, *Los moriscos y la medicina. Un capítulo de la medicina y la ciencia marginales en la España del siglo XVI* (Barcelona: Labor, 1984).

19 Soriano, *Methodo y orden* (cit. n. 13), p. 92; Pérez Cascales, *Liber de affectionibus puerorum* (cit. n. 2), ch. XXXV, p. 11.

20 Mercado, *De Puerorum educatione* (cit. n. 3), p. 26.

21 Soriano, *Methodo y orden* (cit. n. 13), p. 51.

22 Pérez de Herrera, *Defensa de las criaturas* (cit. n. 10), p.8.

23 Pérez de Herrera, *Defensa de las criaturas* (cit. n. 10), p. 9.

24 Carbón, *Libro del arte de las comadres* (cit. n. 17), fol. II.

25 Pérez de Herrera, *Defensa de las criaturas* (cit. n. 10), p. 5; Soriano, *Methodo y orden* (cit. n. 13), p. 9.

Christian, the doctor has a greater obligation than would a non-Christian to do what is right and just in order to restore health. Among his Christian duties, he is obliged to spread his knowledge to other doctors and medical students who, for lack of experience in the field, might require it,[26] and also to the layman in order to avoid as many mistakes as possible.[27] The latter case refers directly, or indirectly through more or less knowledgeable intermediaries, to midwives, mothers and wet-nurses. The use of the vernacular proved to be most appropriate in conveying information to the layman.[28]

In all these tasks the doctor is not alone, as he can count on the best of all assistance, that of God and the Holy Mother,[29] the Virgin Mary. The doctor finds his true dignity within the religious context, as God himself decided that human nature is prone to illness, and thus the doctor is needed in order to discover causes and ascertain the correct treatment.[30] The role of the doctor in society is enhanced precisely by this divine support.[31] On the other hand, he is much more guilty if, through ignorance, greed or simple lack of interest, he makes mistakes, especially if these lead, as can easily happen given the fragility of the infant, to the death of the patient.

26 Mercado, *De Puerorum educatione* (cit. n. 3), p. 26; Soriano, "Al lector," *Methodo y orden* (cit. n. 13); Carbo, *Libro del arte de las comadres* (cit. n. 17), fol. II; Pérez de Herrera, "A los Caballeros Procuradores de Cortes de los Reyes de Castilla," *Defensa de las criaturas* (cit. n. 10).

27 Soriano, *Methodo y orden* (cit. n. 13), p. 51.

28 J. Alonso y de los Ruizes de Fontecha, *Diez previlegios para las mujeres preñadas... Con un diccionario médico (de los nombre de piedras, plantas, fructos, yerbas, flores, enfermedades, causas y accidentes)* (Alcalá de Henares, 1606); E. Perdiguero, "The popularization of medicine during the Spanish Enlightenment," in *The popularization of medicine 1650–1850*, ed. R. Porter (London/New York: Routledge, 1991).

29 Soriano, *Methodo y orden* (cit. n. 13), ch. XI, p. 124; Pérez de Herrera, "A los señores Procuradores," *Defensa de las criaturas* (cit. n. 10). Pérez Cascales, F. "Ad lectorem," *Liber de affectionibus puerorum* (cit. n. 13).

30 Carbón, *Libro del arte de las comadres* (cit. n. 17), fol. XV, CXXXX.

31 "Estando Natura sugeta a enfermedades fue necesario el medico para entender las causas y proveer en la cura dellas," Carbón, *Libro del arte de las comadres* (cit. n. 17), ch. XII, pp. 138, 229.

The doctor in the moral upbringing of the child

The nature of infancy in the classical world included the capacity of the infant to be directed and educated. The doctrines of the Christian faith, especially in connection with the Patristic tradition, introduced new elements. The child was of unquestionable value as one of God's creatures, but his ignorance, uncontrollable passions and lack of judgment made him weak and liable to sin. Adults must therefore treat children both pragmatically and with moral zeal in order to place them on the path to virtue. Discipline and punishment are part of this process, as they are necessary for the good of the child. Instruction, habits and discipline make up the traditional fundamental pedagogical triad.

In opposition to this scholastic framework, the pedagogues,[32] who leaned more and more toward the natural sciences, opened a new path with a complete *Doctrina pueri* initiated by humanists such as Erasmus of Rotterdam and Luis Vives. This doctrine would eventually help produce the ideas of the Enlightenment. One of the characteristics of modernity may be found in the change of social attitudes toward infancy. It is now considered a "tabula rasa" with the possibility of improvement due to its plasticity, and as the genuine source of the future of humanity.

The medical literature which deals with the care of children[33] clearly reflects the prevailing ideologies in a way which respects plurality and is not without contradictions. This can be seen, for example, in traditionally-oriented works such as those of Pérez Cascales and above all those of Luís Mercado, which include modern features of doctor-patient relations.

What role should the medical professional play in the upbringing of infants? The title of a book by Luís Mercado, *De puerorum educatione, custodia et providentia*, provides some indications as to his role. The

32 Th. Ballauf, *Pädagogik. Eine Geschichte der Bildung und Erziehung. Band II. Vom 16. Jahrhundert bis zum 19. Jahrhundert* (Freiburg/München: Verlag Karl Alber, 1970); I. Gutierrez Zuloaga, *Historia de la educación* (Madrid: Eiter, 1970).

33 E. Seidler, "El desarrollo de la Pediatra moderna," in *Historia Universal de la Medicina*, ed. P. Laín Entralgo, 7 vols. (Barcelona: Salvat, 1981), vol. VI, pp. 203–212.

doctor takes part both in the correct care and feeding of the child and also in his training, instruction and teaching. His role as guardian includes vigilance and action in the preservation of health and is closely linked to providence, which involves the prevention of those things which threaten the harmony of nature and which may lead to illness. The doctor must instruct, protect and care for the life of the child from the very moment of birth or even before. This idea appears in the works which belong to the mother-infant tradition, where emphasis is placed on the care of the pregnant woman. However, references to hygiene during pregnancy also appear in books which deal only with pediatrics, where emphasis is placed on the child. The doctor is to care for the health of both the body and the soul. The doctrinal basis for his actions is the dietetic tradition, above all the works of Galen. In order to preserve the health of the child, the doctor must maintain the balance between the qualities of the child's constitution, and therefore ensure the normality of the functions conditioned by this balance. This balance is achieved through the regulation of the *sex res non naturales*, which have special connotations in the case of infants.[34] The Christianization of these doctrinal assumptions includes a series of moralizing components which are discussed below and a certain perspective on the child's soul. The soul is immortal due to its divine origins: "at the very moment that the creature is formed, God endows this body, shaped in His own image and likeness, with an immortal soul."[35] The human soul, with its faculties of memory,

34 On this classical concept, see H. Schipperges, *Lebendige Heilkunde* (Olten/Freiburg, 1962); S. Jarcho, "Galen's six non naturals: a bibliographic note and translation," *Bulletin of the History of Medicine*, 1970, *44*:372–377; L.J. Rather, "The Six Things Non-Natural. A note on the origin and fate of a doctrine and a phrase," *Clio Medica*, 1968, *3*:337–347; L. García-Ballester, "On the Origin of the 'six non-natural things' in Galen," in *Galen und das Hellenistische Erbe*, ed. J. Kollesch and D. Nickel (Stuttgart: Franz Steiner Vg., 1993). pp. 105–115. The most systematic and learned exposition on this topic is L. Mercado, *Tomus primus Operum... De veritate et recta ratione principiorum ac theorematum, et rerum omnium, quae in Medica Facultate tractantur: in tres libros divisus... Liber secundus, De sanitate et de arte ipsam conservandi ac praecavendi* (Pintiae, 1604), pp. 743–882. Mercado uses both "rebus non naturalibus" and "causa conservans sanitatis."

35 Carbón, *Libro del arte de las comadres* (cit. n. 17), fol. XV.

understanding and will, is still undeveloped in these first stages of life, and the role of education is to induce the consolidation of these faculties.

The close interactions between body and soul make it necessary to be especially careful in controlling one of the six non-natural elements: the passions of the mind. All of the works studied include recommendations on how to acquire virtues and avoid vices. During breast-feeding, the fundamental question is how to avoid a tendency to overeating. This tendency makes children demanding, and an excessive fullness of the stomach may harm them.[36] It is also important to provide peace and tranquillity in the form of music and gentle rocking in the cradle rather than in the arms of mothers or wet-nurses.[37] This will prevent children from becoming accustomed to excessive pampering and affection.[38] Once the breast-feeding phase is finished, it becomes necessary to act with greater vigor, as "at these ages when they accept neither warning nor reason, it is vital to accustom them to obeying, as in this way the passions of the mind submit to reason. It is necessary to create new habits and discipline and above all to develop modesty and obedience." The behavior of the children and their acquisition of skills must be corrected in accordance with their constitutions and social status so that they may fulfill their roles as human beings and as God's creatures.[39]

The advice given by doctors for the care of children over two years of age includes education for proper behavior and correct relations with adults. It ranges from table manners (children must eat what they are given without complaint, not be greedy, nor ask for more food) to the way children should be treated[40] by the teachers to whom they are entrusted starting at the age of seven. Some authors explicity base this part of their work on the new pedagogical trends, and include a highly detailed prescriptive orientation. The pedagogical concern for infancy

36 Soriano, *Methodo y orden* (cit. n. 13), ch. IV.

37 Mercado, *De Puerorum educatione* (cit. n. 3), p. 22; Pérez de Herrera, *Defensa de las criaturas* (cit. n. 10), p. 13, 42; Carbón, *Libro del arte de las comadres* (cit. n. 17), fol. LV.

38 *Ibid.*

39 *Ibid.*

40 *Ibid.*, fol. LXXXVIII, LXXXX.

had important representatives in Spain of the modern era, as in the works of Hervás y Panduro[41] and especially those of Huarte de San Juan[42] and his theory of 'talent' as an individual attribute of man for a certain activity. Among the recommendations of the latter is to "maintain the ingenuity of children after creation and birth." His reasoning, however, is orthodox Galenism following Galen's own treatise as analyzed by García-Ballester, *Quod animi moris corporis temperamenta sequantur*, or the faculties of the soul originate from the humoral constitution of the body.[43]

The moral education of those who care for the child

The role of the doctor also includes dealing with the people who participate in the care of children, particularly parents, wet-nurses and midwives. Without their collaboration it would be difficult to achieve not only that perfection of body and soul which is the goal of education, but even, in many cases, the very survival of the child. The doctor is thus needed to protect the life of the child against calamities caused by adults. Condemnations of negligent parents, careless wet-nurses and inept midwives and surgeons who lack a Christian conscience frequently appear in the texts. The moral aspects of maternal or mercenary breast-feeding are especially relevant in the case of mothers and wet-nurses, and the subject is raised in all of the texts studied. This question is of crucial importance as it deals with religious and cultural issues in addition to the strictly medical ones.

The mother has a fundamental role in the moral upbringing of her child, and should follow the example of the Virgin Mary, who personally fed and cared for her divine Son. God wished to be born as a child,

41 L. Hervás y Panduro (1735–1809), *Historia de la vida del hombre o idea del Universo* (Madrid, 1789).

42 J. Huarte de San Juan (1529-1588), Examen de ingenios para las sciencias, en la qual el lector hallara la manera de su ingenio para escoger la sciencia en que mas a de aprovechar. Y la differencia de habilidades que hay en los hombres y el genero de letras y artes que cada uno responde en particular (Baeza, 1594).

43 L. García-Ballester, "Soul and body. Diseases of the soul and diseases of the body in Galen's medical thought," in *Le opere psichologiche di Galeno*, eds. P. Manuli and M. Vegetti (Naples, 1988), pp. 117–158.

and became incarnate in a specific woman at a particular time. His humanity comes from His mother; through her He became human. The importance of both spiritual and biological maternity are emphasized. Breast-feeding plays an important role in both aspects, as mother's milk is not only the sole natural and proper food for the child, but also forms the beginning of its Christian education. Physical maternity is extolled as essential in the civic and Christian training of the child. It is the vocation of every woman, and especially that of every virtuous Christian woman who as such must serve God and her husband.[44]

The defense of maternal rather than mercenary breast-feeding is an important subject which recurs in all the texts and indicates an important social problem in Europe during the modern era. Foster mothers or wet-nurses took care not only of the children of the more privileged classes, but also of those of the urban small business and artisanal middle class. These women were also needed for the care of abandoned children in orphanages, where the mortality rate was very high.[45]

The medical explanation used to persuade mothers to feed their own children is the principle of likeness. The menstrual blood retained during the months of pregnancy provides the material substratum from which the new being is formed. The milk flowing from the mother's breasts after childbirth also comes from this blood after a transformation in which it undergoes a double process of concoction. Maternal breast-feeding is thus more conducive to the development of the child, as this nourishment is more easily converted into a substance of the child's nature. The doctors supplement this theoretical argument with empirical criteria, for experience clearly shows the advantage of mother's milk over any substitute, including another woman's milk.[46]

44 C. Atkinson, *The Oldest Vocation. Christian Motherhood in the Middle Ages* (Ithaca/London: Cornell University Press, 1991).

45 A. Carreras Panchón, *El problema del niño expósito en la España Ilustrada* (Salamanca: Universidad de Salamanca, 1978); J. Sherwood, *Poverty in Eighteenth Century Spain. The Women and Children of the Incluse* (Toronto: University of Toronto Press, 1988), especially "The exposito as a patient: the medicalization of the Incluse," pp. 150–173.

46 L. Mercado, *De Puerorum educatione* (cit. n. 3) p. 2; Alonso y de los Ruizes de Fontecha, *Diez previlegios para las mujeres preñadas* (cit. n. 28), p. 170; Pérez Cascales, *Liber de affectionibus puerorum* (cit. n. 2), p. 3; F. Flores, *Regimiento de Sanidad* (Sevilla, 1541); F. Nuñes de Oria (*fl.* 1569–1580) *Regimiento y aviso*

These scientific arguments provide decisive support for the theological, moral and social arguments. The references in the texts are unanimously and strongly in favor of maternal breast-feeding. With the passing of time, this advice is given with ever greater firmness, and women who do not follow it are explicitly criticized. The very titles of some books or chapters are highly expressive, such as the works of Gutiérrez de Godoy, *Three discourses to show that women of good health are obliged to feed their children at their own breast (1629)* and Jaime Bonells, *Harm occasioned to the human race and to the condition of mothers who refuse to breast-feed their children (1786).*[47]

This moralizing discourse includes numerous testimonies of ancient authors and famous historical figures in favor of breast-feeding and uses strong language to condemn those women who neglect it. The most frequently used adjectives are impious and cruel, and these women are placed below the brute animals which care for their offspring; they are more savage than the cruelest beasts. They leave their children in the hands of strangers; the milk of others can cause illness; these are depraved customs and sinful habits.[48]

Medicine provides biological arguments which were accepted by theologians and moralists. At the same time, religious discourse also had a great influence on the question of breast-feeding. Religion and science join forces to achieve the same end, and in this way reinforce their mutual objective. There is thus a more or less detailed list of

de Sanidad que trata de todos los géneros de alimentos y del regimiento della. Agora nuevamente añadido y corregido... Tratado del uso de las mujeres y como sea dañino y como provechoso (Medina del Campo, 1586), ch. 49, p. 157; B. Alvarez de Miravall (*fl.* 1597), *Libro intitulado de la conservación de la salud del cuerpo y del alma para el buen regimiento de la salud...* (Salamanca, 1601), ch. IX, p. 37; Mercado, *De mulierum affectionibus* (cit. n. 3), pp. XVI, 533; Mercado, *De Puerorum educatione* (cit. n. 3), Lib. I, p. 4; Pérez Cascales, *Liber de affectionibus puerorum* (cit. n. 2), p. 3.

47 J. Gutiérrez de Godoy (1579–1656), *Tres discursos para probar que estan obligadas a criar a sus hijos a sus pechos todas las madres quando tienen buena salud, fuerças y buen temperamento, buena leche y suficiente para alimentarlos* (Jaen, 1629); J. Bonells (*fl.* 1779–1800), *Perjuicios que acarrean al genero humano y al Estado las madres que rehusan criar a sus hijos* (Madrid, 1786).

48 T. de Montalvo, *Práctica politica y económica de expósitos* (Granada, 1701), ch. XXVIII, pp. 291–295.

legitimate and illegitimate causes[49] for exempting women from the obligation of breast-feeding. The latter include two different types. One is the social mores among "Queens and illustrious ladies" which lead them to use a wet-nurse so as not to harm their dignity through the "indecency" or "lack of decorum" in exposing their breasts. The counter-example is the Virgin Mary, Queen of Queens and Lady of Ladies, whose dignity was increased by breast-feeding her Son. The practice of lactation is not only an act of virtue, but is also an act of justice and charity for the weak. Another unacceptable reason is the suppression of lactation so that the woman may become pregnant again, as it is forbidden to obtain good through a morally reproachable act.

Despite the general condemnation, there are legitimate causes which exempt a mother from breast-feeding her child. In this group of causes, the bond between medical and moral doctrines is even stronger. For example, one legitimate cause is the illness or weak constitution of the mother,[50] but this concept is broadly interpreted; if the father is Catholic and the mother an infidel or heretic, he must prevent her from breast-feeding the child, as she is spiritually ill. Moral arguments and questions of social convenience are also given when breast-feeding might provide a "source of scandal," as in the case of maids or widows "of honest reputation." The literature on foundlings devotes ample space to this subject, especially those texts written by members of religious orders. The degree of guilt also varies according to personal circumstances and cause. Thus, the sin committed is mortal in all cases of illegitimate causes, but only if the parents' obligations toward the child are completely abandoned. On the other hand, if the choice of wet-nurse is correct and the welfare of the child is taken into consideration, then the sin is venial. The Church completely forgives all the cases where there is a legitimate cause, but the parents must still be aware that a bad wet-nurse may corrupt a child born to virtuous parents.

Luís Mercado[51] authoritatively affirmed that while women who have no justifiable cause for not wishing to feed their children are guilty, this guilt is diminished if they at least take the trouble to find a

49 *Ibid.*
50 Carbón, *Libro del arte de las comadres* (cit. n. 17), fol. LVI.
51 Mercado, *De Puerorum educatione* (cit. n. 3), p. 3.

proper wet-nurse. All of the doctors agree, and it seems that they go farther than do the theologians in defence of maternal breast-feeding, as for them medical arguments and those in defense of young children are more important than questions of social convenience.

Despite their objections to the practice, the social importance of *mercenary breast-feeding*[52] was such that the doctors offer scientific arguments to help the parents in the important task of choosing a wet-nurse. They had the last word in this decision as experts in practice and because of the rich medical tradition which had developed since ancient times.

The advice of these experts again offers a series of practical rules based on the doctrines of Galenic-traditional medicine, in which physical qualities such as strength, build, skin color, smell and youth are combined with highly detailed moral qualities. These latter qualities include being acquiescent, modest, prudent, calm, gentle and kind, and not being irascible, sad, or excessively merry; above all, emphasis is placed on honesty and the avoidance of lust.

Control of the wet-nurse's sexuality during the period of breast-feeding is another important point in all of these sources. She should avoid all sexual practice during this time, as her milk will otherwise be of poorer quality since nature uses the purest blood in the formation of the fetus. The need for abstinence is also related to non-natural elements such as the passions of the mind, since sexual encounters arouse the emotions and affect the milk, which is then no longer suitable for the child. In this case, the food is not assimilated, the milk becomes putrid, irritates the expulsive faculty of the organ and easily produces vomiting. The doctor must not trust the word of the wet-nurse but must personally verify that the development of the child is normal. Ignoring the medical advice relating to the management of the wet-nurse, which includes a minutely detailed description of the regulation of the six non-natural elements of these women, represents a serious and sinful act of irresponsibility because of the harmful effects this negligence might have on the child. A systematic study of medical texts for all the illnesses which affect children indicates that almost all of the

52 Carbón, *Libro del arte de las comadres* (cit. n. 17), ch. XXXIIII; Mercado, *De Puerorum educatione* (cit. n. 3), pp. 519–528; Soriano, *Methodo y orden* (cit. n. 13), ch. XXX; Lobera de Avila, *Libro del regimiento de salud* (cit. n. 9).

ailments connected to the period of breast-feeding and even later are attributed directly or indirectly, as the sole cause or as a contributing cause, to the incorrect life-style of the wet-nurse, particularly to an incorrect diet. This list ranges from serious ailments such as epilepsy to less important problems, such as chafing of the skin. The following paragraph sums up the situation: "there are some wet-nurses who are so gluttonous and greedy... that they do not hesitate to eat whatever (they want), be it garlic, onions, salted fish, and then afterwards they drink as they will, not a drop of water (but wine). No wonder the milk they give is bitter and pungent and the urine of the children corrodes and chafes the skin."[53]

In addition to mothers and wet-nurses, midwives also required the advice of doctors. In this context, I make use of the three ways or paths which a person may take in order to solve his health problems.[54] The first path, extremely important in the present case, is that which deals with the domestic environment. This path includes not only the family but also the advice and actions of people close to the patient who have no professional medical status but who offer first aid based on existing empirical traditions. In this period, most decisions on problems of infant health are made in this environment, and this area is directly involved in the making of ethical decisions. It is also fundamental in the contacts the child patient may have with the other two paths: the highly complex popular sector, which includes a wide range of non-institutionalized empiricists and healers, and the professional medical sector.

In recent years, a number of historical studies have dealt with this subject, and have revealed that important changes were made in the

53 Soriano, *Methodo y orden* (cit. n. 13), p. 233; Pérez Cascales, *Liber de affectionibus puerorum* (cit. n. 2), pp. 3, 48, 51; F. Nuñez de Oria, *Libro del parto humano en el qual se contienen remedios muy utiles y usuales para el parto dificultoso de las mugeres. Con otros muchos secretos a ello pertenecientes y a las enfermedades de los niños* (Alcalá de Henares, 1580), pp. 240–241, 246–247; R. Ballester, "La utilización de los clásicos en la obra pediátrica de Luís Mercado," in *Actas V Congreso Nacional de Historia de la Medicina* (Madrid: Sociedad Española de Historia de la Medicina, 1978) vol. II, pp. 307–318; López Piñero, Bujosa, *Los tratados de enfermedades infantiles* (cit. n. 1).

54 A. Kleinman, *Patients and healers in the context of culture* (Berkeley: University of California Press, 1980).

health care of mothers and children during the modern era in Europe. These changes led to the almost complete medicalization of their care. The third medical path achieved growing and today almost complete hegemony over the care for sick children to the detriment of the other two paths, which traditionally played an important role.

This growing medicalization provided the context for the relations between doctors and midwives. The latter women belonged to the domestic environment and were traditionally in charge of both childbirth and the care of the newborn. J. Gélis[55] has described for France and Spain how the competences which society attributed to these women were eventually taken over by the doctors. The latter controlled the activities and training of the midwives, either directly in the hospitals or indirectly through works designed to teach this occupation, which was considered a "trade belonging to the mechanical arts, because the operation is manual." The sixteenth and seventeenth-eighteenth centuries demonstrate the initial stage of this attempt at control, and the texts often consider this struggle for professional competencies. There are constant allusions to the lack of skill, lack of knowledge and all types of errors made by the midwives. However, there is also an attempt to redirect their activities and even, in some cases and not always explicitly, to let the midwives use traditional remedies which cannot harm the patients. The authors hope that the expert advice of the doctor will bring the midwife to understand the necessity of certain operations with which she is not familiar and of scientific explanations for procedures which she has previously employed. It was important that the midwives understand that their cultural and social proximity to the families they treated allowed them to gain the trust of the families and made them excellent allies for the doctors.[56]

55 J. Gélis, *L'arbre et le fruit. La naissance dans l'Occident moderne XV–XIX siècle* (Paris: Fayard, 1984); J. Gélis, M. Laget, M.F. Morel, *Entrer dans la vie. Naissances et enfants dans la France traditionelle* (Paris: Gallimard, 1980); J. Gélis, "L'évolution de la conscience de la vie et du corps en Espagne aux XVI et XVII siècles. La protection de la femme et du nouveau-né," in A. Redondo, *Le corps dans la société espagnole des XVI et XVII siècles* (Paris: Publ. de la Sorbonne, 1990), pp. 15–25.

56 Carbón, *Libro del arte de las comadres* (cit. n. 17); Alonso y de los Ruizes de Fontecha, *Diez previlegios para las mujeres preñadas* (cit. n. 28).

If there is a prototype of the good doctor, the good mother and the good wet-nurse, there is also one of the good midwife. The catalogue of moral conditions again goes hand in hand with that of the technical skills which are needed; among the former are devotion to the Virgin Mary and all "the Saints in Heaven above"[57] and a clear warning to avoid any type of superstitious practice.[58]

If the midwives make mistakes, even if through ignorance rather than malice, they are not free from sin, as their profession requires them to ask the advice of the doctor and consult the works written for their guidance. Negligence here would be culpable negligence, especially as the relevant works were published in Spanish rather than Latin. The language of publication was a much debated subject. Some doctors believed that such serious matters as childbirth and child-care should not be within reach of the layman, as the latter might interpret them incorrectly due to his ignorance of the scientific principles on which they are based. Nevertheless, general opinion was in favor of the vernacular and was based on the argument that works of every type were being written in Spanish. Sermons were also in this category, "even though the material is more serious insofar as the soul is more important than the body." The main reason which the doctors had for revealing their knowledge was "to serve God by fulfilling the needs of the midwives for knowledge."[59]

In short, as has been demonstrated in general for all the areas of medicine, the doctor consolidated a legal and practical monopoly over the health of mothers and children. They established control over the nature of orthodox practice and persecuted all types of deviations.[60]

57 Carbón, *Libro del arte de las comadres* (cit. n. 17), fol. XIIII.

58 For example: "Las mujeres y el vulgo creen que la fascinación de los niños cura mediante higas o esmeraldas, lo cual no es motivo sino de superstición y de demonio y demuestra gran ignorancia," in Pérez Cascales, *Liber de affectionibus puerorum* (cit. n. 2), pp. 120–125.

59 Nuñez de Oria, *Libro del parto humano* (cit. n. 53).

60 D. Gracia, *Fundamentos de bioética* (Madrid: Eudema Universidad, 1989).

Ethical Problems in Pediatric Care

The clinical encounter with the child patient reflects all the problems found in the relations between adults and children in general and, in turn, is a corollary of all the theories and practices inherent in this relationship.[61]

The ethics of pediatric diagnosis in Christian societies of the modern era were strongly influenced by the traditions of Ancient Greece. Thus, the moral rule was that of the "natural order"[62] as God, the Creator of Nature, established it. Nevertheless, the emerging modern states imposed another series of civil and religious duties on doctors. The doctor had to fulfill three different types of obligations: those arising from his own personal conscience, the civil obligations and those relating to the requirements of religion.[63]

In reference to the latter, it has been shown that a good children's doctor is a Christian, as he draws many qualities such as charity or compassion in the treatment of the patient from his religion. His advice to parents and others close to the child must reflect his Christian beliefs. He therefore has unavoidable obligations such as that of baptizing a newly-born child facing death, even though this provisional baptism must later be endorsed in a religious ceremony should the child survive.[64] Nonetheless, the later texts of the eighteenth century indicate a more secularized attitude, and, though the rules are still respected, these works give the impression that the rules are less dogma than customs to be observed. For example, there are fewer references to theologians and jurists than in earlier periods, especially than in the Counter-Reformation, when there were abundant quotations from Hippocrates, Galen, Paul of Egina, Avicenna and others, but also from religious authorities such as Saint Thomas Aquinas or Saint Augustine.

61 H. Müller, H. Olbing, *Ethische Probleme in der Pädiatrie und ihren Grenzgebieten* (München: Urban & Schwarzenberg, 1982).

62 Gracia, *Fundamentos de bioética* (cit. n. 60).

63 A. Albarracín, "The Ethics of Diagnostic in the Modern and Contemporary Worlds," in *The ethics of diagnosis*, ed. J.L. Peset and D. Gracia (Dordrecht/Boston/London: Kluwer Academic Pub., 1992), pp. 29–39.

64 Montalvo, *Practica politica y economica* (cit. n. 48), pp. 229–230.

The process of moral decision making

Before discussing the nature of doctor-patient relations and the ethical dilemmas raised in the relationship between doctor and child, family and society, it is necessary to refer to the fundamental aspect of the intrinsic value of the infant. During the sixteenth, seventeenth and eighteenth centuries there was an ambivalence over the value of human life.[65] The positive side was an ever greater awareness of the social value of infancy as a transforming agent of society and states, while the negative reality was that of wretched living conditions (an extreme example is that of the increased number of foundlings)[66] and an appalling mortality rate, often due to lack of care or even to infanticide. The question remains as to how the medical world confronted and cared for those children who were under professional care. The schemas of the historians of medical ethics indicate that in this period the prevailing orientation was the principle of beneficence, which took the form of paternalism.[67] The idea to treat the patient as a parent would treat his child is, if possible, even more marked here due to the special nature of the child care.

To specify the form which this general principle took in medical practice, I will refer to three ethical constants which appear in all the sources. They represent orientations and criteria for diagnosis and therapy.[68]

To secure the good of the child

The first topic is the existence of a special inequality in the doctor-patient relationship. In the first stages of life, adults are the point of reference, and they interpret what is good for the child and the best way to achieve it. In the medical decision-making process, people

65 Ph. Ariès, *L'enfant et la vie familiale dans l'Ancien Régime* (Paris: Seuil, 1960).

66 Carreras Panchón, *El problema del niño exposito* (cit. n. 45); Sherwood, *Poverty in eighteenth century Spain* (cit. n. 45).

67 Gracia, *Fundamentos de bioética* (cit. n. 60).

68 E. Seidler, "Ethische Probleme in Umfang mit den Kind," in *Ethische Probleme* (cit. n. 61), pp. 45–56.

other than the patient make the decisions according to a certain system of values by which they measure the decisions of the professional. How did the doctors in this period deal with this question? The answer to this question may be found in something that is discussed above; the doctor himself resolves the situation, as he is better suited than anyone else, including the parents themselves, to decide on the best option. He has this right because of the moral authority conferred on him by his profession. Nevertheless, there are still conflicts, especially with mothers, who are accused by the doctors of following popular traditions rather than their own expert advice.[69] In these conflicts, paternal authority is often brought in to reinforce the position of the doctor.[70] In order to achieve the best for the child, to preserve his physical and moral well-being, the doctor must maintain a proper balance of the child's nature; his tendencies to excessive heat and humidity are the main pitfalls, together with the difficulty in diagnosis. "Children do not know how to explain their illnesses nor demonstrate them by complaints, nor show them exactly through their pulse, tongue, urine or by other signs or excrements which (in adults) usually give some indication."[71]

The doctor uses two fundamental tools to face these difficulties: dietary rules,[72] which are applied to each particular case, and the drawing up of a doctrinal and practical *corpus* on the treatment to be carried out on the patient. The general procedure includes two important rules: the first is to emphasize prevention in order to avoid illnesses which were difficult to control; if pharmacological or surgical treatment was necessary, it should also be accompanied by a controlled diet. In addition, the therapeutic principles themselves should be modified in the case of pediatric patients, including the denial of the general Hippocratic principle of *contraria contrariis curantur*. In ac-

69 "Suelen tener los niños diversas enfermedades de las quales acostumbran a morir y es por culpa de sus padres y madres porque en lugar de pedir consejo al medico, lo demandan a la comadre y ella no sabe las causas y ansi se pierden y es pecado grande." Carbón, *Libro del arte de las comadres* (cit. n. 17), fol. LXII.

70 Soriano, *Methodo y orden* (cit. n. 13), p. 121.

71 Pérez de Herrera, *Defensa de las criaturas* (cit. n. 10), pp. 5–6.

72 The works of Galen, especially *De sanitate tuenda* (cit. n. 6), provided the first framework for children's dietetics. Galenic concepts were expanded by Aetius, Paulus of Egina and Avicenna.

cordance with Galenic assumptions, it was considered necessary to use remedies similar to the nature of the child.[73]

The criterion of *preserving life* leads to a central issue at the time: attitudes toward death. The preservation of the life of children was, for the doctors who treated them, a religious and social duty and the *raison d'être* for their professional activity. The appearance of a wide variety of monographic literature on childhood illnesses, particularly from the beginning of the modern era, clearly reflects this situation. The preservation of the lives of infants is both a necessary duty imposed by Christian ethics and useful for a society ever more aware that its collective survival largely depends on the fulfillment of this aim.

The protection of life begins even before birth, which raises several ethical questions which cannot be considered here, as a more thorough analysis would require an extension of the number and types of sources. As a general rule, the doctor must place the life of the child before the life of the mother, although the texts state that the aim is the preservation of both lives. "The doctor must restore the mother to health, for if she is lost, the child will also be lost, so in conclusion, whenever mother and child may be saved, everything possible must be done."[74]

The pregnant woman must take maximum care of her health because of the repercussions it may have on her fetus, and she sins grievously if she fails to do so. The chapters discussing the etiology and pathogeny of natural miscarriage[75] include a series of factors which the woman must check. Among these are the passions of the soul; fear, sadness and anger produce a reduction in the heat of the uterus. This weakens its movements and can easily produce a miscarriage. Mother and child suffer the same illnesses at this stage as a result of the connection between them, and therefore she must take extra care. There are many discussions of the use of specific medicines during pregnancy and of the recourse to bloodletting. The usual curative practices are restricted or withdrawn during pregnancy, for fear of the damage which they may cause to the fetus. The preservation of the life of the child is so

73 Mercado, *De veritate et recta ratione* (cit. n. 34), Lib. I, p. 1.

74 Carbón, *Libro del arte de las comadres* (cit. n. 17), fol. XXVIII, XXX.

75 Pérez Cascales, *Liber de affectionibus puerorum* (cit. n. 2).

important that in extreme cases no cautions are taken and an interventionist attitude is adopted.[76]

Social history and its different approaches, such as the history of mentalities, have in recent years become interested in social attitudes toward infancy and among them those related to *the death of children*. The medical texts provide a wide range of reactions to death, from total indifference to genuine sadness and pain. There are frequent references to deaths caused by more or less culpable negligence, such as children who are asphyxiated while sleeping in the same bed as their mother or wet-nurse, and to those caused by abandonment. At the same time, there are many indications of a desire to take care of children: "the questions related to children's illnesses are so important... for the good of so many children, who for want of treatment... die in these kingdoms, causing pain and affliction to their parents and to the people who cared for them and knew them."[77]

What then were the attitudes of the doctors? Their role as special witnesses of the different social attitudes of which they offer interesting testimony has been discussed, but we need to know personal positions. In their role as protectors of infancy, the loss of the life of a child arouses a double sense of grief both for the fragility of the life lost and for the feeling of professional failure. These feelings can scarcely be diminished by the lack of confidence on the part of the doctor and the society around him that these problems, which are considered to be the most difficult ones confronting a doctor, expert though he may be, can be cured.[78] However, I believe that this lack of confidence does not mean that they had a fatalist attitude and were reluctant to take measures. I consider instead that one of the characteristics of modernity in pediatrics is the adoption of a more active approach based not only on theories inherited and scarcely modified, but especially on the

76 *Ibid.*

77 Pérez de Herrera, *Defensa de las criaturas* (cit. n. 10), p. 7.

78 "Cuando Dios asigna el término de la vida a una persona, ningún remedio humano puede hacer nada. El médico debe actuar con toda diligencia, pero si la vida peligrase aún le queda el consuelo de la esperanza que debe proporcionar a los que se la piden." C. Pérez de Herrera, *Brevis et compendiosus Tractatus de Essentia, Causis, Notis, Praesagio, Curatione et Praecautione faucium et gutturis anginosorum ulcerum Morbi suffocantis, garrotillo Hispane appelati* (Madrid, 1615).

accumulation of practical experience. These texts usually include descriptions of real clinical cases and practical advice on infant pathology, although such features are more common in some works than in others.

This last question seems to me to indicate a modern attitude toward nature. A respectful monitoring of the changes in the infant's nature very often is replaced by direct action on the part of the doctor in order to change the course of the illness. "Let (the doctors) not wish that nature cure all, when nature always requests help and support."[79] The weakness of the patients and the rapid development of illnesses in children make it necessary, even more than with adults, for the doctor to take action in order to try to save the life of his patient.

Do no harm to the patient, or the principle of non-malice,[80] is one of the oldest ethical precepts. It requires that the doctor carefully judge his knowledge and techniques in order to ensure that his actions are more beneficial than harmful. This principle is especially important here, as the life and future of the child are in the hands of the adults and professionals who will decide between the different options. This criterion was the one most clearly dealt with by doctors, and the one which received the most space in the texts. Therapeutic strategies were generally decided on in accordance with the availability of resources, the type of illness and the circumstances of the child (constitution, physical condition). However, the most important factor was a profound knowledge of the beneficial and harmful effects which a certain therapeutic procedure might have on the infant, and much of the energy of the doctors was directed toward this matter. The guiding principles of medical assistance (diet and the use of medicines which were similar to the nature of the child) have been indicated, and now it is necessary to consider the application of specific remedies. The *theriaca*[81] was the subject of debate, but the most controversial therapy was universal evacuation. In the case of blood-letting,[82] the decision-

79 Soriano, *Methodo y orden* (cit. n. 13), p. 51; Carbo, *Libro del arte de las comadres* (cit. n. 17), fol. LXXIX.

80 D. Gracia, *Primum non nocere. El principio de no-maleficiencia como fundamento de las obras médicas* (Madrid, Instituto de España, 1990).

81 Soriano, *Methodo y orden* (cit. n. 13), ch. XXIII.

82 Pérez de Herrera, *Defensa de las criaturas* (cit. n. 10), pp. 10–37; Soriano, *Methodo y orden* (cit. n. 13), ch. X, p. 121.

making process began by evaluating whether or not a given child could be bled. The determination was made on the basis that the treatment should not produce unwanted effects on the health of the child, either at the time or later, for some opinions stated that the debilitating effects of blood-letting would influence the development of the child. If, in the end, the doctor decided to let blood, he should consider the various techniques. In the case of small or weakened children, leeches or small cupping glasses were suggested. The decision as to the method of treatment was not made only on the basis of medical arguments (age, type of pathology, constitution), but also took into account what today would be called quality of life. For example, both the pain which might be suffered by the patient and which should be avoided as far as possible and the marks left by the incisions during bleeding were considered. "Scars and blemishes on the skin of young girls who must one day be wed should be avoided as far as possible, for otherwise they are marked and disfigured for life."[83]

Once the doctor has made a decision and after he has considered the possibilities in order to cause the least possible suffering, nobody has the right to prevent him from acting, not even the parents. In various texts, mothers are urged not to oppose bleeding on the grounds of misplaced maternal love, as doctors, with the help of God, know what is best for the child.[84]

The example of blood-letting applies to many other therapeutic procedures[85] where it is necessary to consider aspects beyond the strictly medical. These procedures may also affect the future of the child and therefore they introduce an element of moral responsibility.

In conclusion, it seems appropriate to offer a series of reflections.

1. Within the historical study of ethical problems in medicine, the special complexity of pediatrics makes it necessary to use various types of sources, including the theological and moral. The exclusive use of

83 Pérez de Herrera, *Defensa de las criaturas* (cit. n. 10), p. 27.

84 Soriano, *Methodo y orden* (cit. n. 13), p. 138.

85 Pérez Cascales, *Liber de affectionibus puerorum* (cit. n. 2), pp. 24, 39; Mercado, *De Puerorum educatione* (cit. n. 3), Lib. II; Pérez de Herrera, *Brevis et compendiosus Tractatus* (cit. n. 78), p. 42; F. de Figueroa, *Dos tratados, uno de las calidades y efectos de la aloxa y otro de una especie de garrotillo o esquinencia mortal* (Lima, 1616).

published medical sources can only paint an incomplete picture, as the texts themselves indicate the limitations of both the number and type of subjects and approaches.

2. Even so, I believe that there are a series of aspects in the written works of doctors which can only be analyzed through the use of such medical texts. A summary of the most significant points includes:

a) The specific nature of the pediatric patient in the doctor-patient relationship. As this object of health care by his very nature lacks the capacity to make decisions, other people, adults, always make decisions for him. In this situation, the doctor assumes the role of the protector of infants and shoulders the responsibility to care for their health.

b) This responsibility extends to the family and to those close to the child. Their behavior will be approved or rejected based on the double authority conferred on the doctor by his Christian principles and by his ever more extensive scientific and social monopoly over questions related to children.

c) During the modern era, a moral code was drawn up which acted as a pattern against which the actions of the doctor would be judged as good or bad, beneficial or harmful. Starting from a background of Christian ideology, but with an increasingly secularizing tendency, a series of guiding principles would be established for those doctors engaged in the care of children.

THE ETHICAL MANIPULATION OF THE PATIENT IN THE ANCIENTS VERSUS MODERNS CONTROVERSY: THE IMPACT OF GIUSEPPE GAZOLA'S *IL MONDO INGANNATO DA FALSI MEDICI* (1716) IN SPAIN

GUILLERMO OLAGÜE DE ROS

Introduction

Texts describing the disputes between medical professionals in the modern world have not received a great deal of attention from historians, and those who have examined these texts have been harsh in their criticisms.[1] Perhaps because of the scarcity of doctrinal arguments, such material has been held in low esteem as a minor genre, or as of questionable value to period literature. During the seventeenth and eighteenth centuries there appeared a number of works of this genre, especially in northern Italy, where conflicts of this sort seem to have been dealt with more openly. I have collected more than fifty such texts published between 1605 and the last quarter of the eighteenth century, most of them written in the vernacular by physicians with no further intentions than to influence some local argument. In nearly all such texts, the unifying theme was the discussion from different standpoints of the capacity of medicine and physicians to deceive and disappoint and, despite this, of the nobility of the profession and its practitioners.

* My thanks are due to Professor José María López Piñero of the University of Valencia, Professor Alvar Martínez Vidal of the University of Barcelona, Professor Jon Arrizabalaga (C. S. I. C., Barcelona), and Mr. Robin Price, Deputy Librarian of the Wellcome Institute for the History of Medicine in London, for their generous assistance and illuminating conversations.

1 The text examined in this study was the object of an ill-founded critique by G. Marañon, *Las ideas biológicas del P. Feijóo*, 4th ed. (Madrid: Espasa Calpe, 1962), *passim*.

In contrast to the negative sense of the word deception characteristic of Baroque literature, where it was interpreted as disillusion or disappointment, during the eighteenth century deception acquired a positive connotation: deception, synonymous with error, was amenable to correction by educating or instructing the deceived.[2] However, deception and the possibility of disappointment in the medical context had a highly significant ethical content, as the physician who deceived was seen as doing the patient harm, and was therefore behaving in a morally incorrect way. The deceived patient could not be expected to be satisfied with being educated about the error, as the physician's lack of expertise could cause harm which might lead to his or her death. The patient should therefore receive instruction at an early stage, and should be advised about situations which might cause him or her to fall ill, and about the little scientific value of the theories applied by other colleagues in their diagnosis and treatment of specific clinical cases. Some texts even went so far as to suggest that the physician was not necessary for the preservation of health and the treatment of illnesses.

Despite the local character of most of these writings, they were widely disseminated at the time throughout Europe. This circulation was directly connected to the crisis in the traditional Galenic paradigm and to the numerous controversies, from the middle of the seventeenth century onward, between the proponents of the ancient and modern approaches to professional practice. In these arguments, the physician's expertise and ability to deceive were among the most important topics.[3] The frequent publications, reprintings, replies and counterreplies to many of these works cannot only be attributed to the interest in their contents, but also to the provocative tone used by the authors. Criticism of the professional conduct of other physicians was motivated by unresolved tensions over the control and practice of medicine. This was not a case where the physicians tried to retain control in the face of intruders from outside the profession such as faith healers or quacks,[4]

2 P. Alvarez de Miranda, *Palabras e Ideas: el léxico de la Ilustración temprana en España (1680–1760)* (Anejos del Boletín de la Real Academia Española, Anejo LI) (Madrid: Imprenta Aguirre, 1992), pp. 612–616.

3 L.S. King, *The Medical World of the 18th Century* (Chicago: The University of Chicago Press, 1958), pp. 227–261.

4 D. Harely, "Honour and property: the structure of professional disputes in

but rather a conflict between professional groups which defended specific medical doctrines, as well as a struggle for the control of the decision-making power in matters relating to practice. Moreover, in Italy, disputes between medical colleges over issues of competence and control of the professional practice of their members were relatively frequent.[5] The authors who participated in these controversies were questioning, from the modern or the traditionalist standpoint, a particular mode of professional conduct which was susceptible to criticism on ethical grounds, and which threatened to supplant the position defended by the author of the work. At the same time, the position held by the other side in scientific and social institutions was sought. In these attempts, the innovators made use of a new professional standard, while the Galenists exalted tradition. The physicians who supported reform considered that the nobility of the profession, on which both sides agreed, required the ennoblement of its practitioners. If the *novatores* (reformers) were more successful than the traditionalists in treating patients, they should be accorded the socio-economic success, and hence the ennoblement, hitherto enjoyed only by the traditionalists.

Once the conflict of views had been established within professional ranks, the patient was reduced to an instrument which would serve the interests of the two groups, Galenists and moderns, although neither group had explicitly intended for this to happen. From the time that modern medicine became widespread, the patient's personal data appeared at the beginning of his or her medical record, but the science-based clinical report nevertheless concealed any further information on the patient's identity. The patient was depersonalized and was treated according to specific theories, with the aim of proving the truth of one and the falsehood of the other. This process led to the ethical manipulation of the patient by those following a certain set of epistemological assumptions. The conflict between traditionalist and modern physicians did not result in legal action, but in attacks on moral

eighteenth-century English medicine," in *The Medical Enlightenment of the Eighteenth Century*, eds. A Cunningham and R. French (Cambridge: Cambridge University Press, 1990), pp. 138–164.

5 I. Ghibellini, *Una secolare divergenza tra i Collegi Medici di Bologna e di Ferrara circa l'esercizio professionale extra territoriale* (Ferrara: Università degli Studi, 1961).

grounds (the ineffectiveness of the "other" was proof of his "immorality"). Each side attempted to demonstrate the ethical inferiority of his opponent, as the opponent's scientific, diagnostic and therapeutic resources were denigrated as inferior.

Few Italian medical works from the beginning of the eighteenth century produced as much fame, fortune, and controversy as *Il Mondo Ingannato da Falsi Medici* (1716) by Giuseppe Gazola (1661–1715). Published posthumously by his brother Giovanni Baptista, it went through a total of twenty-three editions in different countries during the eighteenth century. Although Gazola was not one of the great medical theoreticians of the Enlightenment, almost all medical and general history texts cite him as a judicious writer who maintained a highly critical attitude toward the medicine of his time, especially with regard to the clinical and therapeutic abuses of his colleagues. Why was this book, written in Italian, containing little of a doctrinal nature, and criticizing the moral conduct of a particular type of physician, reprinted and translated so widely? Which individuals identified themselves with its contents, and which others therefore felt maligned? Finally, why did it become even more notorious in Spain than in Italy?

Some biographical background on Gazola may help to provide a partial answer to these questions.[6] He was born in Verona and studied

6 *Biographisches Lexikon der hervorragenden Ärzte aller Zeiten und Völker*, 6 vols., eds. A. Hirsch, E. Gurlt and A. Wernich (Berlin-Wien: Urban and Schwarzenberg, 1929–1935; rpt. München-Berlin: Urban and Schwarzenberg, 1962), Vol. II, pp. 702–703; F. Ballestrasse, *Studi sul Settecento Medico. "Contro i Dommatici e i Galenisti" del Dott. Giuseppe Gazola (1716)* (Scientia Veterum, n. 153) (Pisa: Casa Editrice Giardini, 1970), pp. 5–47; "Copia dell'articolo quinto del Tomo Ventesimosettimo del Giornale de'Letterati d'Italia. Anno MDCCXVI," in G. Gazola, *Il mondo ingannato da falsi medici* (Trento, 1718), pp. 201–251, on pp. 203–212; S. de Renzi, *Storia della Medicina Italiana*, 5 vols. (Napoli, 1845–1848; rpt. Bologna: Forni Editore, 1966), Vol. IV, *passim; Dictionnaire historique de la Médecine Ancienne et Moderne*, 4 vols., eds. Dezeimeris, Ollivier and Raige-Delorme (Paris-Bruxelles, 1828–1839), Vol. II/2e., pp. 510–511; N.F.J. Eloy, *Dictionnaire Historique de la Médecine Ancienne et Moderne,* 4 vols. (Mons, 1778; rpt. Bruxelles: Culture et Civilisation, 1973), Vol. II, pp. 319–320; F. Sánchez Blanco, *La prosa del siglo XVIII*, in *Historia de la Literatura Española*, 50 vols., ed. R. de la Fuente (Madrid: Ediciones Júcar, 1992), vol. 27, p. 68; J. Sarrailh, *La España Ilustrada de la segunda mitad del siglo XVIII* (México-Madrid-Buenos Aires: Fondo de Cultura Económica, 1974), *passim.*

at the Faculty of Medicine of Padua, where he obtained his doctorate in 1683. In Verona in 1686 he founded, together with Sebastiano Rotario, Girolamo Allegri and Francesco Bianchini, the *Accademia degli Aletofili* (Friends of the Truth).[7] The *Accademia* was active for a relatively brief period until the beginning of the eighteenth century. Silvano Benedetti has shown that this academy was the center from which modern physicians issued their doctrinal and professional opposition to the city's College of Physicians, whose members were followers of obsolete Galenic precepts.[8] Its members succeeded in obtaining from the Venetian magistrates an authorization allowing all the physicians of the city, and not only the members of the Venetian College of Physicians, to practice their profession freely. In December 1688, Gazola travelled to Spain as personal physician to the Venetian Ambassador. After three years in Madrid, where he met with reformists and where he published his *Enthusiasmos médicos, políticos y astrológicos* (Medical, political and astrological delights, 1690),[9] he travelled widely in France and Italy, then returned to Verona, where he died in 1715. Three years before his death, he published the *Origine preservativo e rimedio del contagio pestilenziale del Bue*, which Alfonso Corradi has called a "very important text in the history of public health."[10]

Gazola was a reformist physician who went from a position of empiricism almost at odds with Galenism in his *Enthusiasmos* to one of antisystematic scepticism regarding clinical practice and treatment in *Il mondo Ingannato*. In his *Enthusiasmos*, Gazola also launched a harsh attack against the *Protomedicato*, the organ responsible for

7 M. Maylender, *Storia delle Accademia d'Italia*, 5 vols. (Bologna, 1926–1930; rpt. Bologna: Arnaldo Forni Editore, *s.d.*), Vol. I, pp. 141–147.

8 S. Benedetti, "L'Accademia degli Aletofili di Verona," in *Accademia e Cultura. Aspetti Storici tra Sei e Settecento* (Biblioteca dell'Edizione Nazionale del Carteggio di L.A. Muratori. V) (Firenze: Leo S. Olschki, 1979), pp. 223–226; F. Scarcella, *L'antico Collegio dei medici di Verona: cenni storici (1000–1959)* (Verona: Ghidini e Fiorini, 1959).

9 J.M. López Piñero, "Los comienzos de la medicina y de la ciencia modernas en España en el último tercio del sigo XVII," in *Actas del Segundo Congreso Español de Historia de la Medicina*, 2 vols. (Salamanca: Sociedad Española de Historia de la Medicina, 1966), Vol. I, pp. 271–292.

10 A Corradi, *Annali delle epidemie occorse in Italia dalle prime memorie fino al 1850 compilati con varie note e dichiarazioni,* 5 vols. (Bologna, 1865–1892; rpt. Bologna: Forni Editore, 1972), Vol. II, p. 322.

controlling the practice of health professionals, and clearly sided with the Spanish *novatores* physicians.[11]

Within the framework of a more extensive study of Italian Enlightenment sources dealing with the expertise of physicians, this study aims to explain the doctrinal, scientific and ethical assumptions contained in Giuseppe Gazola's *Il mondo Ingannato*, and to account for its widespread dissemination in Spain during the eighteenth century.

Medicine, Physicians and Patients in Giuseppe Gazola's *Il Mondo Ingannato da Falsi Medici* (1716)

The different editions of Gazola's book contain some slight variations which deserve comment. The fifth Italian printing (Trent, 1718) and all subsequent editions include an extract from a work which had been published in the *Giornale de'Letterati d'Italia* and two *Lettere* from Galenist physicians. The extract accurately describes the contents of Gazola's treatise, while the authors of the two letters, who were aware of the discredit and danger the work posed to Galenic medicine and who were threatened by the headway the moderns were making, were unable to effectively refute Gazola's writings.[12] Peripatetic philosophy, the basis of traditional medicine, was also Mosaic philosophy and that cultivated by the Patriarchs, the Prophets, and the Great Sanhedrin. In opposing traditional thinking, modern philosophy, corpuscular and Cartesian in nature, "makes war against all... dismantling and ruining Society, Commerce, Religion and Divinity."[13] The author of this letter was fully aware of the controversy between the two models of medical practice, which was based on the doctrinal differences between ancients and moderns. On the one hand, the peripatetic view was still the predominant philosophy, and was not amenable to change.

11 J.M. López Piñero, "Juan de Cabriada y las primeras etapas de la iatroquímica y de la medicina moderna en España," *Cuadernos de Historia de la Medicina Española*, 1962, *2*:129–154.

12 "Copia dell'articolo quinto..." (cit. n. 6), pp. 201–251; "Lettere di due Medici Galenici Veronesi sopra il Libro intitolato Il Mondo ingannato da falsi Medici del Dottor Giuseppe Gazola Veronese Medico Cesareo," in G. Gazola, *Il mondo ingannato* (cit. n. 6), pp. 253–272.

13 *Ibid.*, pp. 270–271.

On the other hand, modern philosophy was open to change, and was submitted to the control of the new scientific academies. Gazola used these arguments in his work, and even went so far as to attribute to Jewish physicians a particular mode of professional practice more characteristic of faith healers or quacks.[14] Despite the fact that Gazola's two critics called themselves Galenists, they were undoubtedly physicians sympathetic to Gazola's thinking, and were very likely members of the *Accademia degli Aletofili.*

The last two Italian editions (Venice, 1746 and 1747) added a sixth dissertation on blood-letting and a treatise on baths and the waters of Caldiero. The only new feature in the Spanish editions was the inclusion in the Valencia edition of 1733, and in all subsequent printings, of two Dialogues on Physicians by the Spanish humanist Pedro de Mexía.

The main body of the work consists of a dedication, *To Good Physicians*, and five dissertations.[15] Despite the apparently iconoclastic title of the first dissertation (*Better no Doctor than a Bad One*), the dedication makes his attitude clear. Gazola states that his intention was to write an apology "for the true medical art and an invective against those who... inhumanely destroy life to obtain gold, although it be at the cost of their many errors." As we will see, beneath this denouncement of those whose only intention was to use their practice to become rich lay veiled accusations of collusion between physicians and pharmacists. Gazola states his position very clearly and concludes: "this booklet, in upbraiding Physicians, upbraids bad Physicians," those for whom "the Art... is a matter to be learned in four days. In their conception, all experience is dogma beyond a shadow of a doubt. Lacking studies and observation, they would pass judgment on the

14 J. Gazola, *El mundo engañado de los falsos médicos* (Sevilla, 1729), on p. 29: "Con esto creo que siempre que os acordéis quan fácil cosa sea hacerse Médico, ya no os causará admiración la multitud de curanderos, que vereís cada día que exercen semejante profesión: Ermitaños, Herbolarios, Cirujanos, Boticarios, Saltimbancos, Judíos."

15 I. *Más vale estar sin médico que no tenerle bueno;* II. *La medicina sirve, pero cada uno puede ser Médico de sí mismo*; III. *De la dificultad de la Medicina y del engaño de las más famosas sectas de Médicos, y particularmente de los Dogmáticos y secuaces de los antiguos;* IV. *Advertencias para vivir, y conservar la salud mucho tiempo*; V. *Si es mejor valerse de médicos Modernos o Galénicos.*

most recondite causes." Gazola did not see himself as an enemy of medicine and physicians, which his contemporaries accused him of being, but questioned how medicine, which had been held in such high esteem in the ancient world, had become the subject of "entertainments by French Comics." In other words, why had medicine fallen "from praise to satire, and from applause to sardonic nicknames?"[16]

The third and fourth dissertations form the foundation of the argument on which the entire work is based. In these sections, Gazola attempts to prove the superiority of the medicine practiced by good, i.e., modern physicians, and the fraud committed against the patient who trusted the Galenists. In the other dissertations, Gazola advises his readers on the best ways to conserve their health and to correctly regulate the Galenic *sex res non naturales* in order to avoid situations which might cause them to fall ill.

I shall first examine Gazola's scientific assumptions, and then analyze the ethical-deontological bases of his defense of modern physicians and his disparagement of the traditionalists.

In Gazola's view, medicine was of divine origin. This origin did not, however, make it invulnerable to criticism, as those who practiced medicine were men who could commit errors. His justification for the necessity of medicine was that the physician was the body's priest, who freed the body from disease. He clearly sided with modern physicians against the dominant Galenist majority, and saw one of the basic doctrinal differences between the two schools as the acceptance by the former of the usefulness of recent contributions from the new sciences in improving medical practice.[17] On the other hand, the Galenist physicians based their practice on four aphorisms, texts by Galen and other classical writers, an essentialist explanation of disease, and a number of complicated prescriptions for the treatment of diseases. The blind acceptance of authority and the following of "false assumptions," such as the scheme of the movement of fluids and blood through the body, were also integral parts of the theoretical basis of traditional medicine. The ancients were therefore bad physicians, but acceptable practitioners. Although their practice, founded on experience, may have been valid, their theories were spurious.

16 Gazola, *El mundo engañado de los falsos médicos* (cit. n. 14), p. 53.
17 *Ibid.*, p. 27.

Gazola, like most other modern physicians, considered the process of treatment to be one of the fundamental points of contention between them and the Galenists. The defense of new medications and the strengthening of the empirical component of treatment advocated by the modern physicians involved a rupture of the theory-practice binomial espoused by the traditionalists. The institutions which controlled professional training and practice thus felt that a major reason for their existence was being questioned. The Schools of Medicine, which had a monopoly on theoretical knowledge, and the Colleges of Physicians, which were the watchdogs of professional practice, were being pushed aside by a new medicine which combined theories opposed to the predominant tenets with a more effective therapeutic empiricism. It is not surprising, therefore, that Gazola frequently warned his readers against the uselessness of any empiricism which was not based on theoretical knowledge. "It is not the same to call one's self a Physician, and to know how to practice medicine, to write out a prescription, and to cure a disease."[18] What distinguished the moderns from the Galenists was "the understanding of the cause of the disease, and thus, the cure of the disease."[19]

Gazola advocated a kind of medicine based on experience and reason. The modern physician relied on the new discoveries in macroscopic and microscopic anatomy, chemistry, medicine and experimental philosophy in order to provide a rational explanation for the functioning of the human machine and disease.[20] Gazola himself was especially partial to mechanistic theories. Following the thesis of Giorgio Baglivi (1668–1707), Gazola considered the body to be composed of innumerable machines whose function was to "distill the humors through whose circulation and nutrition the individual human lives."[21] Life was governed by the correct circulation of the blood, and health depended on the harmony between the humors and their correct circulation through the body. Illness, on the other hand, was a "force

18 *Ibid.*, p. 8. "En el número de los empíricos entran también todos aquellos que no entendiendo más que Chímica pretenden con cualquier medicina que han manipulado curar algunas particulares indisposiciones por haver experimentado una o más veces buenos efectos."

19 *Ibid.*, p. 158.

20 *Ibid.*, pp. 165–166.

21 *Ibid.*, p. 123.

of nature against health, attempting to accumulate harmful humors against it."[22] In accordance with classical Hippocratic precepts, Gazola differentiated between curable diseases, which were the majority, and incurable diseases, which required more care and caution on the part of the physician. The main curative agent was the patient's own natural healing power (*vis curatrix naturae*). The good physician was a servant of nature, who devoted himself to study and hoped to attain fame only through virtue. If he should by chance forget that he was a servant of nature, the patient's life could be in grave danger.[23]

Gazola wondered how Galenist physicians, who were not as well trained in theory or, at times, in practice, had so many followers, while the better trained modern physicians encountered so many difficulties in their professional practice. He offered several explanations. One was the outstanding ability to deceive shown by the "liars, who trap the most trusting [and] the most wise in their nets."[24] The most ignorant physician, backed by undeserved fame, could be the "Protomedico of a city." Another reason for the success enjoyed by the Galenists was that people were generally very conservative and ignorant.[25] The patients had no medical training, and therefore they were not able to succeed in suits against a physician who made a mistake, because the physician could always find some justification for his treatment which the patient could not refute.

However, the main reason for the success of the Galenists was their questionable ethical behavior. Gazola clearly decried the collusion between traditional "physicians, apothecaries, and surgeons" who supported each other in order to become rich, and increased their prestige by deceiving the ignorant patient. According to Gazola, this practice had been recommended by Galen himself, and his followers had followed his advice to the letter.[26] The pharmacists obtained the greatest economic benefit from this practice, as Galenist physicians recommended treatments involving numerous drugs.[27]

22 *Ibid.*, pp. 174, 191.

23 *Ibid.*, pp. 9–13.

24 *Ibid.*, pp. 1–2.

25 *Ibid.*, p. 155.

26 *Ibid.*, pp. 13, 32–33.

27 "Los enfermos, no tanto estimulados de dolor, quanto lisongeados de la esperanza, viendo tanta salud en perspectiva, exponen a la fortuna la vida en manos de los

The Dissemination of Giuseppe Gazola's *El Mundo Engañado de Los Falsos Médicos* in Spain (1729–1788)

Il Mondo Ingannato had an enormous influence on Spain, becoming even more widely known there than in Italy or the rest of Europe.[28] Between the appearance of the first translation in Valencia in 1729, barely ten years after it appeared in Italy, and 1788, when the last edition was published, Gazola's text appeared in eleven different Spanish editions: six in Valencia, three in Madrid, and one each in Valladolid and Seville.[29] Two parts of the *Diálogo de los Médicos* by the Sevillian humanist Pedro de Mexía (1497–1551) were appended to the 1733 Valencia edition.[30] Mexía's text was undoubtedly the most intelligent

Médicos, cuyas recetas son las letras de cambio de aquellas tiendas" (*Ibid.*, pp. 44–46). "... Los cordiales... no tienen más virtud que ganancia a los boticarios" (*Ibid.*, p. 170).

28 In addition to the Italian and ten Spanish editions, French and Dutch translations were published in Leyden in 1735. The translator of the French edition was A. F. de Coulange. The Italian editions were published in 1716 (Venice, Perugia and Prague), 1717 (two in Trent), 1718 (two in Trent), 1728, 1746 and 1747 (Venice).

29 Of these, the Valencian editions of 1745 and 1751 are probably identical. According to F. Aguilar Piñal, *Bibliografía de autores españoles del siglo XVIII* (Madrid: C.S.I.C., 1981–1993 [in progress]), Vol. V, p. 576, the 1729 Valladolid edition may not exist, as the printer's notice at the foot of the title page is the same as that of the Valencian edition of the same year. However, a copy of the Valladolid edition exists in the National Library in Madrid (R–25454). In contrast to the claim of M.L. López Terrada, *Libros y folletos científicos en la Valencia de la Ilustración* (Valencia: Edicions Alfons el Magnànim, Institució Valenciana d'Estudis i Investigació, Institut d'Estudis Juan Gil-Albert, 1987), p. 106, there is no Valencian edition of 1721 with the same printer's notice as in the 1729 edition.

30 J. Gazola, *El mundo engañado de los falsos médicos. Obra póstuma traducida fielmente del Toscano. Va añadido un diálogo del Magnífico Caballero Pedro Megía* (Valencia, 1765), pp. 193–251 [*Diálogo de los Médicos. Compuesto por el Magnífico Caballero Pedro Megía, vecino de Sevilla. El argumento de este Diálogo es introducir dos caballeros leídos, que el uno dice mucho mal de Médicos, i tiene por opinión que no los avia de aver, ni Arte de Medicina, sino que se curassen los hombres por uso, i esperiencia, sin Maestro conocido. El otro alaba, i defiende la medicina, i Médicos, como se platica oi. Introducesse así mismo un doto hombre, llamado el maestro Velázquez, que dice la sentencia, i opinión que se deve tener. En lo qual se tocan, i tratan muchas cosas notables de erudición, i dotrina* (pp. 193–219)*; Segunda parte del Dialogo de los Médicos, en que se acaba i concluye el Diálogo* (pp. 220–251)].

and best documented satire on the medical profession which had appeared in Spain since the Renaissance.[31] Gazola's publisher, the erudite Valencian Gregorio Mayáns y Siscar (1691–1788), clearly intended the inclusion of Mexía's text to remind the reader of the deeply-rooted tradition of criticism of medicine and physicians in Spain. This criticism was far removed from the frivolous writings of Diego de Torres y Villarroel (1693–1770) and other eighteenth century writers, and thus clearly in line with Gazola's stance.[32] Moreover, other Spanish texts critical of physicians which had been published at the same time as *Il Mondo Ingannato*, for example, the works of Father Benito Jerónimo Feijóo (1676–1764), may not have been well received by some of the contemporary advocates of reform of the training and control of medical practice in Spain.

I believe that the different Spanish editions of this work appeared as a result of concrete socio-scientific circumstances. Almost all of the editions were printed in Valencia, Seville, and Madrid, cities where the tensions between traditionalists and moderns had become intense during the final decades of the seventeenth century. In addition, the publication of Gazola's *Il Mondo* in Spain coincided with the appearance of the earliest antisystematic tendencies which followed the failure of iatrochemistry, the first system of modern medicine.[33] The support which the members of the Royal Sevillian Society of Medicine and Other Sciences (*Regia*) offered in 1733 to Juan José García Romero, a Sevillian priest who criticized Gazola's work on strictly religious grounds, should be understood within the context of these tensions.[34]

31 L. Sánchez Granjel, "Las ideas antropológico-médicas del 'Magnífico Caballero' Pedro Mexía," in *Humanismo y Medicina* (Salamanca: Seminario de Historia de la Medicina Española, 1968), pp. 75–99.

32 L. Sánchez Granjel, "La Medicina y los médicos en la obra de Torres Villarroel," in *Ibid.*, pp. 245–313. To these antimedical writings should be added what Sánchez Granjel has called *picaresque literature*.

33 J. M. López Piñero, "La mentalidad antisistemática en la medicina española del siglo XVIII. La influencia de la Alte Wiener Schule," *Cuadernos de Historia de la Medicina Española*, 1973, *12*: 193–212.

34 During the 1720s, the *Regia* was torn by internal dissention between supporters of iatrochemistry and followers of antisystematic eclecticism. For example, there was a dispute between Juan Gil Sanz (d. 1728), representing the former approach, and Martín Martínez (1684–1734), defender of the latter. See L. Sánchez Granjel,

I will examine the situation in Valencia and Seville, as well as the belated response of Giovanni Francesco de Bartolomeis, an Italian physician living in Madrid, who in 1762 published a piece in which he refuted some of the points discussed in Gazola's treatise.

1. The Valencian editions (1729–1788)

> E che direm noi, o Signori, dell'Accademie tutte delle Spagne, da quella di Valenza in fuori, la qual sola, e constantemente, di non dipartirsi giammai in cosa niuna dal suo Ipocrate, e Galieno si da vanto? Costoro certamente han seguito sempre, e seguon tuttavia per solo titolo i medesimi Greci maestri...[35]

Gazola's work was published in Valencia in six different editions between 1729 and 1788. It has repeatedly been shown that Mayáns was not only the publisher but was also responsible for the Spanish translation of *Il Mondo Ingannato*. Juan Sempere y Guarinos first made this claim in his *Biblioteca*,[36] and no one has yet contested it[37]. However, Mayáns is not credited with the translation in any of the Spanish editions of Gazola's work. It appears that Mayáns did translate part of the work, but, unsatisfied with the final results, decided not to assume responsibility for the Spanish version.[38]

Why did *El Mundo Engañado* become a best-seller, its first edition selling out in scarcely six months?[39] Why were Mayáns and Valencia so

"El pensamiento médico de Martín Martínez," *Archivo Ibero Americano de Historia de la Medicina y Antropología Médica*, 1952, *4*: 41–74, on p. 74.

35 L. di Capoa, *Parere del Signor... Divisato in otto Ragionamenti, Ne'quali partitamente narrandosi l'origine, e' l progresso della Medicina, chiaramente l'incertezza della medesima si fa manifesta. Terza impressione* (Napoli, 1695), on p. 28.

36 J. Sempere y Guarinos, *Ensayo de una Biblioteca Española de los mejores escritores del Reynado de Carlos III*, 6 vols. (Madrid, 1785–1789; rpt. Madrid: Editorial Gredos, 1966), Vol. IV, p. 20.

37 See, for example, Aguilar Piñal, *Bibliografía de autores españoles del siglo XVIII* (cit. n. 29), Vol. V, pp. 576–577.

38 A. Mestre, "Correspondencia Feijóo-Mayáns en el Colegio del Patriarca," *Anales del Seminario de Valencia*, 1964, *4*: 147–186, on pp. 156, 157 and 179.

39 "El Dr. Gazola ha tenido tan buen despacho que solo quedan catorce copias, i luego se habrá de reimprimir" (*Ibid.*, p. 156). Mayáns' endorsement of this edition is dated 1 March 1729.

interested in the writings of the Veronese physician? Whom did the dissemination of his opinions favor in Spain?

The publication of numerous editions in Valencia can only be explained in terms of the socio-scientific changes mentioned above, more specifically the attempts to modify the regulations governing the training of physicians at the School of Medicine and the problems surrounding the career of Andrés Piquer y Arrufat (1711–1772) during the 1740s. A supporter of the new medicine, Andrés Piquer had to overcome the obstacles set in his path by the traditionalists who controlled the *Hospital General*, the largest medical center in the city.

At the end of the seventeenth century, Valencia attracted supporters of the novator movement.[40] Among the members of this small group of reformists were Mayáns and Antonio Bordázar (1671–1744), printer of the 1729 Valencia edition. In addition to being a bookseller, Bordázar was connected to the notable figures of the *novator* movement in the city. In 1687, he attended the mathematical academy organized by Baltasar de Iñigo (b. 1656), and also participated in the lectures organized by the Marquis of Villatorcas (d. 1722). He founded another *Academia Mathemática* during the 1730s; this institution, however, was little known and relatively short-lived.[41]

The University of Valencia was founded under municipal auspices, and was therefore a secular institution. Its authorities required that the professors of the medical school adhere strictly to its statutes. The conflict between the traditional teaching mandated by the University

40 V. Peset, "La Universidad de Valencia y la renovación científica española (1687–1727)," *Asclepio*, 1964, *16*: 214–231; J. M. López Piñero, *La introducción de la Ciencia Moderna en España* (Barcelona: Ediciones Ariel, 1969); idem, "Valencia y la Medicina del Renacimiento y del Barroco," in *Actas del III Congreso Nacional de Historia de la Medicina*, 3 vols. (Valencia: Sociedad Española de Historia de la Medicina, 1971–1972), vol. III, pp. 95–108.

41 V. Ferrán Salvador, "Antonio Bordázar de Artazu. El impresor erudito. Ensayo bio-bibliográfico," *Boletín de la Sociedad Castellonense de Cultura*, 1964, *49*: 119–147; A. Mestre, *Despotismo e Ilustración española* (Barcelona: Ediciones Ariel, 1976), pp. 22–28; V. Navarro Brotóns "Inventario de los Manuscritos que figuran en la Biblioteca Mayensiana," in *Primer Congreso de Historia del País Valenciano*, 4 vols. (Valencia: Universidad de Valencia, 1974–1976), Vol. I, pp. 591–606; idem "Noticia acerca de Antonio de Bordázar y la fundación de una Academia Matemática en Valencia," in *Ibid.*, Vol. III, pp. 589–595.

by-laws *(Constituciones)* and the incorporation of new scientific doctrines frequently generated tension in the university's governing board *(Claustro).* Vicente Peset showed some years ago that at the end of the seventeenth century, the School of Medicine in Valencia displayed a critical attitude toward Galenic medicine and was relatively open to new approaches. Some notable teachers, including Tomás Longás (d. 1722), a moderate Galenist from a long dynasty of physicians who was connected with both the Medical School and the *Hospital General,* obtained authorization in 1722 to use modern authors in their teaching.[42] The reformation of the *Constituciones* in 1733 finally allowed the introduction of a certain degree of eclecticism, including the incorporation of the works of Hermann Boerhaave.[43] It was thus not coincidental that the first edition of Gazola's work appeared in Valencia in 1729, while reformists were proposing changes in the curriculum of the School of Medicine. Nor is it surprising that the final two Valencia editions, published in 1765 and 1788, appeared at the same time as proposals for an ambitious reformation of the program of study, which affected the university's future and government. For example, the 1765 edition featured a dedication by the printer, Salvador Fauli, to Manuel Martínez de la Raga, President of the *Protomedicato*; this dedication was a paean to the past and present glories of the University of Valencia. However, the hopes for reform, toward which Mayáns had worked since 1761, were not to be realized until 1767.[44] The program of study developed in 1786 by Vicente Blasco, Chancellor of the University, meant the end of municipal patronage. His plan called for important changes in medical teaching, such as the inclusion of clinical training and chemistry. The physicians of the *Hospital General*

42 V. Peset, "Informe del Claustro de Medicina de Valencia sobre renovación de estudios (1721)," *Archivo Ibero Americano de Historia de la Medicina y Antropología Médica,* 1961, *13*: 143–156; "La Universidad de Valencia" (cit. n. 40), p. 221.

43 Peset, "La Universidad de Valencia" (cit. n. 40); J.M. López Piñero, *La Facultad de Medicina de la Universidad de Valencia. Aproximación a su historia* (Valencia: Facultad de Medicina, 1980), p. 25.

44 M. Peset, J. L. Peset, *Gregorio Mayáns y la reforma universitaria. "Idea del Nuevo Método que se puede practicar en la enseñanza de las Universidades de España." 1 de abril de 1767* (Valencia: Artes Gráficas Soler, 1975).

strongly opposed the inclusion of the former, and during the 1788–1789 academic year this subject was not yet offered.[45]

The *Hospital General* was also a secular institution, administered and governed in part by the city of Valencia. The medical staff was usually drawn from the professors of the School of Medicine, at first by direct designation by the hospital administrators, then by competitive examination from the second half of the seventeenth century onward. The administrators did not receive a salary, were usually members of the local oligarchy, and divided their time between the hospital and other posts in the municipal administration. In contrast, the physicians were the best-paid members of the hospital staff. For these reasons, during this period there was intense competition for such posts among the recently certified physicians of the medical school in Valencia. The Crown introduced the Royal Inspector *(Visitador Regio)* in 1666 as a means of limiting the excessive independence of the Hospital.[46]

A position at the *Hospital General* became the prime objective of medical students who wished to achieve fame, prestige, and wealth. Alvaro Martínez Vidal has recently reconstructed the early career of Andrés Piquer y Arrufat (1711–1772), one of the key figures in medicine during the Spanish Enlightenment. Martínez Vidal clearly shows that Piquer's attempts to join the staff of the hospital during the 1730s were motivated by two basic goals: to achieve fame, and to become part of the city's professional elite.[47] After concluding his studies in Valencia with brilliant results — although, according to his son Juan Crisóstomo, he was very disappointed with the quality of teaching because of the predominantly Galenic beliefs of the faculty — Piquer

45 J.L. Peset, "Reforma de los estudios médicos en la Universidad de Valencia. El Plan de estudios del Rector Blasco de 1786," *Cuadernos de Historia de la Medicina Española,* 1973, *12*: 213–264, on pp. 226–227; R. Gago, G. Olagüe, J.L. Carrillo and L. García Ballester, "El Plan de Estudios del rector Blasco (1786) y la renovación de las disciplinas científicas en la Universidad de Valencia: la química y la enseñanza clínica," *Estudis*, 1977, *6*: 157–169.

46 M. Peset Reig, J.L. Peset Reig, "Felipe V y el Hospital Real y General de Valencia," *Medicina Española,* 1969, *61*: 405–414; M. Vilar Devis, "El Hospital General de Valencia en el siglo XVIII (1600–1700)," *Estudis*, 1991, *17*: 213–227.

47 A. Martínez Vidal, "La vinculación de Andrés Piquer al Hospital General de Valencia," *Medicina e Historia*, 1987, n. 20, I–XVI.

devoted himself to preparing for the competitive examination which he hoped would lead to an appointment at the *Hospital General.* Despite having been a disciple of Juan Bautista Longás (d. 1742), who belonged to the dynasty of Aragonese physicians connected with the University of Valencia's *Claustro* and with the *Hospital General,*[48] Piquer failed disastrously in all his attempts. After Longás' death, he was appointed Professor of Anatomy at the University in 1742, thanks in part to the support of Gregorio Mayáns, who remained a close friend from that time.[49] Piquer's failure to pass the competitive examinations during the first years of his career, despite his growing prestige, should be understood as an attempt by the local oligarchy to keep such ambitious but unknown young men out of their circle. The hospital administrators, members of the same oligarchy, were also members of the boards of examiners which chose new staff members for the hospital. Only when Piquer had the support of Mayáns, a prestigious intellectual, was he able to gain a certain entry into the circle by obtaining one of the coveted posts left vacant by the death of Longás. Within this context, it is easier to understand why Juan Crisóstomo, Piquer's son, was anxious to connect his father with a long dynasty of physicians, and why Piquer himself, having become a highly respected physician in Madrid, published an aristocratic family tree in 1767.[50]

2. The Sevillian edition of *El Mundo Engañado* (1729) and the reply by the priest Juan José García Romero

2.1. The Royal Sevillian Society of Medicine and Other Sciences (Regia) (1697): An institution at the service of the renovation of knowledge and the

48 Tomás Longás (1620–1690) studied medicine in Valencia and was *Protomédico* of Aragón; Tomás Longás y Pascual, his son, became Professor of Anatomy at Valencia in 1698; Juan Bautista (d. 1742), Piquer's mentor, was also Professor of Anatomy at Valencia, although he did not obtain the post through the compulsory competitive exam (Peset, "La Universidad de Valencia" (cit. n. 40), p. 220; J. Soriano Faura, "La obra de Tomás Longás (1620–1690) como aportación al movimiento 'novator'," *Medicina e Historia,* 1977, n. 70, I–XVI).

49 Martínez Vidal, "La vinculación de Andrés Piquer" (cit. n. 47), pp. V–VI.

50 A. Piquer, *Hidalguía de Sangre de Don Andrés Piquer, Médico de Cámara de su Magestad, justificada con escrituras auténticas, Testimonios verídicos, y Historiadores dignos de fé* (Madrid, 1767). (Martínez Vidal, "La vinculación de Andrés Piquer" (cit. n. 47), p. II).

professional practice of the physicians.

> Ya, Sociedad, es llegado el tiempo que triunfes. Tu, que eras el escuadrón de la ignominia, serás la que enarboles el estandarte triunfante sobre los muros de la envidia. Quien te dió este triunfo? El sufrimiento. Quien la nobleza? La humildad. Quien el aplauso de docta? El estudio. Quien el nombre por toda Europa? El trabajo. Quien el premio a tus obras? El bien del próximo. Y quien, por último, te ha dado la protección Real? Tus méritos.[50*]

The *Regia* (1697) started as a series of meetings at which new scientific principles were discussed, and was soon brought under the auspices of the Spanish monarchy, first by Charles II (1700), and a year later by the first Bourbon monarch, Philip V (1701). In 1729, the *Regia* obtained the highest level of recognition from the court, and Philip V awarded it generous privileges and a substantial financial endowment, allowing the Society to carry out its scientific activities without economic restrictions.[51]

I nonetheless believe that the *Regia* had other objectives, in addition to its scientific goals. I think that the Society was a political instrument which advocated technical innovation in medicine under Charles II, the last of the Austrian monarchs. It also served the interests of the *Protomedicato*, the institution responsible for controlling the practice of health professionals in the Kingdom of Castile. Members of the *Regia, novatores*, were used by the Crown to limit the power of the University of Seville over medical training and practice.[52] In contrast

50* J.J. García Romero (1773), p. 16. See note 55.

51 G. Sánchez de la Cuesta, *Momentos estelares de la medicina sevillana* (Sevilla: G.E.H.A., 1967), pp. 79–84; J. Arriaga Cantullera, "Historia de la Regia Sociedad de Medicina y demás Ciencias de Sevilla," *Archivo Hispalense*, 1951, *14*: 373–441; A. Hermosilla Molina, *Cien años de medicina sevillana. La Regia Sociedad de Medicina y demás Ciencias, de Sevilla, en el siglo XVIII* (Sevilla: G.E.H.A., 1970); B. Ponce de León Almazán, "La Química en la Real Sociedad de Medicina de Sevilla," *Archivo Hispalense*, 1951, *15*: 195–240; López Piñero, *La introducción de la Ciencia Moderna en España* (cit. n. 40), pp. 45, 115–117.

52 The Crown later initiated an ambitious program of reforms in the teaching and practice of surgery. The Colleges, such as that of Cádiz (1748), became centers of teaching outside the universities, and were charged with the training of military surgeons. An analysis of these Colleges during the process of reformation in teaching and professional practice can be found in M. Astrain Gallart, *La*

to book learning and the scholastic teaching of medicine with emphasis on theory, which the Galenist or traditionalist professors at the university supported, the *Regia* introduced its members to a much more dynamic and technical type of training which included dissections and chemical experiments as prime elements. Clashes between the Sevillian College of Physicians, whose members were part of the *Claustro* of the Medical School of the University of Seville, and the members of the Society, most of whom were *revalidados*, physicians who had received a more empirical training, or those who eventually obtained permission to practice, were common almost from the start. The social differences between the two groups were also significant; the members of the *Claustro* formed an elite which was closed to the *revalidados*. One of the latter who supported the creation of the *Regia* was Juan Muñoz y Peralta (d. 1746), the first president of the Society, who was eventually named personal physician to Philip V. Both Muñoz and Diego Mateo Zapata (1644–1738), who urged Charles II to give his wholehearted support to the young organization,[53] were *conversos*, which was an obstacle in entering the university and severely limited their chances of social success. However, despite being persecuted by the Inquisition, neither of them suffered severe punishment, owing to their significant social and scientific prestige.[54]

The confrontations between the Sevillian *Galenists* and *revalidados* reached their peak in 1729, the year in which the Seville edition of Gazola's *El Mundo Engañado* was published. These confrontations

medicina del Mar. Sanitarios y Sanidad Naval al servicio del Rey: de Utrecht a Trafalgar (1715–1805) (Granada: unpublished Ph. D., 1992).

53 In his youth, Zapata was an ardent follower of the traditionalist physicians. At the urging of the University of Alcalá he published in 1690 a harsh criticism of Gazola's *Enthusiasmos*. This "respuesta" led to his social ascent at Court (V. Peset, "El doctor Zapata [1664–1745] y la renovación de la medicina en España," *Archivo Ibero Americano de Historia de la Medicina y Antropología Médica,* 1960, *12*: 35–93; López Piñero, *La introducción de la ciencia Moderna en España* [cit. n. 40]).

54 For an account of the proceedings against them, see J. Caro Baroja, *Los Judíos en la España Moderna y Contemporánea,* 3 vols. (Madrid: Ed. Arion, 1961), Vol. II, pp. 71–77; A. Domínguez Ortiz, "Dos médicos procesados por la Inquisición: I. El doctor Juan Muñoz Peralta. II. El proceso inquisitorial de Diego Mateo Zapata," in *Hechos y figuras del siglo XVIII español* (Madrid: Siglo XXI Editores, 1973), pp. 159–191.

revealed the different approaches to the training of physicians, and especially the different attitudes toward the control of professional medical practice. These conflicts ended with a victory for the *Regia*, which was awarded full autonomy from the University of Seville by the Crown.[55] The situation became so extreme that Madrid, in order to protect the interests of the Society, designated the *Assistente*, the highest civil authority in the city,[56] as defender, *socio protector*, of the *Regia*.[57]

The *Ordenanzas* (by-laws) of the Society — approved by the Royal Warrant of Charles II on May 25, 1700, clearly indicated that the Society had the power to authorize any of its physician members to practice in Seville, if they moved to the city *(Ordenanza XII)*. The Society also controlled, both within and outside the city, health professionals working in more empirical and experimentally-oriented fields, such as pharmacists and surgeons *(Ordenanzas I, II* and *III)*.[58] In the first Royal Warrant, the Society's full name was *Sociedad Médica de los Rebalidados (sic) de la Ciudad de Sevilla*; in a subsequent Royal Warrant, issued by Philip V on August 27, 1729, the society's name was *Regia Sociedad de Médicos, Cirujanos y Boticarios de la Ciudad de Sevilla* (The Royal Society of Physicians, Surgeons and Pharmacists of the City of Seville).[59]

The Sevillian College of Physicians clashed with the *Regia* as soon as the latter was annexed to the Castilian *Protomedicato*, thus placing it above the College of Physicians in the administrative and political hierarchy. Any provisions enacted by the Crown which favored the

55 The King gave the *Regia* permission to publish books without endorsement, and also granted the *Assistente* the exclusive authority to arbitrate in disputes between members of the *Regia* and doctors of the *Claustro* (J.J. García Romero, *Triumpho de la Regia Sociedad Hispalense y Diálogo de Medicina* [Sevilla, 1733], p. 42).

56 The *Assistente* was the Sevillian equivalent of the *Corregidor* in other cities, the Crown's representative in the City Council. See E. Terreros y Pando, *Diccionario de la Lengua Castellana, en que se explica el verdadero sentido de las voces, su naturalez y calidad, con las phrases o modos de hablar, los proverbios o refranes, y otras cosas convenientes al uso de la Lengua. Compuesto por la Real Academia Española,* 5 vols. (Madrid, 1726–1739; rpt. Madrid: Editorial Gredos, 1969), Vol. I, p. 447.

57 García Romero, *Triumpho de la Regia Sociedad* (cit. n. 55), pp. 42–43.

58 *Ibid.*, pp. 19 *ss*.

59 *Ibid.*, p. 49.

Regia were harshly contested by the physicians of the university. It was therefore no coincidence that consultations, which included members of both institutions, and the presidency of the *Claustro*, which was traditionally held by a *revalidado* despite the strong opposition of the members of the university governing board, were the points of most intense conflict between the two organizations.[60] Similarly, the *Regia* only recognized the City Courts and the City Council, but not the College of Physicians, as the authorities to whom they were responsible. Behind these disputes seem to have been a struggle for the control of the professional activity of the physicians. However, the *Regia* had highly influential supporters in Madrid among the physicians of the Court, who were usually members of the *Regia* and had important posts within the *Protomedicato*.[61] These advocates consistently defended the interests of their colleagues in the *Regia* before the Crown.[62]

To decentralize their activities, the Castilian *Protomedicato* delegated to the *Oidores*, the Judges of the Royal Courts, the job of controlling professional practice. In order to do so, the judges were to consult with reputable physicians. In Seville, this job was given to Pedro Ramos, who the following year was named President of the newly-created Subdelegation of the *Protomedicato* in Seville. It was no coincidence that Ramos had been a consultant to the *Regia* since 1739, and that the members of the Society were named examiners of this subdelegation.[63]

60 *Ibid.*, pp. 41 *ss.*; Arriaga Cantullera, "Historia de la Regia Sociedad" (cit. n. 51), pp. 378–380; Ponce de León Almazán, "La Química en la Real Sociedad" (cit. n. 51), p. 221.

61 M.C. Calleja Folguera, *La reforma sanitaria en la España Ilustrada* (Madrid: Editorial de la Universidad Complutense, 1988), pp. 24–25.

62 In 1729, the physician members of the *Claustro* of the University of Seville, now superseded in authority on all matters by the members of the *Regia*, presented their criticisms of the *Regia* to the Crown in a *Memorial*. The Crown's response could not have been more clear: it gave the *Regia* even greater autonomy, awarded it ample economic support, and increased its membership by permitting the physicians, surgeons and apothecaries of the Royal Household to join. Finally, it required the "physicians and surgeons of the Academy" to be "present and accountable" at all contacts between members of the *Claustro* and patients.

63 Calleja Folguera, *La reforma sanitaria* (cit. n. 61), pp. 37–38, 151; Hermosilla Molina, *Cien años de medicina sevillana* (cit. n. 51), p. 242.

2.2. ***Nobility through work/Nobility from the cradle:*** *Juan José García Romero's* ***El Triumpho de la Regia Sociedad*** *(1733) and his critique of Giuseppe Gazola (1729)*

In 1729, the same year in which the *Regia* had obtained its considerable privileges from the Crown, Jacobo de Herve, a Sevillian printer, published Gazola's *El Mundo Engañado* from the 1729 Valencia edition. The Sevillian text contained the five dissertations written by Gazola, his prologue entitled *To Good Physicians*, and the prologue of the Spanish translator. Although the title page noted that the edition was published with royal permission, there was no official statement of approval. Moreover, the contents of the five dissertations were literally the same as in the previous editions of Gazola's work. There was nothing to suggest who was ultimately responsible for the Seville edition. I believe that it may have been sponsored by a Galenist member of the College of Physicians (a representative of the *Claustro*) in a final attempt to halt the Crown's unconditional support of the *Regia*.[64] The purpose of this edition may well have been to publicize the view that the Sevillian Academy, while proposing the "new medicine" as an alternative, was actually denouncing the social superfluity of this approach. In addition, it should be recalled that at the time, the *Regia* was in the midst of a profound doctrinal crisis, a fact which Gazola's Sevillian publisher no doubt used to good advantage.

Juan José García Romero, a Sevillian "clergyman and priest,"[65] was the son of Francisco Pablo García, a former Professor of Method and Anatomy at the University of Seville, a physician member of the *Regia*, and, according to his son, one of its founders.[66] In 1733, García Romero published in Seville a work traditionally considered to be one of the first historical analyses of the Sevillian Academy. The *Triumpho*

64 The Valencia edition of 1729 contains the endorsement of Gregorio Mayáns, dated 1 March. In the Royal Warrant of August 1729, Philip V gave his wholehearted support to the *Regia*. This Seville edition may therefore have been published immediately before or after the Royal Warrant was issued.

65 A. Hernández Morejón, *Historia Bibliográfica de la Medicina Española*, 7 vols. (Madrid, 1842–1852; rpt. New York-London: Johnson Reprint Co., 1967), Vol. VII, pp. 37–38.

66 García Romero, *Triumpho de la Regia Sociedad* (cit. n. 55), pp. 29, 52.

de la Regia Sociedad Hispalense was also the first published work in Spain to openly refute Gazola's *El Mundo Engañado*. In the final section *(Chapter XV)*, the author strongly attacked Gazola's first dissertation, which maintained that both medicine and physicians could be done without. Other aspects of Gazola's text, such as his defense of the modern physicians against the traditional practitioners, were side-stepped, as they were of little use to the arguments García Romero attempted to use. The "triumphant" *Regia* could not countenance a text which disparaged the social necessity of physicians just when its members had finally received the Crown's recognition and support. Gazola's work was considered an insult to the efforts of the Society during the previous thirty years to impose a new professional standard opposed to the type which was then socially dominant, the Galenist physician who was a member of the Sevillian *Claustro*.

García Romero's wrath at the new printing of Gazola's text must have been great, as he completed his rebuttal within a few days of its appearance. However, his text was not printed until 1733, when it appeared as the second part of the *Triumpho*.[67] One of the reasons for García Romero's irritation was the unethical conduct of Gazola's Sevillian publisher, who brought out his edition without complying with the necessary legal requirements. According to García Romero, Gazola was no more than a pseudonym, probably that of a local clergyman or physician, and the publication of *El Mundo Engañado* was probably meant to discredit the noble medical profession. In marked contrast, García Romero's work appeared with a number of official endorsements, most of them signed by members of the *Regia*.[68] However, this work had not been submitted to the Society for approval, as was generally done, because García Romero was not a full member. As a result, when the *Regia* became aware of its publication, it named a

67 The publication of the *Triumpho* was apparently delayed, as according to some of the previous endorsements, the text was completed in 1731 (*Ibid.*, p. 137).

68 The *Aprobaciones* were by Juan de Náxera, Juan Bartolomé González Moreno, and Fr. Pedro Andrés de Velasco; the *Licencias* were by Antonio Fernández Raxo and Gerónimo Antonio de Barreda y Yebra, and the *Censura* was signed by Fray Antonio de la Ssma. Trinidad. All of the official endorsers except for those who issued the two *Licencias* were members of the Sevillian *Regia*.

commission to forestall possible conflicts with the governing board of the University.[69]

García Romero marshalled a number of subtle arguments to refute Gazola's text. The first part of the work, containing the history of the *Regia*, skillfully presents several of them. The main argument was based on the sanctification of medicine and the medical profession, which would protect them from malicious critiques.[70] To make his point, García Romero resorted to a quaint tale about the origins of the Society. His goal was to demonstrate the antiquity and divine origin of medicine and the medical profession in Spain, and particularly in Seville, where the *Regia* flourished.[71] It was therefore not surprising that García Romero dedicated his work to Saint Luke, "Protophysician among holy physicians, Evangelist, one of the Sixty Disciples of Christ, Bishop and Martyr," whose conversion to Christianity had been greatly influenced by his profession as a physician, when he was impressed by the healing powers of Christ. Thus, "if he was able to heal after his conversion, he healed as a Saint."[72]

According to García Romero, the sciences and medicine appeared in Spain before any other country. "The sciences were present in Spain before Athens, Mainz and Paris, because the Spanish people were more ancient."[73] Hercules founded an Academy of Sciences in Seville, where Galen, a Galician from Mondoñedo, and Avicenna, an Andalusian, studied. These considerations led García Romero to conclude: "I believe no other society older than the Sevillian Society can be found, nor can any other kingdom be found in this part of Europe superior to Spain in the sciences."[74]

The antiquity and divinity of medicine found their expression in nobility. However, for García Romero the word *noble* had other connotations with reference to medicine which should be emphasized, and which fully justified the special privileges awarded to the *Regia* by Philip V in his Royal Warrant of August 1729.[75] García Romero was

69 Hermosilla Molina, *Cien años de medicina sevillana* (cit. n. 51), p. 188.
70 García Romero, *Triumpho de la Regia Sociedad* (cit. n. 55), p. 60.
71 *Ibid.*, p. 35.
72 *Ibid., Dedicatoria, s.* p.
73 *Ibid.*, p. 35.
74 *Ibid.*, pp. 36–39.
75 *Ibid.*, pp. 44 *ss.*

not referring to honesty,[76] no the mere certification of *purity of blood*, obligatory for all physicians, surgeons and apothecaries. According to Miguel Eugenio Muñoz (1751), it was not required in order to practice other activities.[77] The author did not refer to the tax exemptions which some cities allowed their local physicians.[78] Nobility was, according to García Romero, the quality sanctioned by the Crown in the 1729 Royal Warrant obtained through the efforts of the members of the *Regia*. It allowed them to form part of the country's aristocracy and to enjoy considerable economic and social privileges. In this sense, the members of the *Regia* were compared to the members of the *Claustro* of the University of Valencia, who had "personal nobleness," although their "presence in the Courts... was within the Royal estate, as befits lay persons."[79] The members of the *Regia* were accorded "the same status as judges and other political and military public servants."[80] However, the privileges awarded by Philip V were limited to the group of founding, or full members, those who had participated in the first circles at the end of the seventeenth century. Thus, the Crown itself established an aristocracy within the heart of the *Regia*. Promises of future titles of personal nobility and of the Presidency of the *Claustros*, traditionally a point of conflict with the members of the Sevillian College of Physicians, together with the consequent repudiation of the latter, led to an increase in the number of applications to join the *Regia*, as noted by García Romero.

Because nobility meant wealth, García Romero felt that it was necessary to demonstrate the relationship between nobility and medicine, citing numerous sources, including many from the Bible, which

76 "Vale también honroso y estimable, como contrapuesto a lo deshonrado y vil" (E. Terreros y Pando, *Diccionario de la Lengua Castellana* (cit. n. 56), Vol. IV, p. 672).

77 M. Eugenio Muñoz, *Recopilación de las Leyes, Pragmáticas, Reales Decretos, y Acuerdos del Real Proto-Medicato hechas por encargo y dirección del mismo Real Tribunal* (Valencia, 1751), p. 28.

78 *Ibid.*, pp. 71–91, 368–372. García Romero lists the privileges enjoyed by some contemporary Sevillian physicians practicing in different places, such as Alonso López Cornejo in the town of Salteras and Manuel Pérez in the town of Santiponce. See García Romero, *Triumpho de la Regia Sociedad* (cit. n. 55), p. 65.

79 Eugenio Muñoz, *Recopilación de las Leyes* (cit. n. 77), p. 381.

80 García Romero, *Triumpho de la Regia Sociedad* (cit. n. 55), p. 50.

upheld this relation.[81] If divinity was beautiful and noble, then medicine, a profession of divine origin, was also beautiful, and hence noble.

However, ennoblement of practice was also based on rigorous control, which protected the noble profession from contamination by unqualified persons. According to García Romero, those who had studied medicine and been examined by the *Protomedicato* were fully capable of healing. Therefore, those who practiced without due regard for these requirements sullied the nobility of medicine. Intruders should therefore be prosecuted, as they represented a risk to the public well-being.[82] The physician should give priority to the ruling social minority, "important persons such as the Bishop and Governor," but he should also not forget the poor, "because the physician has a different obligation to tend the poor in places where there is no hospital, [but] in Seville there are twelve, nine for men and three for women."[83] For García Romero, the hospital had negative connotations; he considered it "shameful." The physician, who was obliged to show charity to the poor, should prevent a ruined "gentleman" or a "churchman" from having to resort to such places. The Holy Spirit would reward them for their pains with freedom on the Day of Judgment.

García Romero devoted the last chapter of his book to refuting the Sevillian edition of Gazola's work. In contrast to the strictly medical text published by Giovanni Francesco de Bartolomeis (1762), which is analyzed below, García Romero's intention was to demonstrate Gazola's ignorance of the Holy Scriptures, which formed the basis of his arguments in favor of the divinity and nobility of the medical profession.

Carried away by his anger, García Romero called Gazola a heretic and a trickster, and said that he was set on discrediting all physicians, including the good ones. This condemnation was impossible, as medicine and physicians, being the works of God, could not be harmful or

81 *Ibid.*, p. 89.

82 "El Rey manda... à los Médicos ser Juezes de las vidas de todos; y así digo... que debe constar de su habilitación en el Real Protomedicato... El Médico que cura faltándole alguno de los requisitos... como son la ciencia o la práctica, peca mortalmente. Las Leyes del Reyno mandan que se inquiera y castiguen a los que curan sin ser médicos. Los que no saben recetar son la peste de una República, son oficiales de Herodes, que es menester esconderse de ellos" (*Ibid.*, pp. 92–93).

83 *Ibid.*, pp. 101–102.

evil. Medicine was divine, and its therapeutic resources, such as bloodletting, should also be considered divine. On the other hand, it was wrong to wait for a spontaneous cure, as the physician could help the patient to recover from his or her illness.

3. A belated Italian reply from Madrid to *El Mundo Engañado*: Giovanni Francesco de Bartolomeis' *Il Mondo s'Inganna nella Medicina* (1762).

Very little is known about Giovanni Francesco de Bartolomeis, an Italian physician, other than the information which he himself provided in his text. *Il Mondo s'Inganna nella Medicina* indicates that he was born in Rome and that he wrote his *Riposte* to Gazola's work in August 1750, when he was a physician in Madrid. His text, published in 1762, was addressed to a non-physician friend from Freiburg who lived in Athens and who had sent him a copy of Gazola's *Il Mondo*. De Bartolomeis, in turn, promised to send his friend the works of Quevedo and of the Neapolitan physician Lionardo di Capoa.[84]

Dedicated to a high-ranking prelate of the pontifical court, *Il Mondo s'Inganna nella Medicina* was subject to the usual censorship and endorsements. One of these notes observes that de Bartolomeis was a *publico profesore* (practicing physician) in Rome. Trained in Turin, he had first-hand knowledge of European medicine, having travelled widely in many countries, especially in Germany. In October 1747 he lived in Freiburg, and later in Lisbon and Alcalá de los Gazules (province of Cádiz, Spain), where his method of curing fevers was highly successful. He had also planned to move to the Basque Country.[85] Among the works on Spanish medicine, de Bartolomeis cited the 1744 Roman edition of Benito Jerónimo Feijóo's *Teatro Crítico* and the work of Vicente Gilabert, who, in his opinion, published an impor-

84 G. F. de Bartolomeis, *Il mondo s'inganna nella medicina. Risposte familiari apologetiche in difesa del domma Fisico-Ippocratico del Dottor... Romano Già Medico in Madrid, ove le scrisse nel 1750. Ad un amico... il quale gli aveva mandata l'opera intitolata Il mondo ingannato da'falsi Medici del Dottor Gazzola* (Roma, 1762), p. 200.

85 *Ibid.*, pp. 151–152, 187.

tant work which was written at the request of José Cervi, president of the *Protomedicato*.[86] According to de Bartolomeis, the followers of the "mechanistic" and "chemical" schools in medicine met with little favor in Spain, though Baglivi was highly respected. Gazola failed completely in Spain, as the universities were opposed to his doctrines.[87] Like García Romero, de Bartolomeis thought that Gazola's book had not been written by him, or at most, that it was written in his youth, as it was impossible to understand how the author of the "*Enthusiasmos médicos, políticos y astrológicos*, a physician famous in Spain... and renowned in France, Germany and Italy" could have written the nonsense found in *El Mundo Engañado*.[88] At the end of the book, de Bartolomeis told his correspondent that he would soon be sending him another book which was then nearing completion: his *Prontuario Médico-Práctico* (Practical Medical Handbook).

3.1. A portrait of the perfect "Hippocratic" physician versus the modernist social climber

De Bartolomeis did not intend to write a treatise on medicine; his purpose was instead to disprove some of the assumptions found in Gazola's five dissertations. In a prologue addressed to his *Amico*, the author explained the reasons which had led him to publish his writings. He disliked the growing sectarianism in medicine, of which Gazola's work was a clear example, and the abandonment of the "physico-Hippocratic dogma" which had proved so effective over the previous two thousand years. He presented himself as a non-systematic physician and as a follower of rational empiricism who was deeply concerned with the curative aspect of medicine.[89] De Bartolomeis was more radical than Gazola with regard to therapy, firmly advocating that the physician not intervene in most illnesses, so as to allow the healing power of nature, *vis curatrix naturae*, to run its course. This was in

86 B. J. Feijóo, *Teatro Crítico Universale... Tradotto... da Marcantonio Franconi* (Roma 1744); V. Gilabert, *Examen medicum, per dialogos, juxta antiquorum, receptiorum placita, ut Tyronibus prodesse queat* (Madrid, 1736).

87 De Bartolomeis, *Il mondo s'inganna nella medicina* (cit. n. 84), pp. 19 and 98.

88 *Ibid.*, pp. 65–66.

89 *Ibid.*, pp. 1–2.

stark contrast to the activist position.[90] From this standpoint, the opinions of de Bartolomeis were similar to those of the German clinician Georg Ernst Stahl (1656–1734).[91] It is not surprising that both Stahl and his follower Ludwig Gottfried Klein (d. 1756) were frequently cited in *Il Mondo s'Inganna*. De Bartolomeis believed that the basic sciences were of no use in medicine, that the microscope was an instrument which distorted reality, and that morbid anatomy had nothing to contribute, given the lack of correlation between symptoms and lesions. He thus felt that the schools of medicine, the mechanists (the Boerhaavenists, as de Bartolomeis called them), and chemistry were false.[92]

As a physician concerned with the daily practice of his profession, de Bartolomeis cited numerous examples of incorrect clinical intervention by his contemporaries, which in his opinion were motivated more by greed than by the noble desire to cure illness. The different doctrines of systematic medicine in vogue during the period were used to cover up professional incompetence and made it easy for practitioners to become rich at the patient's expense. Treatment was therefore the aspect of medical practice in which the good physician proved his skill. Fevers, which were then one of the central topics in pathology because of the frequent errors in treating them, were used as the basis of his criticisms of modern physicians, especially the "mechanistics" and "chemists."[93]

This criticism was shared by those physicians more concerned with

90 E.H. Ackerknecht, *Therapeutics. From the Primitives to the 20th Century* (New York-London: Hafner Press, 1973), p. 78.

91 The origins of therapeutic nihilism in the Enlightenment, the topic of an excellent article by E. Lesky, "Los orígenes del nihilismo terapeútico," *Asclepio*, 1962, *14*: 3–21, will be investigated in a future study. Another significant author is Jean Emmanuel Gilibert (1741–1814), a follower of Sauvages and the Hippocratic method. In 1772, Gilibert published his three-volume work, *L'anarchie médicinale ou la médecine considérée comme nuisible à la société* (Neuchâtel), in which he harshly criticized the quackery and ignorance of the physicians, the tendency to use multiple drugs, and the neglect of the *vis curatrix naturae* principle in treatment.

92 De Bartolomeis, *Il mondo s'inganna nella medicina* (cit. n. 84), pp. 122, 159 and 166–170.

93 J. Geyer-Kordesch, "Fevers and other fundamentals: Dutch and German Medical Explanations c. 1680 to 1730," in *Theories of Fever from Antiquity to the Enlightenment,* eds. W. F. Bynum and V. Nutton (London: Wellcome Institute for the History of Medicine, 1981) pp. 99–120, on p. 119.

curing than with the theories of medicine. According to de Bartolomeis, ninety-five per cent of all fevers were essential or benign and represented nature's own curative forces; they required no treatment. Symptomatic fever, on the other hand, did require the attention of a physician, who should act cautiously and prudently.

Most fevers were benign, and thus it made no sense for the physician to intervene. He should trust the patient's own curative powers instead. As a result, the therapeutic triad of blood-letting, purging and quinine, which was then in use, should, according to de Bartolomeis, be used with prudence. Bleeding was recommended at the very beginning of an illness because it removed the febrile ferment in the blood, but it was not indicated in the paroxysmal phase. Purgatives were to be used only in the case of mesenteric fevers. De Bartolomeis had a low opinion of quinine, and believed that the overuse of this agent had caused changes in benign fevers; by acting against nature, it made a cure more difficult to achieve. Quinine was thus not an antipyretic, but an anti-medical agent. The key to health lay in the proper regulation of the *sex res non naturales*, to which the author devoted numerous hygienic and health rules.[94]

Conclusion

On many occasions, the fortuna of medical text has depended not only on its theoretical grounds but also on its critical and polemic contents. Giuseppe Gazola's *Il mondo ingannato da falsi medici* (1716) had a wide audience in Spain at the beginning of the XVIIIth Century, even more than in other European countries. At that time in Spain clashes concerning doctrinal and professional aspects between traditionalist and innovator *(novatores)* physicians achieved its climax. In denouncing the strengthening of medical power upon patients, Gazola's text became a commonplace in which those conflicts were developed. Valencia and Seville lodged the bitterest arguments. Remarkably these were the cities where innovator physicians attained a significant scientific and social role. As soon as these clashes were over, the medical interest in Gazola's text declined, as indicated in *Il Mondo s'Inganna nella Medicina* (1762) by Giovanni Francesco De Bartolomeis.

94 De Bartolomeis, *Il mondo s'inganna nella medicina* (cit. n. 84), pp. 141–144.

Elements of Moslem Forensic Medicine

Yaakov Meron

The Moslem law which prevailed in Spain under the Arabs was its brand emanating from North Africa and known as Maliki Moslem law. This brand has its importance locally but was and remains quite distinct[1] and different from Moslem law prevalent in other parts of the Moslem world, most notably in its foremost center of culture and civilization in the Near East.[2] Throughout most of the period Spain remained under the Arabs, the center of the latter civilization was in Iraq, the cradle of Hanafi Moslem law.

There were contacts between East and West, so that Spain was, to some extent, subject to influence from the East.[3] During the reign of 'Abd al-Raḥman II (822–852), Spain opened its gates to influences from the Abbasid Orient and from the civilization of Baghdad. This enlightened prince ordered books to be brought from Iraq, but medical practice at that time was restricted to the more or less able use of potions, elixirs and pomades. One of the physicians practicing in Spain was an immigrant from northern Iraq, Yûnus ibn Aḥmad al-Harrânî. He was born in Harrân, which was for a long time a center of learning in philosophy and sciences.

It was only during the reign of 'Abd al-Raḥman III (912–976) that the study of medicine from the books of the Orient began.

1 On the relationship between Maliki law and the other brands of Moslem law, see my "Parents and Children under Moslem Law," in *Jewish Law Annual*, vol. X (1992), pp. 213–234, especially p. 215 note 15 and pp. 219–220.

2 On doctors and medicine in the eleventh century, under the Mamluks (1250–1516) and in medieval times see in the bibliography note 49 below.

3 See H.P.J. Renaud, "Les origines de la médecine arabe en Espagne" dans: *Bulletin de la Société française d'histoire de la médecine* 29 (1935), pp. 321–332; Danielle Jacquart et Françoise Micheau, *La Médecine arabe et l'Occident médiéval*, Paris, Maisonneuve et Larose, 1990, pp. 137–138.

Two sons or grandsons of the above-mentioned Yûnis ibn Aḥmad al-Harrânî went to Baghdad, where they spent ten years with Thâbit ibn Qurra (about whom see below in the text before note 41) and Ibn Waşif. They were back in Cordoba in 962. They were not the only ones to cross the Mediterranean in order to benefit from the teachings of Iraqi or Egyptian masters and then to enrich their country of origin with the knowledge and the books from the Orient.[4]

Less than half a century after the death of Al-Râzi, the influence of his *Kitâb al-Ḥâwi* may be seen on the *Kitâb al-Taşrîf* written in Spain by al-Zahrâwî (died shortly after 1009) a noted surgeon.[5]

The eleventh century saw the entrenchment of the science of medicine in Spain: the teaching and practice of medicine was carried on in Granada, Seville, Almeria, Murcia, Cordoba and Toledo.[6] Medicine reached its zenith in Spain in the twelfth century with Ibn Rushd, known in the West as Averroès, who was born in Cordoba in 1126 and died there in 1198. The same century also saw the great work of translation from Arabic into Latin led by Gerard of Cremona (1114–1187), who came to Spain for this purpose.[7] The two most important texts thus translated into Latin were the above-mentioned text of Al-Râzi (Razès) and the *Canon* by Ibn Sina' (Avicenna) (*ibid.* p. 150). The translation activity, which started in Toledo after it was taken by the Christians in 1085, has been called "the forerunner of Oriental studies in the modern sense of the word."[8]

According to Jacquart and Micheau the decline which set in the thirteenth century was "mainly" due to the departure of the Jews "who played a major role," but for whom Spain became an inhospitable country.[9] However, the little known so far about Moslem forensic

4 Jacquart et Micheau, *op. cit.*, p. 139.

5 (*Ibid*, p. 140). Moreover, a history of physicians which appeared in Spain in 987 contains the biographies of 57 individuals: 15 from the ancient Greek world, 16 from the Moslem Orient, 3 from the Maghreb, but 23 from Spain (*Ibid*, p. 141).

6 *Ibid*, p. 141.

7 *Ibid*, pp. 142–144, 150.

8 Mustashriḳûn, in the *Encyclopedia of Islam*, New Edition, vol. VII, p. 738a *in fine*).

9 (*op. cit.* p. 145). On the "Position of Jewish Physicians in Medieval Muslim countries" see the "Note" by Moshe Perlmann in JOS (1972) 315–319 in note 45 below. "According to an Ottoman document written ca. 1607–1608, the Palace

medicine is mostly limited to the area dominated by Ḥanafi Moslem law, that is, the Middle East. The following remarks are therefore restricted to Ḥanafi Moslem law.

Restrictions on free exercise of the medical profession

"The physician is allowed to look at her diseased place."[10] This dispensation follows a general prohibition: "A man is not allowed to look at a strange woman except for her face and her hands."[11] The liberty of action enjoyed by the doctor is apparently unlimited, as can be seen a fortiori from the following text: "If a person hires a man (*insan-an*) to cut off a member [of his body] this is permissible because this can be achieved, for the object is known. He can thus put the knife on it and cut it off."[12] If an ordinary "man" is allowed to perform surgery, a qualified doctor would certainly be allowed to do so.[13]

medical staff consisted of forty-one Jewish and twenty-one Moslem physicians. By the mid-seventeenth century, the numbers and proportions had shrunk to four Jews and fourteen Moslems." Bernard Lewis, *The Jews of Islam*, in note 45 below.

Jews in North Africa considered as "custom" provisions which were in fact culled from Ḥanafi Moslem law, which probably reached them through contacts with the Jewish spiritual leadership which was then centered in Iraq. See Abraham L. Udovitch, "*The Jews in the Middle Ages: A Case of the Moslem Views of Difference*", in: *Settimane di Studio del Centro Italiano di Studi Sull'Alto Medievo* XXVI. Gli Ebrei Nell'Allto Medievo 30 Marzo — 5 Aprile 1978, Tomo Sicondo, Presso la Sede de Centro, 1980, p. 665.

10 "*Wa-yajûzu lil-ṭabîb an yanẓur ilâ mawḍi' 'l-maraḍ min-hâ*, Aḥmad bn-u Muḥammad al-Qudûrî, *Matn*, Halabi Edition, 3rd impression, Cairo, 1957, p. 119, 1.2.

11 Qudûrî, *op. cit.* p. 118, l. 24–25.

12 Abû Bakr bn-u Mas'ûd al-Kâsânî, *Badâi' 'l-Ṣanâ'i' fî Tartîb-i 'l-Ṣharâ'i'*, Cairo, 1910, vol. III, p. 189, 1. 19–20.

13 The last of the thirty volume encyclopedia of medicine composed by the Spaniard Abû al-Qâsim Khalaf al-Zahrâwî (see above note 3) is devoted to surgery (English translation and commentary: M.S. Spink and G. Lewis, Albucasis: *On Surgery and Instruments*, London, 1973). It shows the influence of Al-Râzî's *Kitâb al-*Ḥâwî (=Razès, Liber ad Almansorem = Al-Manṣûri) but largely based on Paul of Egina, who studied and practiced medicine in Alexandria and remained there after the Arab conquest in 640. He was considered in the Moslem World as one of

There are, nonetheless, a number of restrictions which may hamper a doctor's work or even prevent him from carrying it out.[14] For example, dissections are presently regulated by secular law in various Moslem countries.[15] However, Moslem law displays considerable reluctance about dissections and it is generally believed that Moslems never performed them.[16] The first modern school of medicine in the Moslem World, the Army Medical School in Istanbul founded in 1827, "has to overcome a strong traditional prejudice against dissections of human bodies."[17] A similar "traditional prejudice" may be seen in the opinions given by Moslem Cadis in Israel when questioned by the Israeli Government during the preparation of the 1953 Anatomy and Pathology Law.[18] These opinions, as well as contrary opinions expressed in Egypt, fail to show any authoritative Moslem texts on dissection. It therefore seems that the opposition to dissection, far from reflecting a religious or legal injunction, stems from an innate prejudice prevalent among people who are devoid of any religious knowledge. An Israeli doctor working among the Bedouin in the Negev confirms this impression:

> I had Bedouin patients whose relatives took them home a few hours before their deaths in order to avoid the possibility of

the principal authorities in medicine (Jacquart et Micheau, *op. cit.* p. 140).

The work of Albucasis, i.e., Abû l-Qâsim, was the basis of the great treatises on surgery from the thirteenth century onward (*ibid*, p. 150) and played a decisive role in European surgical art (*ibid*, p. 150 and the bibliography given there).

14 See "Religious Prohibitions" below.

15 In Jordan, section 8 of the 1966 Public Health Law provides for places where dissection may be carried out. In Syria, Legislative Decree No. 227 of 10.5.1953 provides for "Permission to open corpses of the dead in certain cases," and Decision No. 36 of 2.10.1975 defines the cases of dissection "for scientific needs."

16 E.G. Brown, *Arabian Medicine*, Cambridge 1921, p. 36. A French edition is E.G. Brown, *La médecine arabe*, mise à jour et annotée par H.P.J. Renaud, Paris, 1933.

17 U. Heyd, "The Ottoman Ulema and Westernization" in: *Scripta Hierosolymitana*, vol. IX, U. Heyd (ed.), *Studies in Islamic History and Civilization*, Jerusalem, 1961, pp. 61–96, 67.

18 Y. Meron, "Medical Treatment Viewed by Moslem Law" in: H. Karplus (ed.), *International Symposium on Society, Medicine and Law*, Jerusalem, March 1972, Amsterdam, Elsevier Scientific Publishing Company, 1973, pp. 43–53, at p. 48.

> dissection. On this very day when I am writing these lines the following has happened: A patient whom I had sent to Kaplan Hospital with a serious renal insufficiency was taken away the next day, brought home and died there within a few hours without any medical care. Had he received the right treatment, he would have lived for months. This, too, happened because of the fear that he would die there and be dissected.[19]

If, despite the lack of source-material, one may speak about "reluctance about dissections," it is because Moslem law is clearly against a somewhat similar surgical procedure: organ transplants.

Human bones must never be used for medical purposes. This view is attributed to Muhammad al-Shaybani[20] (d. 804), the first man who wrote down Moslem law. The same view is expressed by Abû Bakr al-Kâsânî (d. 1191), who represents the summit of legal thought in Islam and was its foremost lawyer in the Classical period (1000–1200 C.E.).[21] This prohibition was later extended to all members of the human body in the late seventeenth century Indian compendium of responsa.[22] However, a certain difference of opinion on a specific application of this prohibition dates back to the early days of Moslem law. It concerns the transplant of teeth — an operation, I am told, which has not been carried out even by modern dentistry.

At that time, the transplanting of a dead man's tooth into the mouth of a living person was unanimously considered to be a bad thing.[23] The difference of opinion was whether it is permissible to reimplant a man's tooth, an operation which can be done today.[24] Abû Ḥanîfa (d. 767)

19 Z. Von-Weisel, "Dissection, Religion and Tradition" in *Eretz Israel* No. 9 (14), January, 1972.

20 *Al-Fatâwî 'l-Hindiya*, the 1350 edition, vol. IV, p. 112.

21 Abû Bakr al-Kâsânî, *op. cit.* (above note 12) vol. V, p 142, l. 29–30.

22 *Al-intifâ' bi-ajzâ 'l-â'damî lam yajuz, qîla lil-najâsa wa-qîla lil-karâma wa-huwa 'l-saḥîḥ (Al-Fatâwî 'l-Hindiya), op. cit.* (above note 20), p. 111. Kâsânî (above note 12) also held that the prohibition was based on protecting the dignity of the corpse although the term he uses is *iḥtirâm*, not *karâma*.

23 In Islam, human actions are classified into five categories: forbidden, blameworthy, neutral, praiseworthy and obligatory. Teeth transplants are blameworthy.

24 Dr. A. Tamir of Israel delivered a paper on this subject at the International Convention of Dentists held in Tel Aviv between 3 and 5 July, 1978. See Avraham Peleg, *Ma'ariv* 4 July, 1978.

and al-Shaybani held that there was no difference between reimplantation and the transplantation of a dead man's tooth, since any separated member of the human body, like the body as a whole, requires burial. Abu Yusuf (d. 798) disagreed and equated the tooth to any other member of the body, which, if cut off and reinstated in its place, may return to its initial state. Abu Yusuf stressed that the consideration of not putting another's body to contempt (*ihâna*) did not apply to a person's own limb if it became detached from the body.[25] Later developments in Moslem law, which prohibited the use of any member of the human body, cannot be reconciled with Abu Yusuf's opinion allowing tooth reimplantation.[26]

A modern challenge to the Moslem prohibition on organ transplants was presented by the 1956 Jordanian Law concerning "Use of the Eyes of Corpses for Medical Purposes."[27] The Responsa Institute (*Dar al-Ifta*) in the Jordanian capital issued a response prohibiting the transplant of a cornea from the eye of a dead man to a living person. The Jordanian Senior Scholar (*Ra'is al-Ulama*), who had probably been consulted in the preparation of the Law, contested this ruling, insisting that his views should prevail by virtue of his position.

This point did not pass unchallenged. The Responsa Institute, in its answer, recapitulated the Senior Scholar's argument as follows: "His excellency contradicts the Imam Muhammad [al-Shaybani] and the author of the *Fatâwî l-Hindiya* (the seventeenth century Indian compendium of responsa) and claims that their words are not based on any explicit text of the Koran or of the Prophetic tradition. This is merely an [arbitrary] opinion (*ra'y*) preferred by a group of sages..."[28] The "group of sages" referred to are the scholars of the religious Al-Azhar University in Cairo who permitted the transplant of corneas and of

25 Kâsânî, *op. cit.* (above note 12), pp. 132–133.

26 However, permission for "plastic" surgery, namely fixing a golden nose to a war invalid, was granted by the Prophet of Islam himself (died 632). The tradition relating it is cited by al-Kâsânî, *ibid*, vol. V, p. 132 and is also found in the *Sunan* of al-Nisâ'î, Cairo 1313, vol. 2, "*Kitâb al-Zina*," p. 286.

27 Law No. 43 of 1956, published in the Jordanian Official Gazette of 16 December, 1956, No. 1310, pp. 2336–2337.

28 *Majallat Hadyi 'l-Islam*, issued by the Department of Islamic Affairs in Amman, Jordan, Sixth year, vol. VI, pp. 57–67.

human organs generally basing themselves on humanitarian considerations.[29] Neither they nor the Senior Scholar of Jordan tried to reconcile their preferred solution with the authoritative Moslem texts, rightly relied upon by the Jordanian Responsa Institute and also substantiated, at least in part, by the International Covenant on Civil and Political Rights,[30] article 7 of which states, "...no one shall be

29 *Magallatu 'l-Azhar [sic!]* (Al-Azhar Magazine), vol. 34, November 1962, pp. 523–524: *Ḥukm naql a'ḍâ mayit ilâ ḥay*. Egyptian practice seems to follow this *responsum*. On 10 May, 1992, Mr. Ṣaleḥ Aziza from the Druze village Abû Snân in the Galilee told an interviewer on the first channel of Israeli television (on the program "Between the Chairs") that he had undergone a kidney transplant in Egypt. He had paid a 26-year-old Sudani man for the kidney. When asked by the interviewer about other Israelis who had failed to obtain organs for transplants in Egypt, Mr. Aziza answered that non-Moslem foreigners cannot obtain such organs in Egypt.

To combat commercialization of human organ tranplantation the World Health Assembly in May 1991 adopted "Guiding Principles on Human Organ Transplantation," in: *Human Organ Transplantation*, A report on developments under the auspices of WHO (1987–1991), Geneva: WHO, 1991, 28 pp.

G. Dworkin, "The Law Relating to Organ Transplantation in England" (1970) *33* Modern Law Review, 356–357.

For the U.S. legal situation, see H. Hansmann, "The Economics and Ethics of Markets for Human Organs" (1989) *14*, *J. of Heath Politics, Policy and Law* 57–85. Both Hansmann and Noam J. Zohar (in his article "Toward Justice in the Organ Trade," *Isr. L. Rev. 27* [1993] 541–565) seem to see nothing wrong in exchanging organs for money. The latter calls, however, for "[e]nforcing a fair price" in this trade.

The trade in organs gave rise to a lively debate in law, Professors Levontin and Weisman holding that a thing which is not transferable must be excluded from the framework of property rights and is no "asset" at all. The late Professor Tedeschi (in his article "Ownership of Organs taken from a Living Person," *Isr. L. Rev. 27* [1993] p. 624), followed by Professor Alfredo Mordechai Rabello ("Gift of Organs — A Note" in *Isr. L. Rev 27* [1993], 661–667), affirms the traditional view according to which organs which have been removed from the body are the object of property right ("movable property") of the person from whose body they are taken. Moreover, this matter would not cause any dispute because Weisman's opinion is "contrary to the prevailing legal position world-wide" (p. 627 in Tedeschi's article, *ibid*). Indeed, this is also the position of Jewish Law: Rabbi Mordechai Halperin, M.D., "Organ Transplants from Living Donors," in *Isr. L. Rev. 27* (1993), 556–587 and Rabello, *ibid.*, p. 664, note 14.

30 Annexed to resolution 2200 (XXI) of the General Assembly, adopted on 16 December, 1966. United Nations Yearbook on Human Rights for 1966, 1969.

subjected, without his free consent, to medical or scientific experimentation," and by article 43 of the 1971 Egyptian Constitution which states, "No medical or scientific experiment may be performed on any man without his free consent."

Contracts

The payment which the doctor receives for his services, its imposition upon the patient and the determination of its amount all bring the relationship between doctor and patient within the realm of contracts. This contract is considered in Moslem law to be that of hire. However, granted that the doctor is hired, it is not always clear who hired him, especially in emergencies, when the doctor intervenes without any prior negotiation. Moslem jurists actually discussed the case of a midwife who delivered a child without being asked to do so.

The ambiguity of the hirer bears directly upon the question: who is to pay for that medical service? This question was raised in connection with medical assistance for pregnant women. The problem of the doctor's fee is particularly acute here owing to the very strict regime of separation of property between husband and wife under Moslem law.[31] Long before Lord Denning saw "no reason why a rich woman's own means should not come into the family pool" in order to meet her personal expenses on hats and dresses, the Moslem wife, whether rich or poor, had to meet her personal expenses from her own purse.[32] In Islam, these personal expenses include, *inter alia*, her medical care.

For centuries Moslem jurists debated the question of whether the husband or the wife should pay the midwife.[33] Since the delivery of the

31 Y. Meron, "A Muslim Solution," in: *Israel Law Review*, (1972) *7*, p. 315.

32 *Fatḥ* (Cairo edition 1316, 3:248) (but should be 328) relying on no source at all; *Baḥr*, Cairo edition 1916, IV:182 relying on the *Tabyîpn* by Zayla'î (d. 1342), chapter *Ṣadaqat al-Fiṭr* ; al-Ḥaṣkafi (d. 1677) author of *Al-Durr* printed on the margins of *Radd* Bulaq Edition 1284/1864 II:704 *in fine* (relying on the *Jawhara*) — 705. See also Y. Linant de Bellefonds, *Traité de Droit Musulman Comparé*, vol. III, Paris, 1973, p. 132.

33 The debate probably started with a *responsum* by Iftikhâr al-Din (died 1147), author of the *Khulâṣa*. He is cited by Ibn al-Humâm (died 1457), author of the *Fatḥ op. cit.* vol. 3, pp. 327–328. The problem is later tackled by Ibn Nujaym (died

child was considered to be essential medical treatment for the pregnant woman, the midwife was to be paid by the woman. However, Ibn 'Abidin, the last great traditional jurist, who died in Damascus in 1836, took the opposite view. He held that the midwife's fee should be paid by the husband, as the father is responsible for maintaining the child and the greater benefit of the midwife's service has accrued to the child.[34] This liberal attitude towards the wife provides no hard and fast rule for the lawyer, as a still-born child can hardly be seen to benefit from the services of a midwife. It is therefore not always easy to determine who is liable for services rendered by a midwife, a gynecologist or any other physician, if a contract was not concluded prior to attendance.

However, even if a contract has been concluded, its existence is fragile. According to an express provision of the Ottoman Civil Code *(Mejelle)* which is still the law in Judea, Samaria and Gaza, as well as in Kuwait,[35] if "a person suffering from a toothache makes a contract with a dentist to extract his tooth for a certain fee" and before the treatment "the pain ceases, the contract of hire (*ijâré*) is cancelled."[36] This case, like the rest of that Civil Code, is culled from Moslem law where, beside the contract with a dentist, a similar contract with a surgeon is cited, to the same effect: "If a person, in whose hand a necrosis has set in, hires a person to cut it off but the pain calmed down

1563), author of the *Baḥr, op. cit.*, vol. IV, p. 177; by al-Ḥaṣkafi (d. 1677), author of *Al-Durr* printed on the margins of *Radd* II:704–705; and by Ibn-'Abidîn (d. 1836), author of the *Radd, op. cit.*, vol. II, p. 1003.

34 Y. Meron, *L'Obligation alimentaire entre époux en droit musulman hanéfite*, Librairie Générale de Droit et de Jurisprudence, Paris 1971, pp. 220–223. Israeli courts do not always uphold the criterion of benefit. A hospital which claimed its fee from a patient had its claim rejected because the benefit obtained by the patient was not considered sufficient ground for imposing the payment upon the patient and because it was not proved that the patient had actually asked for the treatment at the hospital. See: (1961) 15(1) P.D. 1238, 1237 *in fine.*

35 C. Chehata, *Etudes de Droit Musulman*, Paris PUF, 1971, p. 41.

36 Article 443. The original text of that Code, known as the *Mejelle*, is in Ottoman Turkish. The above citation is taken from the English translation by C.A. Hooper, *The Civil Law of Palestine and Trans-Jordan*, Jerusalem, 1933, with which the present writer humbly concurs.

and later his hand recovered"[37] "the contract of hire (*al-ijâra*) is cancelled (*tantaqid*) by itself (*bi-nafsi-ha*)."[38] These two cases, of the dentist and the surgeon, had appeared already in the *Mabsût* by al-Sarakhsi (died 1097).[39]

Both of these cases are cited to substantiate the argument that there is no need for an act of rescission to bring a contract to its end. The opposite view, held by al-Shafi'i (died 820), is that "in the same way as the contract was concluded by their mutual consent (*bi-ittifaqi-himâ*) so can it be dissolved only by their mutual consent."[40] As shown also by the above citation from the Ottoman Civil Code, the latter opinion has been totally rejected. The *Mejelle* loaded on these cases the sweeping conclusion that, "if any event happens whereby the reason for the conclusion of the contract disappears so that the contract cannot be carried out, such contract is cancelled."[41]

In fact, Moslem law, at least as al-Kâsânî presents it, reveals a more refined attitude. The contract is cancelled not by "any event whereby the reason for the conclusion of the contract disappears" but by weighing of the benefits (*maṣlaḥa*) against the damage (*maḍarra*)[42] in executing the contract. When the toothache has disappeared and the necrotic hand has recovered, the damage in carrying out the contract is certainly greater than the benefit. It is as if a condition is implied in every such contract that it is concluded only for the benefit of the patient.

It remains, however, that the decision as to whether the illness is gone or not is left to the discretion of the patient. This unilateral power of one side to the contract explains the fragile nature of such contracts.

Torts

In sixteenth-century Turkey, doctors used to require from their patients an undertaking in court that they will not sue them in case the treatment

37 Kâsânî, *op. cit.* (above note 12), vol. IV, p. 197, 1. 26–27.
38 *Ibid.*, p. 200, l. 30.
39 Vol. XVI p. 2, l. 17–18.
40 Kâsânî, *op. cit.* (above note 12) p. 197, l. 19 and again p. 200, l. 28–29.
41 Article 443 of the *Mejelle* (above note 36).
42 Kâsânî, *op. cit.* (above note 12) vol. IV, p. 198, 1. 8.

or the operation fails. A famous case at that time was that of a circumciser who was condemned in 1535 to pay the enormous sum of 42,000 akçe to the father of a child who became an invalid as a result of the circumcision.[43]

Moslem law includes measures to protect the public from incompetent physicians. During the Classical Period in Moslem law (1000–1200 C.E.), an author by the name of al-Sarakhsî stated an opinion which he dated to the beginning of Moslem law. The same dating also appears in later sources.[44] According to this opinion, which is ascribed to Abû Ḥanîfa, a sane adult could never be subjected to legal interdiction unless he fell into one of three specific categories:

> Interdiction is inapplicable except for three [persons]: the frivolous jurisconsult, the ignorant physician (*al-muṭabbib al-jâhil*) and the bankrupt public carrier, because of the grave damage [which ensues] if they are not interdicted. The frivolous jurisconsult harms people's religion. The ignorant doctor harms their bodies and the bankrupt public carrier wastes their possessions. Therefore, they are restrained from doing so, in order to avoid damage.[45]

The two disciples of Abû Ḥanîfa, Abu Yusuf and al-Shaybani, disagreed with their master, arguing that as a rule interdiction can be applied to certain sane people, other than those specifically indicated by Abû Ḥanîfa. They added the bankrupt (not only the bankrupt public carrier) and the prodigal.

The discussion in the eleventh-century text centers on legal interdiction and incapacity and the ignorant doctor was mentioned only briefly. It is therefore not surprising to discover that this text does not

43 U. Heyd, *Studies in Old Ottoman Criminal Law*, Oxford, 1973, pp. 308–309.

44 Kâsânî, *op. cit.* (above note 15) vol. VII, p. 169, cited by Chafik Chehata, *Etudes de Droit Musulman*, Vol. 1, Paris, PUF, 1971, p. 112, and by Y. Linant de Bellefonds, *Traité de Droit Musulman Comparé*, vol. 3, Paris, Mouton & Co., 1973, p. 289, who also cites Zayla'î, *Tabyîn* V, 190 and Ibn 'Abidîn (above note 33) *Radd* "V, 102–103," Joseph Schacht, *An Introduction to Islamic Law*, Oxford 1964, also mentions "the ignorant physician" but gives no sources. The ignorant physician also appears in sections 964 and 26 of the *Mejelle* (above note 36). A similar provision is now contained in section 325 of the Penal Law in Israel.

45 Al-Sarakhsî, *Al-Mabsûṭ*, Cairo, 1331/1913, vol. XXIV, p. 157.

clarify how the doctor's knowledge or ignorance is to be determined by the judge.[46] However, from other sources, it is well known that official medical diplomas were instituted in the Moslem World as early as the tenth century by Sinan, son of the great geometrician, mathematician, physician and philosopher Thâbit b. Qurra (836–901). While attending to the Caliph Qâhir (932–4),[47] Sinan made aspirants to the medical

46 Linant de Bellefonds (above note 44) states that "in Abû Ḥanîfa's time an ignorant doctor was he who administers bad medicines or good medicines but in excessive doses" (p. 290). No classical source is given.

However, as already mentioned, in Spain too, in the ninth century, the science of the doctors was limited to the more or less skillful use of potions, elixirs and pomades (Jacquart et Micheau, *op.cit.* above note 3, p. 137). Even later in the Middle Ages, both within the Moslem World and outside it, the proficiency of physicians was measured by their skillfulness in prescribing medicaments. Thus, in the thirteenth century Ibn Rushd (=Averroès) wrote: "He who will possess the Generalities (i.e. his *Kitâb al-kulliyat fî 'l-ṭibb*, a critical edition of which was published in 1987 in Madrid by J.M. Forneas Besteiro and C. Alvarez de Morales, 2 vols. (Consejo Superior de Investigaciones Cientificas, Escuela de Estudios Arabes de Granada) will be able to understand what is right and what is wrong in applying and prescribing medicaments, in the therapeutic of the authors of the Compendiums," (Jacquart et Micheau, *op.cit.* p. 144, relying on vol. 1, pp. 517–518 of the above-mentioned critical edition). Also in the middle of the 13th century Roger Bacon wrote: "[The degree of a composed medicament] cannot be determined except by the method taught by the *De Gradibus* of al-Kindi. This method is very difficult and totally unknown in our times by Latin physicians, as everybody knows. Indeed, anyone trying to apply this philosopher's art must [first of all] possess the foundations of mathematics, because the categories of greater and smaller inequalities of proportions, the rules of the fractions which are used by this author are very difficult" (cited by Jacquart et Micheau, *op.cit.*, pp. 152–153.) According to these last two authors, al-Kindi's treatise depends as much on mathematics as it does on medical theory (*ibid, p. 153*).

The 28th volume of Abu 'l-Qâsim Khalaf al-Zahrâwî (known as *Liber servitoris*) is devoted to the preparation of simple medicaments. A partial critical translation is S. Hamarneh and G. Sonnedecker, A *Pharmaceutical View of Abulcasis al-Zahrâwî in Moorish Spain with special reference to the Adhân*, Leiden 1963, *Janus* suppl. V. According to Jacquart and Micheau, this volume "reveals an enrichment of the *Matière médicale* and presents in the most concrete fashion the operations which are preliminary to the preparation of the drugs" (p. 140).

47 This was Qâhir's second period in power. The first one lasted sometime during his brother's lifetime who died in 932. It is possible that Sinan's innovation was introduced during Qâhir's first period in power.

profession pass examinations. Certificates were awarded to those who passed, defining the limits of their medical practice. In Baghdad alone there were at that time over 800 physicians who held this certificate, not including the physicians who had been exempted from the examination because of the renown they already enjoyed.[48]

It is possible that when al-Sarakhsi, in the eleventh century, cited the opinion about the ignorant doctor he had in mind the certificates of proficiency in medicine which had been in circulation for at least a century. These certificates cannot, however, explain what was in Abû Ḥanîfa's mind when he spoke, if he indeed did so, about interdicting the ignorant doctor sometime in the eight century. That was almost two hundred years before Sinan introduced his diplomas and about a century before the science of medicine "reached its maturity" in the Moslem World.[49]

48 Baron Carra de Vaux, *Les Penseurs de l'Islam*, II, Paris, 1921, pp. 261–262. See also the same author's article "Ṭibb" in: *The Encyclopedia of Islam*, vol. IV, 1934, pp. 740–741, p. 741a.

49 "The history of the development of Arabian Medicine...reached its maturity in the ninth century." See D. Campbell, *Arabian Medicine* vol. 2, London, 1926, vol. I, p. XIII; J.S. Graziani, *Arabic Medicine in the Eleventh Century as represented in the works of Ibn Jazlah*, Karachi, Hamdard Academy, 1980; Doris Behrens — Abouseif, *Fath Allah and Abu Zakariyya, Physicians under the Mamluks*, Le Caire, Institut Français d'Archéologie Orientale, 1987; Penelope Johnstone (ed.), *Studies in Medieval Arabic Medicine*, London, Reprint 1984; S. Ammar, *En souvenir de la médecine arabe. Quelques-uns de ses grands noms*, Tunis, 1965; Manfred Ullmann, *Islamic Medicine*, Leiden, Brill, 1978; Ahmad 'Isâ, *Tarîkh al-bîmaristânât fî l-Islam*, 2nd ed., Beirut, 1981; A.Z. Iskandar, *A Descriptive List of Arabic Manuscripts on Medicine and Science at the University of California*, Los Angeles, 1984; Franz Rosenthal, *Science and Medicine in Islam: A Collection of Essays*, Aldershot, Variorum, c. 1990; Zouhair, M. Agha, *Bibliography of Islamic Medicine and Pharmacy*, Foreword by Abdullah Omer Nassief, London, 1983; Y.K. Hitti, *Hitti's English-Arabic Medical Dictionary*, Beirut, American University of Beirut, 1967, 2nd. rev. ed., 1972; H. Kamal, *Encyclopedia of Islamic Medicine, with a Graeco-Roman Background.* A compendium to the history of Near Eastern medicine, with terms in Latin, Arabic, English and French, Cairo, General Egyptian Book Organization, 1975; X. Ryckmans, *Les droits et les obligations des médecins ainsi que des dentistes, accoucheuses et infirmières*, 2e ed. Bruxelles, Larcier, 1972; W.A.J. Farndale, *Medical Negligence*, rev. ed., Beckenham, Ravenswood, 1976; John Kenyon French Mason, *Law and Medical Ethics*, 3rd ed., London, Butterworth, 1991.

Religious Prohibitions

So far, Moslem religion had little to contribute in shaping the provisions regulating the relations between doctor and patient. There is, however, one field where religion plays an important role: may a Moslem patient receive medical treatment from a non-Moslem doctor? This question occupied many Moslem minds throughout the late Middle Ages[50] as Jewish and Christian doctors catered to Moslems, especially Moslem notables.[51] The question was still discussed as late as the 1960 volume of the *Al-Azhar Magazine*, where a *responsum* followed a minority opinion of the past[52] in allowing a Moslem patient to rely on guidance from a non-Moslem doctor.[53]

The doctor's advice referred to blood transfusions, a problematic procedure because of the Koranic prohibition of the use of blood.[54]

50 From about the twelfth century onward, see: E. Strauss, "The Social Isolation of *Ahl adh-dhimma*" in: O. Komlos, *Etudes Orientales à la Mémoire de Paul Hirschler*, Budapest, 1950, pp. 73–94.

51 Moshe Perlmann, "Notes on the Position of Jewish Physicians in Medieval Muslim Countries," in: *JOS* 2 (1972), 315–319. Uriel Heyd, "Moses Hamon, Chief Jewish Physician to Sultan Süleyman the Magnificent," in *Oriens* 16 (1963), 156–157. Bernard Lewis, *The Jews of Islam*, Princeton, N.J., Princeton University Press, 1984, pp. 130, 214 n. 29.

52 The *responsum* states that the Ḥanafîs and Shâfi'îs as well as the Ḥanbalîs are all of the opinion that a non-Moslem doctor should never be consulted. Even some of the Mâlikîs, who allow a Moslem to call in a non-Moslem doctor, add the reservation that there is no Moslem doctor in the vicinity. The authors of the modern *responsum* substantiate their conclusion by citing two traditions attributed to the Prophet, and, from among the legal writings, only one opinion stemming from the very independent, and therefore isolated, Ḥanbali jurist: Ibn Taymiya (died 1328).

53 *Majallatu 'l-Azhar* (Al-Azhar Magazine) vol. 41, June 1969, p. 316. This reference and others from the Al-Azhar Magazine were first collected by Professor Ḥava Lazarus-Yafeh in her article "Is there today a new religious thinking among the Al-Azhar scholars?" (in Hebrew), in: G. Baer (ed.), *The Ulema and Problems of Religion in the Muslim World*, Jerusalem, 1971, pp. 276–292.

54 Koran XVI:115 — "He hath only forbidden you that which dieth of itself and blood and swine's flesh..." (The Koran, translated into English by George Sale, with an Introduction by Sir Edward Denison Ross, London, no date, p. 269). Yet "[b]lood transfusion is the oldest form of 'transplantation'" (Rabbi Mordechai Halperin, M.D., "Organ Transplants from Living Donors" [*supra* note 29] relying

The religious scruples in this case no doubt were that a non-Moslem doctor might not give sufficient weight to this Koranic prohibition in considering a blood transfusion against some other possible treatment not within the religious prohibition. There could not be any objection to the donation of blood as cupping was in use among Moslems and was even recommended in normal cases.[55] The problem was how to permit the introduction of the blood into the receiving body.

The Egyptian authors of the *responsum* overcame this difficulty by basing themselves on a dispensation found in the late seventeenth-century Indian compendium of *responsa*[56] which allowed a sick man to drink blood if the doctor ordered him to do so. Thus, modern Moslems

on R. Arnon, "Karl Landsteiner, Discoverer of Blood Groups" *Madda* (1969) *14*, 177).

According to the London *Times* of July 25, 1992, blood transfusions are problematic also for the "Jehovah's Witnesses." A case of a "Jehovah's Witness" refusing to accept a blood transfusion occurred also in Jerusalem (*Ma'ariv* 23 March, 1994). Their opposition to blood transfusions claims to be based on Leviticus III:17, "It shall be a perpetual statute for your generations throughout all your dwellings that ye eat neither fat nor blood," and Acts XV:29, "That he shall abstain from meats offered to idols and from blood." Settled law in England solves the problem of children in need of blood transfusions, much the same as the problem of anorectic children, by applying the principle that the welfare of the child is paramount, overriding anything else, even the parents' wishes. The *Times* rightly points out the contradiction created by section 37 of the 1990 Human Fertilization and Embryology Act in allowing late abortions, in total disregard for the supposedly overriding principle of the welfare of the child. How can a Court in England protect "Jehovah's Witness" children, in allowing them to receive blood transfusions against the parent's wishes, while at the same time the law disregards the welfare of the children in cases of abortion?

55 A pregnant woman was not allowed to practice cupping on herself during certain stages of her pregnancy because of the supposed risk to the fetus in her womb. See *Al-Fatâwî 'l-Hindiya* (above note 14), p. 111. Loss of blood by a pregnant woman may be due either to excessive force of the woman who may then begin a second pregnancy in addition to the ongoing pregnancy as taught by Hippocrates and Galen. Alternatively the loss of blood may be due to a weakness or illness in the fetus, resulting generally from a weakness or illness in the mother. These are the observations of Averroès (Ibn Rushd). See: Robert Brunschvig, "Averroès Juriste" in: Id. *Etudes d'Islamologie*, Paris, Maisonneuve et Larose, 1976, pp. 167-200, at p. 196.

56 *Al-Fatâwî 'l-Hindiya, op. cit.* (above note 20) p. 112.

who allow blood transfusions may be said to be not so far removed from their medieval predecessors. Interestingly enough, the same reference in the Indian compendium of *responsa* also contains a very clear prohibition of organ transplants, but the same al-Azhar scholars somehow failed to find it when they were dealing with the permissibility of organ transplants.[57]

As far as treatment by non-Moslem doctors is concerned, the majority opinion in Moslem law which prohibits such treatment coincides with a natural tendency among Moslems. Moslem women who used to be treated by Jewish doctors in Israel, preferred, after the Six Day War in 1967, to call on Moslem physicians in the territories formerly occupied by Jordan. This I learned from nurses serving in "communal dispensaries" in Arab villages in Israel. On 27 April, 1979, after talking to them about "Moslem approaches to family planning and medical treatment," I was told by one of them, who served in a village containing a mixed population of Moslems, Druze and Christians, that she had advised a patient to turn to the woman doctor who lived and practiced her profession in that locality and who had followed her medical studies and training in France. The patient answered her: "If I have to go to a non-Moslem doctor, I would prefer a Jewish one rather than that Christian doctor." Religious affiliation is thus very much a determining factor in the choice of a doctor even today.

57 Note 22 above and the text relying on it.

Contemporary Trends in Medical Ethics

David Heyd

Medicine is an ancient art or science; ethics is equally old as a field of philosophical concern. Ethical problems in the practice of medicine have always attracted the attention of both physicians and philosophers, as can be seen from the history of medicine. However, medical ethics as a distinct discipline is surprisingly new. Thus, the use of the term "medical ethics" with regard to medieval Spain is slightly anachronistic. I hope that it will not sound presumptuous on my part to argue in a forum of historians of ideas and of medicine that much of the interest in, and the delineation of, ethical problems related to the practice of medicine in various societies in the past is significantly dependent on the way we view medical ethics *today*. This suggestion might justify the exploration of some of the major trends in contemporary medical ethics as part of the effort to better understand the ethical dimensions of medieval theories of medicine. The main aim of this short survey is to stress the novelty of much of the concern with contemporary medical-ethical issues, which partly explains the amazing recent upsurge in the investment of intellectual energy and institutional resources in this field. Obviously, I am not denying the continuity and universality of some of the fundamental issues of medical ethics throughout history, but I think we could also profit from an attempt to focus our attention on those aspects of contemporary medical ethics which make it so different from what it used to be in the past.

Many signs demonstrate the recent expansion of the field of medical ethics: public awareness and intense discussion in the mass media, professional debates by both medical practitioners and philosophers, academic journals wholly devoted to medical ethics, rapid growth in medical legislation and government regulation, the establishment of ethical committees in hospitals and research institutes, the introduction of medical ethics as part of the curriculum in medical schools, etc. The term "medical ethics" itself has undergone a radical shift in meaning from a narrow concern with the ethics, or even the etiquette, of a well defined profession to a wide-range concern with everything pertaining to the normative principles governing medical practice in all its ramifications. It has gone from the rules of proper behavior for the members of a guild to the overall assessment of the purpose and value of medical treatments. The effect of this shift can be seen in the decline of the role of the physician's *oath*, which in ancient times reflected the epitome of "medical ethics." In today's complex medical scene the doctor's oath has become marginal, and given the elaborate systems of legal rules and regulations, the oath has become purely ceremonial and symbolic. These indicators highlight the revolutionary aspects of the change which has occurred in the field of medical ethics during the past couple of decades.

Three major trends explain the shift from traditional to modern medical ethics: first, the tremendous growth in the role of the state in medical affairs; second, the loss of shared ethical values in modern western societies; third, the unprecedented advances in medical science and technology. These three factors are closely interrelated, and it is regrettable that most medical ethicists are content in addressing the third, often ignoring the first two.

Consider the expansion of the role of the state in medical practice. In the past century or so, modern medicine has become one of the main areas in which governments play a direct role.[1] The main vehicle for political intervention in medical affairs is the allocation of resources. Medical treatment has become expensive, and cannot be directly financed by the private individuals seeking medical services. Only the state, with its re-distributive powers of taxation and the budgetary allocation of resources, can finance the costs of modern medicine. The constantly rising costs in medicine are due not only to the growing costs of medical treatment as such, but also to the dependence of treatment on long-term investments in medical institutions, machinery, research, development of new technologies, and the long training of a

1 In a well-documented, though highly controversial study, Ivan Illich illustrates in great detail the growing role of society and the state in the management of medicine and health. See I. Illich, *Limits to Medicine* (Harmondsworth: Penguin, 1977), chap. 2.

new generation of medical practitioners. The state has inevitably become the major factor in all these areas, or rather the only body which is able to carry the tremendous financial burden. This situation is most clearly manifest in welfare states, where the government assumes responsibility for almost all medical services, but we should not ignore the central role of the state in societies in which much of the medical sphere is left to the free market, including the United States.

Today, the state also controls medical life through legislation. It licenses institutions as well as individual practitioners, reviews the ethical aspects of medical research, criminalizes certain forms of medical practice, rules on matters of life and death, mental health, and forced treatment, empowers doctors to decide on the ability of citizens to do military service, drive a car, take a job, and even regulates parenthood through the tight control over the access to aritificial reproductive technologies. These are all well known examples of a process which amounts to the politicization of medicine. Medical practice is no longer a matter of individual encounters between patient and doctor, left to voluntary engagement and the forces of the free market. It has become heavily regulated by the state, both economically and legally.

The deeper meaning of this development can be seen in the idea that health has become a *public good.*[2] Health is not only a desired condition sought by the individual, but also a social goal, a primary good of societies. Like freedom, security and education, which beyond their value for the individual are now considered public goods, health is also a matter in which society as such has an interest. The health of individuals should be promoted regardless of their interest in it and independently of their ability to pay for it, both because it is their right and because it affects the lives of other individuals and society at large.

The trend to greater state interference in medical matters has created a new relationship between medicine and the state. On the one hand,

2 The historical sources of this development are traced by Foucault back to the eighteenth century, especially to post-revolutionary France, where society assumed responsibility for the health of the citizens, for their treatment in public institutions (hospitals), and for the struggle against plagues (by means of state control over sanitation, isolation of the sick and the quality of food and water). See M. Foucault, *The Birth of the Clinic: An Archaeology of Medical Perception* (New York: Random House, 1975), chap. 2.

the state has gained unprecedented control over the medical profession by exercising its legal and economic regulating powers in the medical sphere; on the other hand, the medical profession itself, through the very process of politicization, has acquired a most powerful position in social life. With the legal support of the state, doctors manage larger parts of the lives of individuals, and affect more than ever before the quality of human life. The medicalization of life in general is a complementary process to that of the politicization of medicine.[3] The state and the medical profession have become dependent on each other. The politicians hold the legislative and financial powers in their hands, and try to subordinate medical practice to social values and political interests; the medical profession adamantly sticks to its monopoly in deciding the modes of medical treatment, and hides behind an increasingly specialized field of knowledge, incomprehensible to anyone not belonging to the guild. The alliance of academic expertise and prestige with political power has led to new tensions between individuals and medical practitioners, and their mutual relationship has gradually become depersonalized. The growing rate of malpractice suits is just one indication of the loss of trust, personal responsibility and gratitude involved in this process.

The second trend which characterizes modern medical ethics is the fragmentation of values in society.[4] By this I mean our recognition of the fact of the pluralism of incommensurable values in modern societies. Liberalism is the political view which both recognizes and hails this moral heterogeneity. In the absence of a shared value basis, modern liberal societies promote the principle of autonomy as a second-order value which legitimizes individual subjective choices which cannot be rationally supported and universalized as first-order values. In medicine, this substitution of personal autonomy for traditional religious and ethical values widely shared by the members of the

3 Ivan Illich has done more than any other theoretician to highlight and criticize the idea of the "medicalization" of modern life, which he argues is reflected not only in the social and political sphere, but also on the general "cultural" level. Illich, *Limits to Medicine* (cit. n. 1), Part 3.

4 Many philosophers have analyzed this idea, but for its particular impact on medical ethics, see A. MacIntyre, "How Virtues Become Vices," in *Evaluation and Explanation in the Biomedical Sciences*, eds. H. T. Engelhardt and S. T. Spicker (Dordrecht: Reidel, 1975), pp. 97–111.

community has far-reaching implications. There is no longer a consensus about what makes life worth living, and hence no medical rules for the treatment of defective neonatals or terminally ill and dying patients can be established. The source of moral values and legitimacy in these issues is left completely to individual choice. The traditional benign paternalism of doctors toward their patients is today considered a blatant attack on individual rights and self-respect. Consent has replaced beneficence as the guiding principle of medical treatment. The best health interests of the patient as defined by medical science are subordinated to his or her will. Contractual relations between doctor and patient have replaced a relationship based on trust and paternalistic responsibility.

Having lost the firm value basis of medical practice, the modern liberal view sharpens the distinction between the responsibility of the patient for the *ends* of medical therapy and the responsibility of the physician for the *means* of therapy. The doctor is not supposed to guide the patient in making choices regarding the desirability of the goals of medical treatment and the rationality of the risks involved in it; he is only expected to provide the patient with the relevant information and carry out as best as he can the patient's wishes. At the same time, individuals in modern society take less responsibility for their health, and expect medicine to supply remedies whenever things go wrong. The traditional joint responsibility of doctor and patient for both the correct aims of medical treatment and the necessary means for their attainment has given way to an uneasy division of authority. Values are left in the hands of the sovereign autonomous patient, while the right means for achieving them are wholly left to the professional medical expert, who acts in that limited sphere in an absolutely paternalistic and often patronizing manner.

The growth in state intervention in medicine and the liberal ethos often stand in direct opposition in modern political reality. This opposition creates particular conflicts and tensions in the medical sphere and in the search for principles of medical ethics. The loss of social consensus on issues such as the definition of health, the beginning of life and its end, the moral status of fetuses, the definition of human beings on the genetic level, the proper ranking of priorities in the allocation of resources, the permitted level of risk in medical experimentation has created a lacuna which is filled by the principle of individual choice, but also by political intervention on the part of the state. For even the most liberal society cannot remain indifferent to issues of the deepest human and social significance. Some matters cannot be left to individual autonomous choice, as they affect others directly or indirectly (e.g. contagious diseases, priorities in the allocation of resources, the treatment of children, the protection of helpless elderly people or the comatose, the health of airplane pilots, etc.). Thus, in medical affairs the state cannot rest satisfied with the role of the proverbial "night guard," since questions such as the definition of the moment of death, the sale of organs, surrogacy agreements, and the active killing of defective neonatals touch the deepest human sensibilities and relate to issues that define the identity of any society, even the most liberal and pluralistic one.

There are, accordingly, two parallel trends in contemporary medical ethics: on the one hand, an emphasis on the role of the individual and autonomous choice in matters relating to his or her treatment, as seen in the central role of informed consent and patients' rights; on the other hand, a gradual expansion of state intervention through legislation and economic means. This intervention puts strict constraints on the options of both patients and medical practitioners. Experimentation on human subjects is an example: while there are very strict rules detailing the requirement to obtain the subject's consent to any experiment, governments are constantly adding conditions limiting the possibility of conducting medical experiments even when full and informed consent is given. Contemporary American medical practice is equally constrained by the fastidiously protected principle of the autonomy of the individual and the very strict regulations of the Food and Drug Administration.

So far I have discussed the political and ethical factors which bear on the development of contemporary medical ethics. The third trend I wish to mention relates to the specifically medical elements in this development, namely the progress in medical science and technology proper. As in the discussion of the first two trends, I suggest that the dramatic leap in medical options in the past couple of decades forces medical ethics to take radically new paths and sometimes to break with long-held traditional values and principles. Euthanasia and abortion are not new issues, though the methods available for the prolongation of human life and the ability to diagnose defects in fetuses in the early stages of pregnancy and to safely terminate it might bring people to reassess traditional ethical approaches to these matters. Genetic screening and engineering are, however, new techniques which call for a completely new ethical discourse and guiding principles. What is the moral status of a human being not yet conceived? Should there be limits on the reproduction of genetically defective couples? On what basis? Are these limits in the best interest of the child? But then, can a child have an interest not to be born at all? Perhaps the reason for restricting the reproduction of genetically defective children lies in the interest of humanity in a good "gene pool?" But then, who is the subject of this interest? I am not raising these questions to illustrate the complexity and chronically contested nature of problems in medical ethics, but rather to argue that some aspects of contemporary medical ethics cannot even be *discussed* in the language and conceptual framework of traditional moral philosophy.[5]

In the past, medical research made very limited use of experimentation on living humans, and derived most of its information from experimenting with animals or studying human cadavers. The nineteenth century introduced the systematic study of human disease through experimentation on large groups of people, including control groups receiving alternative treatment. This practice created new ethical problems, albeit of a less dramatic nature than those connected to genetic screening and engineering. These problems relate to the ethical basis for the obligation of people to take part in medical experiments. What is a reasonable level of risk? Why should an individual take part in an experiment from which he is not likely to benefit? Can we say that our generation should undergo some medical risk for the sake of the next generation since we are benefitting from the experiments of the previous generation? The inter-generational aspect of medical practice is definitely new, and the traditional tools of ethical discourse provide only a poor clue as to the way to approach these issues.[6]

5 I have elaborated on the need for a completely new conceptual framework for the analysis of choices regarding the creation of new people in *Genethics: Moral Issues in the Creation of People* (Berkeley: University of California Press, 1992). The critical thread of the book's argument is that all attempts to apply traditional ethical theories such as Kantianism or utilitarianism are bound to yield serious paradoxes.

6 For a classical discussion of the ethics of medical experimentation, see H. Jonas,

Finally, consider the ethically prosaic practice of the immunization of large sectors of society to diseases like whooping cough. There is a very slight chance of brain damage following the inoculation. In addition, the chances that an unimmunized individual will get whooping cough are extremely low in Western society, where universal immunization has extirpated the disease. Even so, if the balance of probabilities leads the rational individual to avoid inoculation, and being the rational choice it is acted upon by many others, there is a significant risk of the recurrence of the disease. This is a typical tension between individual and collective choice. Can the state force people to act against their best interests in order to guarantee the collective good? Again, no answer is provided by traditional discussions in medical ethics, which have usually been individual-oriented.

As in other fields of practical reason, the expansion of the repertory of medical options in the treatment and use of medical resources leads to a growing sense of the loss of criteria for making choices. The money used for one organ transplant could support a whole program of preventive medicine; the limited number of dialysis machines forces the doctor to arrange the patients according to some sort of order of priorities; situations of "triage" are much more widespread in modern warfare than they have ever been. Traditional ethical concepts are put under strain in dealing with these typically modern circumstances, so aptly called "tragic choices."[7]

Even worse, there are aspects of modern medical practice for which it is claimed that medicine "backfires," that is to say, the harm caused outweighs the benefits. The three trends which have been sketched here as characterizing modern developments in medicine are in different ways responsible for what has been called the "iatrogenic effect" of medical practice and policy. Modern drugs are certainly more effective than their traditional counterparts, but they also have much more dangerous side effects. The same applies to surgical treatment, to the widespread use of diagnostic instruments and means, to aggressive treatments of mental diseases. Beyond the debate on Illich's controversial thesis of "medical Nemesis," the counterproductive effect of mod-

"Philosophical Reflections on Experiments with Human Subjects", in *Bioethics*, ed. T. A. Shannon (New York: Paulist Press, 1976).

7 G. Calabresi, *Tragic Choices* (New York: Norton, 1978).

ern medical treatment, there is definitely a growing awareness that the old dictum of "primum non nocere" can hardly serve as a guiding principle in modern medicine. The curative power of modern medicine is so strong as to tempt us to replace the priority of the avoidance of harm with the more shaky principle of a cost-benefit analysis.

Reproductive technology is making fast progress, forcing the redefinition of well-entrenched concepts of parenthood. Organ transplantation is going to raise cruel questions regarding the relative value of the quality of life of an individual versus the life saving potential of his separate bodily organs which can already be transplanted to five people or more. The aggressive treatment of premature babies can save their lives, but only at the cost of retardation or other serious defects. Mental diseases can be relieved, if not cured, by drugs which cause changes in the patient's personality. These are all well known examples of advances in medical science where it is not clear whether they are a blessing or a curse for lack of an appropriate ethical theory.

By way of conclusion, let me suggest the following generalization, which captures an essential shift in the ethics of medical practice in modern liberal society. Medical practice contains an inevitable paternalistic component, but a comparison of the older and the more recent approaches to medical paternalism shows an interesting inversion. Traditional medicine held to a strongly paternalistic view of the very definition of health, but advocated a non-paternalistic model of trust, personal concern, and friendship for the doctor-patient relationship. The modern liberal ethos leaves decisions about health and the desirable life-style of people to individual discretion, but at the same time opens the way to professional paternalism and to asymmetrical and alienated relations between practitioners and patients. Although the modern doctor is not paternalistic in the deep sense of having an articulated conception of the proper ends of life and the value of physical health, he is sometimes domineering in his medical paternalism. Liberal agnosticism regarding basic values of human life has become an ally for professionalized, technical medicine, transforming the traditional paternalism of ends to a modern paternalism of means.[8]

8 I have developed this comparison between traditional and modern conceptions of medical ethics in the context of an analysis of Plato's view of medicine in "The Medicalization of Health: Plato's Warning," *Revue Internationale de Philosophie*, forthcoming (1995).

Modern Medicine, Ethical Dilemmas, and the Impact of the Medieval Jewish Codifiers

David W. Weiss

Advances in science and technology, from the wheel to atomic energy and genetic engineering, must often be regarded, in moral terms, as representing a double-edged sword. Science is morally neutral. It is a potential. Its usages can improve human welfare categorically. Its usages can also serve the demonic.

In our time, the ante has been raised. The technological and organizational skills at hand have vastly escalated science's potential for good as well as its potential for destruction. There is little need to specify the obverse, antithetical possibilities. It is self-evident that if existing knowledge and resources were directed morally, the specter of hunger and starvation cast over much of the world would recede, disasters of nature could be contained, infant mortality reduced and life span lengthened. Neither are the glaring misuses of science a secret, not the fatal ravages of the biosphere by nuclear and chemical pollution, nor the application by scientists of scientific methodologies to programs of genocide.

But beyond the manifest dangers of science conducted blindly, in gross indifference to its foreseeable consequences, or in unabashed service to immoral policies — science without compassion[1] — there are other, more subtle dangers that often attend endeavors which are benevolent in purpose. Masked by the permissibility of the works' intent, these attending dangers can compromise the ethical integrity of science the more seriously for their insidiousness. The aim of this

1 Friedlander, R.C. and Müller-Hill, B., eds., *Medical Science Without Compassion, Past and Present*, Proz. No. 11 (Hamburg: 1992), Hamburger Stiftung für Sozialgeschichte des 20. Jahrhunderts; Weiss, D.W., "Science and values," *Tradition*, 1989, *24(2)*: 150–160.

article is to bring them into focus in the area of biomedicine, where the approval given by society to designated ends tends to blur, perhaps more so than in any other area, the ethical concerns pertaining to their larger implications and to the means employed. The following paragraphs cite several recent instances in illustration of this dimension of ethical concern as medicine and medical science rush towards new conquests.

Means, Ends, and Implications: Biomedical Research and Clinical Trials

The individual's dignity, well-being, and life itself are not infrequently placed at risk by individual investigators and by medical and public health organizations in the pursuit of studies whose general aims are indeed laudable. This is not a matter of the past only, nor is it limited to patently criminal human experimentation by criminal governments, as took place in German concentration camps and Japanese prisoner-of-war camps in the years preceding and during World War II. Science in democracies, and even in our period, is not alien to the design of studies in which human life is given an arithmetical value and the morality of the work — to the extent that it is given much thought — is based on numerical equations that juxtapose lives placed at risk against lives that might ultimately be helped.

A case in point is the infamous Tuskegee Experiment[2] conducted under the auspices of the United States Public Health Service. Begun in 1932 and terminated only in 1972, the study set out to examine the course of syphilis in Afro-Americans, on the doubtful supposition that the pathogenesis of the disease differs appreciably in Caucasians and Blacks. Treatment with antibiotics of established efficacy was withheld from many of the patients, without their knowledge. The experiment was essentially a matter of scientific curiosity... shades of Hallervorden and Mengele.[3]

2 Brandt, A.M., "Racism, research and the Tuskegee syphilis study," *Hastings Cent. Rpts.*, 1978, **8**(6): 21–29.

3 Müller-Hill, B., *Tödliche Wissenschaft. Die Aussonderung von Juden, Zigeunern, und Geisteskranken 1933–1945* (Rowohlt: Reinbeck bei Hamburg, 1984).

Shades of Hallervorden again, much more recently, in investigations of the molecular biology of Alzheimer's Disease, as described by Müller-Hill:

> Recently two papers appeared which describe *in situ* hybridizations with amyloid DNA as the probe in normal and sporadic Alzheimer brains. One group used brains from sporadic Alzheimer patients obtained 1 (!) to 7 hours after death... I would not like to repeat these experiments nor would I encourage anybody to do so. *Post mortems* of this type raise the spectre of Hallervorden et al... And the conditions were not even the ideal ones used on monkeys... deep sedation followed by transcardial transfusion with paraformaldehyde. It remains to be seen whether an ethics committee will in a suitable case allow such treatment. Then it may be time to leave the field forever.[4]

The picture that leaps to mind as one reads the papers on which Müller-Hill's comments are based is of the dying patient surrounded by a vulturine pathology team, waiting. Waiting until the last flicker of life has ceased. One hour from life to the brain's harvesting. Has life really ended? What of dignity during its last moments?

A second instance: The Human Genome Program (HUGO) currently under way, the single largest biomedical research effort yet undertaken in the United States, promises to provide an inclusive mapping of the genetic make-up of our species, and thereby the identification of genes that cause, or contribute to, a variety of abnormalities. HUGO may accordingly come to sharpen and expand the scope of genetic counseling and the identification of individuals genetically prone to severe diseases. Such early, preclinical diagnosis can be of significant prophylactic import. And precise information of specific susceptibility loci in the genome might, eventually, lead to new developments of gene therapy. HUGO is a fascinating intellectual endeavor and the medical applications of the knowledge gained may well prove to be important. But HUGO's ethical implications are not necessarily innocuous. The

4 Müller-Hill, B., "Molecular biology of Alzheimer's Disease." Lecture presented at Cold Spring Harbor Symposium, Cold Spring Harbor, N.Y., 1988; published as Müller-Hill, B. and Beyreuther, K., *Ann. Rev Biochem.*, 1989, **58**:287–307.

reservations raised by leading molecular biologists are exceedingly apt. Müller-Hill expresses this concern in the following words:

> The considerations of Nazi eugenics are not only a matter of history. They are particularly relevant for the future of the human genome project.
>
> Through this project some differences in human phenotypes will be scientifically proven to be due to different genotypes. Some of these genotypes will correctly be seen as the cause of disablement or nonfunction of the carriers in the industrial society of the twenty-first century.
>
> What will have prevalence? Scientific truth or the dignity of the afflicted person? Will bioethicists... approve the idea that employers, insurance companies or just anybody will have the right to ask a person about his genotype? Will they agree that employers or insurance companies have the right to deny employment or insurance to those who refuse to have their genotype revealed?
>
> Will they condone the notion that a woman should be punished because she had an abortion for reasons they do not approve of, and punished again when she refuses to have an abortion when they forecast high costs and no return?[5]

S. E. Luria raises the question in similar terms:

> The phantom promise of early diagnosis of a few hereditary diseases is being replaced (Editorial in *Science*, Oct. 13, 1989, p.189) by hints of a eugenic program targeted to "the poor, the infirm, the underprivileged." Are they to be transformed (or perhaps altogether eliminated) by eugenic applications of genetic technology?
>
> Ten years ago, I battled against the unreasonable fears that genetic engineering might create unnatural forms of life. The real danger today is the possible emergence of an establishment program to invade the rights and privacy of individuals, whether

5 Müller-Hill, B., "Eugenics: The science and religion of the Nazis," in *When Medicine Went Mad. Bioethics and the Holocaust*, ed. A.L. Caplan (Totowa, N.J.: 1992), The Humana Press, pp. 43–52.

> in the area of sexual preference, or right of abortion... under cover of beneficient eugenic intervention.
>
> Will the Nazi program to eradicate Jewish or otherwise "inferior" genes by mass murder be transformed here into a kinder, gentler program to "perfect" human individuals by "correcting" their genomes in conformity, perhaps, to an ideal, "white, Judeo-Christian, economically successful" genotype?[6]

Apart from the ill-use to which agencies of society could bring information deriving from HUGO, Luria points to a still more disturbing issue: How far may science rightly go in attempting to alter the personality and character of individuals or of the human species by genetic manipulation?

A third instance of ethically uncertain ground in modern medicine pertains to the area of "reproductive technology." Writing in a paper entitled "Engineering a molecular nightmare," Edwin Chargaff asks:

> The term "reproductive technology" is a designation covering many activities, some of them perhaps not very pretty... It would seem to cover even such heart-rending cases as that reported in *Nature* (June 5, 1986, p. 553) in which a pregnant schizophrenic woman was persuaded or forced to consent to an abortion so that the physicians could examine the fetus in great detail... The manufacture of human embryos with the only purpose of crushing and extracting them?[7]

There are coming into sight other purposes, too, for "manufacturing" embryos. Early findings suggest that implantation of embryonic brain tissue might alleviate the symptoms of Parkinson's Disease. It is not improbable that pluripotential embryonic cells may also find therapeutic application in other diseases.

It would not seem too far-fetched, accordingly, to imagine a future scenario in which young women will be enticed to enter pleasantly appointed holiday institutions where they will be impregnated and their fetuses suitably "harvested" for sound, benevolent medical causes. After all, even modest financial rewards for their efforts would outstrip

6 Luria, S.E., "Human Genome Program (Letter)," *Science*, 1989, **246**:873.
7 Chargaff, E., "Engineering a molecular nightmare," *Nature*, 1987, **327**:199.

the income attainable from more pedestrian employments to women from economic strata below established poverty lines. The word "neomortarium" has already been coined for facilities in which bodies judged to be dead by one criterion or another can be maintained for prolonged periods of time in a state of cooled, intubated suspended animation until their organs can be... harvested... for implantation into patients who are still more convincingly alive. On the other end of the spectrum of life there might, then, arise in a brave new medical world "fetariums" for corresponding ends.

There is no essential ethical objection to utilizing such tissues medically, where termination of fetal and adult existence is an undesigned episode in the natural history of individual life. But when life is intentionally made, or life stopped before its final moments, or the neomortal state frozen in time... have we then not killed as well any remaining notion of the sanctity of human life?

A steadily increasing variety of human organs and tissues can be transplanted to others. For the recipient patient, the implant is often the last and only chance for survival. But there the matter does not end, all on the side of the angels. Questions clamor for resolution: What must be done to mitigate the conceptual corollary of this growing and medically vital exchangeability of human components, that our valuation of the human being will evolve to that attaching to a repository of spare parts. Shall our new card of identity be the HLA profile? How do we preserve the notion of the inviolable integrity of person and *persona*? The advances in genetic and reproductive engineering give the questions added urgency.

As medical science has progressed over recent decades, it has forged a progressively closer association with an entity that should, ideally, be kept at a far remove. The partner is commercialism. The relationship may be unavoidable in modern mercantile societies, but its inevitability the more enforces biomedical ethicists to cry "Havoc!" The erosions of ethical medicine, and, more fundamentally, of core Judaeo-Christian principles, that are brought on by the splicing to research and clinical medicine of the value construct of economics are forbidding.

Proposals have been tendered at recent ethics convocations for a redefinition of death that would include the terminally ill, the irreversibly demented, and those in a permanent vegetative state. The semantic adaptation would permit a painless expediting of such patients to neomortarium or grave, in innocence of any ugly connotation of murder. And the redefining not only makes good economic sense, so its proponents argue, but has in fact become economically imperative. Society can no longer afford the costs of caring for the growing numbers of such persons, it is held. The occasional misdiagnosis of what is terminal, irreversible or vegetative will be more than offset by the funds becoming available as the huge burden of maintaining such patients is lifted from society's shoulders. These monies will then be freed for a plethora of life-affirming programs — mass immunization, pre- and peri-natal care, nutrition for the undernourished, new and better hospitals, etc., etc.

The arithmetic here not only places in competition the value assigned to material resources and the supreme value of individual human life, of the state of aliveness. It is also a mindless arithmetic. The costs involved in the custody of the terminally ill and the insentient represent only a small part of the total medical budget of technologically advanced nations and only a very small fraction of their gross national product. Would such societies really be hamstrung economically by not resorting to murder of their sick, under one lexicology or another? And, if one can judge by experience, any savings accruing from effectuation of the new definition are more likely to go to the agencies of Mars than to those of the public health services.

Indeed, there is an additional semantics that is added to sweeten the putative economic imperative. It is sympathy and compassion: Those to be cast aside live lives of suffering, lives of no use to themselves or society, lives not worth living. Relieving them of such lives should be regarded as an act of mercy, all around. Life's value is thus made conditional on its supposed quality and worth to the community. The terminology in this context bears a chilling resemblance to that fabricated by the German geneticists and psychiatrists who played so seminal a role in the exclusion from society and subsequent annihilation of the severely afflicted and the "racially undesirable": *Ballastexistenz, leere Menschenhülse, lebensunwertes Leben.*[8,9] How far down

8 Müller-Hill, B., "Psychiatry in the Nazi Era," in *Psychiatric Ethics*, 2nd edition, eds. S. Bloch and P. Chodoff (Oxford: Oxford University Press, 1991), pp. 461–472.

9 Müller-Hill, B., "Human genetics and the mass murder of Jews, gypsies and

the slope to moral perdition shall we find ourselves if we now countenance the killing of the useless and unwanted under pretexts of the common good and individual commiseration?

The instances cited above must not be read as an indictment of science. Science must proceed without hindrance, but one. That is the constraint imposed by ethical imperatives.

Culpability rests, rather, with the doers of science and it rests as well with the agencies and public who support science blindly, as if it were in all its manifestations and engagements untouchable, a sacred cow.

It is a particularly disturbing fact that many of the scientists who have been involved in ethically dubious or outright criminal undertakings appear in all other regards to be ordinary, law-abiding individuals. They cannot be dismissed as exceptions to a moral rule, as villains or sadists or bigots. Even the German scientists who conducted savage experiments on Jewish prisoners brought as articles of defense when standing trial after the war that they never harbored anti-Semitic sentiments.

The moral defect is elusive; it evades facile explanation, and there are no ready signs to warn of its expression. J. Robert Oppenheimer was intellectually quite right in describing the development of the atomic bomb as "that technically sweet problem."[10] The gentlemen scientists of the United States Department of Defense Research and Engineering who testified in 1970 before a Congressional committee on their program of research and development of biological weapons were cooly prudent in referring to the exigencies of self-defense:

> I will first restate the constraints... that we have put on ourselves as a matter of policy to prevent exactly what people have been saying — that there will be a world-wide scourge, or a black death type of disease that will envelop the world if some of these materials were to accidentally escape. That could not possibly happen with the biological agents that we have... However, to

others," in *The Holocaust: An International Conference of the Known, the Unknown, the Disputed and the Reexamined. Proc. Conf. U.S. Holocaust Memorial Museum*, Washington, December 5–8, 1993, in press.

10 Oppenheimer, Robert J., cited in Csikszentmihalyi, M., "Reflections on enjoyment," *Perspect. Biol. Med.*, 1985, **28**(4): 489–497.

> keep the record straight, we have done a small amount of research on a few agents that do not satisfy this restraint — the reason for this is that a potential enemy might use them against us and we have to be prepared to defend ourselves — so we try to develop vaccines and rapid identification systems, for example, for defensive purposes... Eminent biologists believe that within a period of 5 to 10 years it would be possible to develop a synthetic biological agent, an agent that does not naturally exist and for which no natural immunity could have been acquired.

The conversation between congressmen and scientist then continues:

> *Congressman S.*: "Are we doing any work in that field?"
> *Dr. M.*: "We are not."
> *Congressman S.*: "Why not? Lack of money or interest?"
> *Dr. M.*: "Certainly not lack of interest."
> *Congressman S.*: "Would you provide for our records information on what would be required, what the advantages of such a program would be, the time and the cost involved?"
> *Dr. M.*: "We will be very happy to. Within the next 5 to 10 years, it would probably be possible to make a few infective microorganisms which would differ in certain important aspects from any known disease-causing organisms. Most important of these is that it might be refractory to the immunological and therapeutic processes upon which we depend to maintain our relative freedom from infectious disease... It was considered possible to initiate an adequate program through the National Academy of Sciences — National Research Council. The matter was discussed with the NAS-NRC, and tentative plans were made to initiate the program. However, decreasing funds in CB, growing criticism of the program, and our reluctance to involve the NAS-NRC in such a controversial endeavor have led us to postpone it for the past 2 years.[11]

It would seem that scientists, like other human beings, know how to spin cocoons that insulate them from unpleasant realities that may

11 Hearings Before a Subcommittee of the Committee of Appropriations, House of Representatives, Ninety-First Congress, First Session, Committee on Department of Defense Appropriations, 1970 (Congressional Record).

accompany their labors. The individual fibers that go into its making are creditable enough — curiosity, the sweet challenge of the problem, its salutary aspects, and the need, too, to create shelters from predators. But within the cocoon there are fashioned instruments of vast power, and too often left outside its protective shell are the regards of humaneness and humanity. Conscience finds a ready refuge in the premise that the uses of science are society's business, not that of its protagonists.

The common archetypes of dereliction in science appear to be personal indifference and a readiness to transfer responsibility. And, too, a proneness to reductionism. A contraction of focus is, of course, an intrinsic necessity in the planning and process of explorations into unknown territories. But a sliding extension from prescriptively narrow dissection of a specified problem to a narrowed perception of the way things are leads to trivialization and distortions of reality. Such reductionism brings with it not only a deconstruction of knowledge and science themselves, but it also proceeds towards moral opaqueness, an erosion of scientific ethics, and, ultimately, to a devaluation of human worth.

The problems and dilemmas that are posed by the adversative polarities of science's potentials are thus largely rooted in the ambiguities and ambivalences of human character. The problems take on different forms at different stages of science's sophistication. They have a greater urgency today than in the past. But in their essence they are timeless. And in their essence they must be addressed.

A Value Framework

The thesis here advanced is that the medieval Jewish *halachists* and codifiers made normative certain value priorities in their jurisprudential conceptions and structures. The values as such precede the medieval period. They derive from the Mishnah and the Babylonian and Jerusalem Talmuds, and some are stated explicitly in the scriptural text. It was the medieval rabbinic scholars who endowed them with sweeping, overriding precedence in the corpus of Jewish law, made them normative and imperative. It is these value imperatives from which guidelines for ethical conduct in modern science and medicine can most effectively be drawn, now, in our time, as then. At risk of oversimplification, they can be delineated as follows:

1. Individual human life is endowed with supreme value, unconditional of its predicted duration or imputed quality; it is a sanctum.
2. Human life and the human body are, as such, invested with incontestable dignity.
3. The guardianship of human wellbeing is an essential purport of the Law.
4. The search for underlying principles and for value priorities is a constant obligation of the Law's interpreters.
5. Compassion is a primary function of the scholar.
6. Individual moral responsibility is not transferable.

The rabbis of the Talmud indicated a series of legislative aphorisms which serve as instrumentalities for bringing these norms to *halachic* reality. Their medieval successors employed them extensively. The writer has discussed these at some length elsewhere;[12] several are here cited in illustration:

"For the sake of peace"[13]
"For the improvement of the world"[14]
"He shall live in them"[15] (i.e., *live* in observing the words of the Torah, not die in their service)

"Her ways (i.e., the Torah's) are ways of pleasance, and all her paths are peace."[16] ("Peace" in rabbinic literature frequently refers not only to an absence of hostility, but, more inclusively, to human welfare)

"It is time to act for the Lord; they have made void thy Torah."[17] (This sentence in Psalms is given a unique reading, to

12 Weiss, D.W., *The Wings of the Dove. Jewish Values, Science and Halachah* (Washington: 1987), B'nai B'rith Books.
13 Mishnah Gittin 5:8.
14 Mishnah Gittin 4:2; Mishnah Gittin 4:3; Mishnah Gittin 4:5; Tractate Ḥagigah (Babylonian Talmud) 2a, b.
15 Leviticus 18:5; Tractate Sanhedrin (Babylonian Talmud) 74a, b; Tractate Yoma (Babylonian Talmud) 85a, b; Maimonides, *Mishneh Torah*, Hilkhot Yesode Ha-Torah, Chap. 5.
16 Proverbs 3:17; also see Reference 26.
17 Psalms 119:126.

serve as a point of departure for rabbinic statutes that contravene established legislation, so as to preserve a community or strengthen its Jewish vitality: "Raba said: The first clause of this verse can be taken as explaining the second, and the second can be taken as explaining the first... Thus: It is time to work for the Lord. Why? Because they have made void Your law... and: They have made void Your law. Why? Because it is time to work for the Lord."[18])

"The hour's exigency"[19], [20]

"To transcend the specified precept"[21] (to transcend its narrow reading)

The application of some of these "catch all" legislative instrumentalities to *halachic* realization of Judaism's value norms is exemplified in the following passages, many from Maimonides (1138–1204). They are chosen for their easy accessibility to the reader not at home in medieval rabbinic literature, much of which is unavailable in translation. In their recognition of the Law's thrust, the passages are representative of the thinking of many of the era's rabbinic leaders. The passages do not specifically deal with issues of medicine. Medieval healing differs greatly from clinical and research medicine in the closing years of our century. The intent here is to demonstrate the universality of Judaism's value imperatives, and for that the topics selected are from situations in the human condition whose externalities are less mutable in the transition of time. It will be apparent, however, that the principles expounded afford guidelines of equal pertinence in the arena of modern biomedicine.

18 Mishnah Berakhot 9:4, and Rashi's commentary on the passage; Tractate Berakhot (Babylonian Talmud) 63a.

19 Tractate Yevamot (Babylonian Talmud) 90b.

20 Tractate Sanhedrin (Babylonian Talmud) 46a.

21 For treatment of the concept of *lifnim mishurat hadin*, see Lichtenstein, A., "Does Jewish tradition recognize an ethic independent of halakha?" in *Modern Jewish Ethics. Theory and Practice*, ed. M. Fox (Columbus: Ohio State University Press, 1975), pp. 62–88.

Medieval Jewish Jurisprudence

Humanity to Other Peoples

The prohibition against idolatry is one of the Noachite Commandments, to which all nations are bound, and there are sentiments of harshness in Scripture and Talmud regarding relationships with heathens. But then one comes across a luminous paragraph in Maimonides' Codex that transcends harshness, transcends it *in* the spirit of the Law:

> ...even with regard to heathens, our sages commanded to visit their sick, and to give burial to their dead as to the dead of Israel, and to provide for their poor as for the poor of Israel, because of the ways of peace, for it is written, "The Lord is good to all, and His mercies are over all His works"; and it is written, "Her ways are ways of pleasance, and all her paths are peace."[22]

And in a similar vein with regard to warfare:

> One may not make war on anyone in the world without first offering peace. This applies to optional war as well as to obligatory war [i.e., for the conquest by the Israelites of the land of Canaan]... If they make peace and accept the Noachite Commandments not a one of them may be killed... And it is forbidden to refute a covenant made with them, or to deceive them. Before Joshua entered the land he sent three messages to the inhabitants. The first message was: Whoever wishes to leave, may leave undisturbed. The second message was: Whoever wishes to make peace with us, let him make peace. The third, and last, message was: Whoever wishes to make war, let him make war... When besieging an enemy city, one may not surround it on all four sides, but only on three, and must leave room to flee for all who wish to save their lives...[23]

Maimonides' view would here seem to be in defiance of the plain scriptural reading. And if it does not meet all the stipulations set in

22 Maimonides, *Mishneh Torah*, Hilkhot Melakhim 10:12.
23 Maimonides, *Mishneh Torah*, Hilkhot Melakhim, Chap. 6.

recent international conventions for limiting the brutalities of modern warfare — stipulations that are brutally violated — this Twelfth Century dictum would not serve mankind badly today in its honoring.

The humanitarian attitude towards the pagan extends to the dimension of etiquette, and here, too, in the spirit of the Law and the very name of God. Thus, Rabbi Shlomo Yitzchaki (1040–1105), known as "Rashi," comments on a Mishnah in the Tractate Gittin that holds "and greetings (*shalom*) may be given to heathens, in the interest of peace":

> [that such greetings may be given] at all times; and even though he thereby places on the heathen the name of heaven, for peace is the name of the Holy One.[24]

Erasure of the Name

In the interests of peace between man and wife, Maimonides would appear to take even greater liberty with the Ineffable Name. The following passage refers to the biblical ritual by which a woman accused by her husband of infidelity can clear her name. She is given a potion into which is dipped a parchment inscribed with an exhortation that carries the letters of the divine name. The writing dissolves. The woman drinks, and if she is innocent she will conceive and give birth to a son, thereby proving her blamelessness and regaining her husband's affection.

> For the very name of God may be erased so as to make peace between husband and wife. Great is peace, for the Torah is given in its entirety to make peace in the world, as it is written, "Her ways are ways of pleasance, and all her paths are peace."[25]

Luminescent Priorities

The obligation to kindle the light of the Sabbath devolves weekly on the household, that of the lights of Chanukkah only once a year. But Maimonides rules that if on the Sabbath that falls in the week of Chanukkah

24 Rashi on Mishnah Gittin 5:9.

25 Maimonides, *Mishneh Torah*, Hilkhot Megillah V'Ḥanukkah 4:14.

> there are at hand in a household sufficient funds to purchase oil for either the lights of Chanukkah or the light of the Sabbath, but not for both, it is the light of the Sabbath that must be lit. For the Sabbath light symbolizes the descending of peace and contentment on the home.[26]

The Abandoned Woman

The canon of peace is recurrent in subsequent rabbinic writings. A classical example of its later application to the resolution of dilemmas encountered when established legislation conflicts with pressing issues of human welfare is seen in the commentary by Samuel Eliezer Edels (1555–1631), known as the "Maharsha," on the Tractate Yevamot of the Babylonian Talmud. The tractate deals largely with family matters, and in its treatment of the situation of the *agunah* the *Amoraim* decisively liberalize accepted regulations pertaining to witness and testimony. An *agunah* is a woman who has separated from her husband but is refused a bill of divorce, or one whose husband has disappeared. In the latter case, even if there is a strong presumption of his demise, she remains an *agunah* until his death is confirmed by reputable testimony. The *agunah* exists in a state of permanent personal limbo; she may not remarry, lest the missing husband should, in fact, be alive. From Talmudic times to the present, rabbinic authorities have struggled with the problem of how, on the one hand, to safeguard the categorical scriptural prohibition against adultery and, on the other, to free the unfortunate woman from the status of marital suspension. Herewith the Maharsha's views of such attempts in the Tractate:

> There appear in this tractate matters that astound, at first sight, in suggesting an uprooting of the Torah... and therefore the Tractate concludes with the *midrash* "the scholars increase peace in the world"... It is not an uprooting of the Torah, but rather a matter that pertains to the attribute of peace... And it is said "may there be great peace to the lovers of Your Torah"... and thus this is not an uprooting but rather of the quality of peace, that a woman not be an *agunah*. It is written [of the Torah] "her ways are ways of pleasance, and all her paths peace"... and "God

26 *Ibid.*, beginning of the passage.

> gives strength to His people," and therefore it is not an uprooting, for the Holy One, blessed be He, gave strength and power to His people, who are the scholars, so that they shall make it light in this matter; for the Lord "blesses His people with peace"... and there is no peace if she will be an *agunah*... In this manner Scripture interprets the verse "the Lord shall lift His face to you," even to the uprooting of a commandment of the Torah...[27]

The Latitudes of Knowledge and Sensibility

The study of Torah is a primary obligation, fulfillment of a cardinal commandment. Understanding of this obligation has at times tended to exclusivity, however, especially during the past two hundred years. The classic formulators of Jewish belief perceived Torah as a vast, secure domain, to which nothing in the appreciation of nature, nor of much of art and literature, is intrinsically alien or hostile. The confidence crumbled in some traditional circles at the advent of the nineteenth century, together with the physical enclosures that had long kept Jews at a distance from Western culture. Some rabbinic authorities strove to replace the ghetto walls with barriers of an ideology that is, in fact, at odds with powerful strains in normative Judaic teaching. The pursuit of all secular knowledge came to be denounced increasingly as frivolous if not outrightly heretical, and cadres of Jewish men and women were persuaded to an obscurantism that barred information of the world at large and also distorted perception of Judaism's fundamental missive. And yet, the opaqueness has throughout been fought. It has not overwhelmed the ethos of enlightenment that has imbued the mainstream of Jewish thought. In the defense of this ethos, the lucidity of vision and sensibility with which Maimonides grasps matters of essence has been a strong point:

> One only loves God with the knowledge with which one knows him... If the former be little or much, so will the latter be little or much... A person ought therefore devote himself to the understanding and comprehension of the sciences and studies which

27 Maharsha, *Ḥidushe Aggadot*, concluding passages on Tractate Yevamot (Babylonian Talmud).

> will inform him of his Master, as far as it lies in human faculties to understand and comprehend.[28]

The inclusiveness of the commission is echoed forcefully by a later Maimonidean follower, the fifteenth century Aragonese rabbi and philosopher Abraham Bibago; the statement is representative of a pervasive mode in Judaism's position to the world of knowledge:

> The reasonable creature, having reason, has to study the sciences. And being a believer, he will study Torah and acquire faith in its roots and dogmas. The first study will be a kind of carrier and vessel to bear the second study. In the same way that life is an assumption and carrier by which humanity and speech are carried, so through the form of reason by whose accomplishment one studies and acquires the sciences, Torah study will be assumed and carried. Thus faith will be complete and without doubt, and the one attitude, faith, will not conflict with the other, philosophy. Therefore did the sages say, "Reason and faith are two lights."[29]

This integrative assessment of man's drive to know himself and the cosmos negates the barriers that would separate and compartmentalize intelligence of the realms of the sacred and the secular, of canon and science. It attests the right of unbridled inquiry. Nothing that man can learn need be at the cost of trampled sancta. It significantly sheltered Judaism from the bitter conflict between science and religion, between the physical and the metaphysical, that has rent Christianity and other systems of faith and thought. And it has been a force against a demeaning of the worth of the individual: Man is a unitary entity of both the material and temporal, and of the spiritual that transcends time. Man is at once a creature of nature and of God, and neither his fabric of flesh and blood nor his spirit may be dealt with lightly. His transcendent dignity is affirmed regardless of his moment's sweep of scientific cognizance and accomplishment.

– – – –

28 Maimonides, *Mishneh Torah*, Hilkhot Teshuvah 10:6.

29 Avraham Bibago, *Derekh Emunah*.

The value imperatives at the core of these indicative passages present guidelines for human conduct. They outline the matrix of a social contract founded on compassion, and they are as such of singular relevance to that sphere of human activity that supposedly is — and that must be — in its very essence a matter of compassion, medicine.

NOTES ON CONTRIBUTORS

Marcelino Amasuno is professor in the Department of Hispanic Studies at McGill University, Montreal. He has edited Spanish medieval medical works. He is currently interested in medieval social history in the Crown of Castile.

Jon Arrizabalaga is research scientist at the CSIC (Scientific Research Council) in Barcelona. He is working on the history of disease in late medieval and early modern European medicine. With R.K. French and J. Henderson he is completing the book *The Coming of the Pox: The French Disease in Sixteenth-Century Europe* (Yale University Press).

Yom Tov Assis teaches medieval Jewish history at the Hebrew University of Jerusalem and specializes in Spanish and Provençal Jewish history. He has published and edited numerous books and articles in these fields. He is director of *Hispania Judaica* and co-editor of the series bearing the same name, editor of the series *Sources for the History of the Jews in Spain* and chairman of the Dinur Institute for Research in Jewish History at the Hebrew University.

Rosa Ballester is head of the Department of Public Health and professor of History of Medicine at the University of Alicante, Spain. She is author of *La historia clinica pediatrica durante el Siglo XIX* (1978) and papers on the history of infant care and pediatrics in modern and contemporary Spain.

Haim Beinart is Professor Emeritus of Medieval Jewish History. Ph.D. hon.causa, The Complutense University Madrid, Spain. Member of the Israel Academy of Sciences and Humanities; Corresp. member of the Real Academia de la Historia, Spain; of the Medieval Academy of America, etc.

Luís García-Ballester is professor of the History of Medicine at the CSIC (Scientific Research Council) in Barcelona. He is now working on the social and intellectual history of medicine in medieval and early modern Spain. He is one of the editors of the collected medical works of Arnau de Vilanova.

David Heyd is professor of Philosophy at the Hebrew University, Jerusalem. His main research topics are ethics and medical ethics. He has published *Supererogation* (Cambridge 1982) and *Genethics* (California Univ. Press 1992).

Samuel S. Kottek is the Harry Friedenwald Ass. Professor of the History of Medicine at the Hebrew University-Hadassah Medical School. He is the author of *Medicine and Hygiene in the Works of Flavius Josephus* (1994) and the editor of the annual journal *Korot*.

Y. Tzvi Langermann, Ph.D. in history of science, has published a number of studies on science and Jewish culture in the medieval period. He is on the staff of the Institute of Microfilmed Hebrew manuscripts in the Jewish National and University Library, Jerusalem.

Etienne Lepicard has written his M.D. thesis on "Several topics in medical ethics, a Christian point of view on Jewish sources." He is presently writing a Ph.D. thesis on the reception of Alexis Carrel's philosophy of life before and after World War II. He is attached to the division of medical history, Hebrew University, Jerusalem.

Yaakov Meron, B.A., M.A. (Jerusalem), Docteur en Droit (Paris), Professor of Law at the College of Management, formerly of Jerusalem and Tel Aviv Law Faculties, member of the Paris Société de Législation Comparée, is Advisor on the Law of the Arab Countries, Ministry of Justice, Jerusalem.

Guillermo Olagüe de Ros is professor of History of Medicine at the University of Granada, Spain. His research is in the field of the history of rising and shaping of medical and scientific language; he has also published on the introduction of modern medicine into Seventeenth and Eighteenth century Spain.

Fernando Salmón is an associate professor (History of Medicine) at the University of Cantabria, Spain. His current field of research is medieval and early modern medicine, in its social and intellectual aspects.

Daniel B. Sinclair, LL.B. (Hons), LL.M., Dr. Juris., is Principal of Jews' College, London; Associate Research Fellow, Centre for Medical Law and Ethics, Kings College, London; Assistant Editor, Jewish Law Annual; Consultant on Jewish Law to the Oxford Dictionary of the Jewish Religion; Director of the Centre for Jewish Medical Ethics, Jews' College, London; author of *Tradition and the Biological Revolution*, Edinburgh University Press, 1989.

David Weiss is Professor and Chairman of the Lautenberg Centre for General and Tumor Immunology and Chairman of the Academic Committee of the Centre for Medical Ethics at the Hebrew University-Hadassah Medical School, Jerusalem. He has published some 40 papers and books on topics related to medical ethics and humanities.

Abortion 78

Euthanasia (and/or suicide) 78f, 177-8, 183

Whether to treat the terminally ill 78f

Sin + sickness 79

Confession + Lateran IV 33, 53, 79-80, 101-102, 133-4

spiritual consolation provided by physicians 80

Ecclesiastical prohibitions of Xtns being treated by Jewish physicians - 46, 59, 101-2, 107-8, 117(?)

Jewish attitudes toward Jews treating gentiles 164-165; 170-172

Jewish distrust of medicine, 166-8; 175, 179-80-81